ANTIBODY THERAPEUTICS

Pharmacology and Toxicology: Basic and Clinical Aspects

Mannfred A. Hollinger, Series Editor
University of California, Davis

Forthcoming Titles

Anabolic Treatment for Osteoporosis, James F. Whitfield and Paul Morley
Antisense Oligodeonucleotides as Novel Pharmacological Therapeutic Agents, Benjamin Weiss
Basis to Toxicity Testing, Second Edition, Donald J. Ecobichon
CNS Injuries: Cellular Responses and Pharmacological Strategies, Martin Berry and Ann Logan
Lead and Public Health: Integrated Risk Assessment, Paul Mushak
Molecular Bases of Anesthesia, Eric Moody and Phil Skolnick
Receptor Characterization and Regulation, Devendra K. Agrawal

Published Titles

Inflammatory Cells and Mediators in Bronchial Asthma, 1990, Devendra K. Agrawal and Robert G. Townley
Pharmacology of the Skin, 1991, Hasan Mukhtar
In Vitro *Methods of Toxicology*, 1992, Ronald R. Watson
Basis of Toxicity Testing, 1992, Donald J. Ecobichon
Human Drug Metabolism from Molecular Biology to Man, 1992, Elizabeth Jeffreys
Platelet Activating Factor Receptor: Signal Mechanisms and Molecular Biology, 1992, Shivendra D. Shukla
Biopharmaceutics of Ocular Drug Delivery, 1992, Peter Edman
Beneficial and Toxic Effects of Aspirin, 1993, Susan E. Feinman
Preclinical and Clinical Modulation of Anticancer Drugs, 1993, Kenneth D. Tew, Peter Houghton, and Janet Houghton
Peroxisome Proliferators: Unique Inducers of Drug-Metabolizing Enzymes, 1994, David E. Moody
Angiotensin II Receptors, Volume I: Molecular Biology, Biochemistry, Pharmacology, and Clinical Perspectives, 1994, Robert R. Ruffolo, Jr.
Angiotensin II Receptors, Volume II: Medicinal Chemistry, 1994, Robert R. Ruffolo, Jr.

Pharmacology and Toxicology: Basic and Clinical Aspects

Published Titles Continued

Chemical and Structural Approaches to Rational Drug Design, 1994, David B. Weiner and William V. Williams
Biological Approaches to Rational Drug Design, 1994, David B. Weiner and William V. Williams
Direct Allosteric Control of Glutamate Receptors, 1994, M. Palfreyman, I. Reynolds, and P. Skolnick
Genomic and Non-Genomic Effects of Aldosterone, 1994, Martin Wehling
Human Growth Hormone Pharmacology: Basic and Clinical Aspects, 1995, Kathleen T. Shiverick and Arlan Rosenbloom
Placental Toxicology, 1995, B. V. Rama Sastry
Stealth Liposomes, 1995, Danilo Lasic and Frank Martin
TAXOL®: Science and Applications, 1995, Matthew Suffness
Endothelin Receptors: From the Gene to the Human, 1995, Robert R. Ruffolo, Jr.
Alternative Methodologies for the Safety Evaluation of Chemicals in the Cosmetic Industry, 1995, Nicola Loprieno
Phospholipase A_2 in Clinical Inflammation: Molecular Approaches to Pathophysiology, 1995, Keith B. Glaser and Peter Vadas
Serotonin and Gastrointestinal Function, 1995, Timothy S. Gaginella and James J. Galligan
Drug Delivery Systems, 1996, Vasant V. Ranade and Mannfred A. Hollinger
Experimental Models of Mucosal Inflammation, 1996, Timothy S. Gaginella
Brain Mechanisms and Psychotropic Drugs, 1996, Andrius Baskys and Gary Remington
Receptor Dynamics in Neural Development, 1996, Christopher A. Shaw
Ryanodine Receptors, 1996, Vincenzo Sorrentino
Therapeutic Modulation of Cytokines, 1996, M.W. Bodmer and Brian Henderson
Pharmacology in Exercise and Sport, 1996, Satu M. Somani
Placental Pharmacology, 1996, B. V. Rama Sastry
Pharmacological Effects of Ethanol on the Nervous System, 1996, Richard A. Deitrich
Immunopharmaceuticals, 1996, Edward S. Kimball
Chemoattractant Ligands and Their Receptors, 1996, Richard Horuk
Pharmacological Regulation of Gene Expression in the CNS, 1996, Kalpana Merchant
Antibody Therapeutics, 1997, William J. Harris and John R. Adair
Muscarinic Receptor Subtypes in Smooth Muscle, 1997, Richard M. Eglen

ANTIBODY THERAPEUTICS

Edited by

William J. Harris, Ph.D.

University of Aberdeen
Aberdeen, Scotland

John R. Adair, Ph.D.

Axis Genetics, Plc.
Babraham, Cambridge, United Kingdom

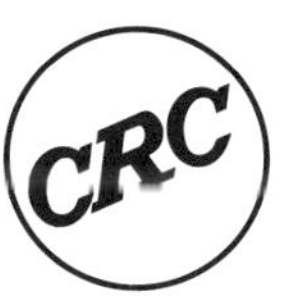

CRC Press
Boca Raton New York London Tokyo

Senior Editor: Paul Petralia
Editorial Assistant Cindy Carelli
Project Editor: Renee Taub
Marketing Manager: Susie Carlisle
Direct Marketing Manager: Becky McEldowney
Cover design: Dawn Boyd
PrePress: Kevin Luong
Manufacturing: Sheri Schwartz

Library of Congress Cataloging-in-Publication Data

Antibody therapeutics / edited by William J. Harris, John R. Adair.
p. cm. -- (Pharmacology and toxicology)
Includes bibliographical references and index.
ISBN 0-8493-8547-4 (alk. paper)
1. Immunoglobulins--Therapeutic use. Monoclonal antibodies--Therapeutic use. I. Harris, William J. II. Adair, John R. III. Series: Pharmacology & toxicology (Boca Raton, Fla.)
[DNLM: 1. Antibodies, Monoclonal--therapeutic use. QW 575.5.A6A629 1997]
RM282.I44A586 1997
615'.37--dc20
DNLM/DLC
for Library of Congress 96-27305
CIP

International Standard Book Number 0-8493-8547-4
Library of Congress Card Number 96-27305
Printed in the United States of America 1 2 3 4 5 6 7 8 9 0
Printed on acid-free paper

Introduction

John R. Adair

Immunotherapy is now into its second century of application.[1] From the early use of serum therapy in the last years of the 19th Century to today when large numbers of monoclonal antibodies[2] (MAbs) and polyclonal antibody cocktails are being tested for efficacy in a variety of medical conditions the concept of the "magic bullet" has never disappeared.

Antibodies have much to offer as pharmaceuticals. Immunoglobulin is a safe, long-lasting, naturally occurring product, present in the blood at 10–15 mg/ml. A vast range of antibody specificities of high affinity can be generated. The affinity of an antibody for antigen, for example, a cell-surface receptor, can exceed the affinity of the natural ligand for that receptor, and so antibodies can be considered for a range of therapeutic opportunities, from simple blockade (which includes entry of pathogens into cells) to sophisticated modulation of intracellular signaling, cell stimulation, anergy, or killing.

Today the ability to generate specific human or human-like binding sites from a number of starting positions is relatively straightforward (see, for example, References 3 and 4). These binding sites can be linked genetically or chemically to a wide variety of effector elements, in a range of size and avidity formats.[5] The products can be produced in a range of expression systems, offering high productivity and accurate processing. This modular approach to design can overcome many of the traditionally posed problems for antibody products, for example, immunogenicity, lack of efficacy, and inappropriate pharmacokinetics.

The development of these engineered products has taken place over the last 20 years, post Kohler and Milstein.[2] Production of MAbs from cell culture increased the specific activity of an antibody preparation, offering a potential reduction in the amount of antibody to be delivered or delivery of an efficacious dose of antibody in a reasonable formulation, thus widening the scope for therapeutic applications. MAbs also removed the problem of transfer of unnecessary blood components in immune globulin preparations and of adventitious infectious organisms.

A number of phases can be identified in this period. Between 1975–1980 murine MAbs were prepared against a range of clinically relevant antigens including tumor-associated antigens, infectious microorganisms, blood proteins, and cell-surface antigens. For example, the murine anti-human CD3 MAb OKT3 was developed in 1979 and subsequently licensed in 1986 as ORTHOCLONE OKT®3 for use as an immunosuppressant for treatment of transplant rejection.[6] In parallel, attempts were made during this time to derive human MAbs, but without much success (reviewed in Reference 7).

During the period between 1980–1985 recombinant DNA techniques and expression technologies were applied to the antibody field. The gene structures of immunoglobulins were revealed and methods for the manipulation of antibody sequences and their expression in heterologous systems were first developed. The first domain swapping experiments to produce chimeric mouse-human antibodies were described,[8,9] the possibility of antibody humanization was proposed,[10] and early experiments to generate transgenic mice expressing human antibody genes were done.[11] The concept of catalytic MAbs was discussed.[12] Several important intellectual property claims were made during this period (summarized in Reference 13), some of which are still being argued over.

Between 1986–1990 commercial antibody engineering began to be taken seriously and many important developments occurred. The range of possible antibody-based products widened with the generation of recombinant antibody fragments,[14-16] antibody binding sites fused to other protein entities (reviewed in References 17–20), and non-antibody binding sites linked to antibody Fc regions (immunoadhesins and receptor globulins).[21,22] Bacterial expression systems became available for the efficient production of these novel entities,[14,15] while mammalian cell[23] and yeast[24] systems were developed for whole antibody production based on other examples from the biotechnology industry. These systems allowed production levels in excess of that produced by hybridomas in cell culture. During this period the first humanized antibodies were produced,[25] and the first recombinant antibodies entered clinical studies.[26,27]

In the period from 1990 to the present, these achievements have been further developed with a wide range of engineered antibodies entering clinical studies. The rate of entry into clinical trials of these product candidates is accelerating; for example, the number of humanized antibodies in the clinic has doubled in the last 12 months.[28,29] One of these engineered antibodies has already emerged as a product. Further developments include: the addition of combinatorial library procedures for the production of novel human antibodies;[3,4] progress in *in vitro* immunization as a means of generating novel specificities (e.g., Reference 30); a clearer understanding of the measures needed to be taken to ensure efficient humanization of the vast range of nonhuman MAbs which now exist;[31] and the use of antibodies as platforms for the presentation of antigenic peptides (reviewed in Reference 32). Explicit links to the pharmaceutical drug development process have been made using antibody[33] or minibody[34] library screening systems, and the use of anti-receptor antibodies to prepare secondary structure mimics of interesting ligands.[35] In addition, large-scale production systems have now progressed to the point where economical production is feasible[36-38] (see also Chapters 9 and 10) which should allow the use of human and humanized antibodies as chronic, as well as acute treatments. Novel expression systems have also emerged that may ultimately challenge the more traditional methods for cost-effective production[39,40] (see Chapter 11).

This book developed from a wish to present a timely summary of the progress of antibody products through development and clinical studies into the market place. Therefore, a focus of the book is with these latter phases of engineered antibody development.

This book is divided into a number of sections. In the first section the chapters describe recent developments in antibody R+D which will provide the platform for further product development. The focus is on how the antibody achieves a therapeutic effect post-binding. M. Clark (Cambridge) has reviewed recent progress in the use of unconjugated antibodies as therapeutics, including their use in antigen blockade, recruitment of antibody-dependent cellular cytotoxicity (ADCC) and complement, and situations where bispecific antibodies might be of benefit. Three chapters then describe the use of antibodies for delivery of toxins (R. Kreitman and I. Pastan, NIH), drugs and radioisotopes (G. Yarranton, Celltech), and enzymes for the activation of prodrugs (I. Benhar and I. Pastan, NIH). These chapters principally deal with the use of antibodies for treatment of cancers, which has been a major focus of antibody therapeutics development. Chapters in the next section identify alternative uses for antibody therapeutics.

The second section provides an insight into areas where antibodies are being considered as products. Recent surveys of antibodies in development[29,41] suggest that while there is still a predominance in the use of antibodies as anti-cancer platforms, recombinant MAbs are being considered for use in a much broader range of indications. The use of antibodies for the treatment of cancer is not dealt with here as a separate subject as it has been reviewed extensively elsewhere and permeates many of the other individual chapters in Sections I and IV. W. Harris (Aberdeen) summarizes the use of immune globulins and MAbs in the treatment of infectious diseases. L. Chatenoud (Oxford) describes opportunities for the use of antibodies in autoimmune situations. ORTHOCLONE OKT®3 has been licensed for use in renal transplantation for 10 years. M. Alegre (Belgium) provides an update on the various ways in which this and other antibodies may, and do, play a role in successful organ transplantation.

In the third section issues relating to the development and manufacture of antibody products are addressed. K. Lambert (Cantab) provides a current view of regulatory issues for the development of antibody therapeutics. D. Robinson of Merck, V. Yabannavar of Schering Plough, and Y. Deo of Medarex have collaborated to describe factors in the manufacture of antibodies by large-scale mammalian cell culture. M. Better and P. Gavit of Xoma Corp. then provide a similar analysis of production of antibody domains in prokaryotes. Finally, in this section A. Porter and colleagues (Aberdeen) review those emerging production systems which may eventually challenge mammalian cell culture and *E. coli* expression for economic manufacture of antibody therapeutics.

The final section includes chapters describing the preclinical and clinical development of a number of recombinant antibodies that are now well down the developmental path and in clinical studies, and which might be expected to be included in the next generation of licensed products. Of particular interest are the approaches taken to demonstrate safety and pharmacokinetics in the preclinical and phase I/II studies. These data, showing long half-lives and minimal immunogenicity, should further increase interest in this type of pharmaceutical product. J. Hakimi (Hoffmann-La Roche) and colleagues describe the use of *Zenapax* (humanized anti-IL-2 receptor antibody) in clinical studies in graft-vs-host disease and in transplantation. S. Stephens and colleagues (Celltech) summarize phase I and II studies of the anti-TNFα antibody, CDP571. RSHZ19 (*SB209763)* is a humanized antibody which recognizes respiratory syncytial virus (RSV), a major cause of morbidity and mortality in infants. S. Dillon et al. (SmithKline Beecham) describe preclinical and early clinical studies with this antibody. Finally, A. Solinger et al. (IDEC) describes the PRIMATIZED® antibody IDEC-CE9.1 and its current clinical status for the treatment of rheumatoid arthritis.

CONCLUDING REMARKS

Today, 20 years after the discovery of MAbs and a century after the concept of the magic bullet, ethical pharmaceuticals built around the basic antibody structure are a reality. Many more products will emerge as the unique qualities of antibodies become more widely appreciated along with the understanding that the major technical hurdles to their acceptance have been overcome. The next few years will be an exciting and productive period for this emerging class of pharmaceuticals.

REFERENCES

1. Cryz, S. J., Ed., *Immunotherapy and Vaccines*, VCH, Verlagsgesellschaft mbH, D-6940 Weinheim, Germany, 1991.
2. Kohler, G. and Milstein, C., Continuous culture of fused cells secreting antibody of predefined specificity, *Nature*, 265, 495, 1975.
3. Winter, G., Griffiths, A. D., Hawkins, R. E., and Hoogenboom, H. R., Making antibodies by phage display technology, *Annu. Rev. Immunol.*, 12, 433, 1994.
4. Burton, D. R. and Barbas, C. F., III, Human antibodies from combinatorial libraries, *Adv. Immunol.*, 57, 191, 1994.
5. Adair, J. R. and King D. J., Reconstruction of monoclonal antibodies by genetic engineering, in *Monoclonal Antibodies: The Second Generation*. Zola, H., Ed., BIOS Scientific Publishers Ltd., 1995, 67.
6. Ortho Multicenter Transplant Study Group, A randomized clinical trial of OKT3 monoclonal antibody for acute rejection of cadaveric renal transplants, *N. Engl. J. Med.*, 313, 337, 1985
7. James, K. and Bell, G. T., Human monoclonal antibody production. Current status and future prospects, *J. Immunol. Methods*, 100, 5, 1987.
8. Morrison, S. L., Johnson, M. J., Herzenberg, L. A., and Oi, V. T., Chimeric human antibody molecules: mouse antigen-binding domains with human constant region domains, *Proc. Natl. Acad. Sci. U.S.A.*, 81, 6851, 1984.
9. Neuberger, M. S., Williams, G. T., Mitchell, E. B., Jouhal, S. S., Flanagan, J. G., and Rabbitts, T. H., A hapten-specific chimaeric IgE antibody with human physiological effector function, *Nature*, 314, 268, 1985.
10. Munro, A., Uses of chimaeric antibodies, *Nature*, 312, 597, 1984.
11. Alt, F. W., Blackwell, T. K., and Yancopoulos, G. D., Immunoglobulin genes in transgenic mice, *Trends Genet.*, 1, 231, 1985.
12. Lerner, R. A., Antibodies of predetermined specificity in biology and medicine, *Adv. Immunol.*, 36, 1, 1984.
13. Crawley, P., Antibody patents, in *Monoclonal Antibodies: Principles and Applications*, Birch, J. R. and Lennox, E. S., Eds., Wiley-Liss Inc., New York, 1995, 299.
14. Better, M., Chang, C. P., Robinson, R. R., and Horwitz, A. H., *Escherichia coli* secretion of an active chimeric antibody fragment, *Science*, 240, 1041, 1988.
15. Skerra, A. and Pluckthun, A., Assembly of a functional immunoglobulin Fv fragment in *Escherichia coli, Science*, 240, 1038, 1988.
16. Huston, J. S., McCartney, J, Tai, M. S., Mottola-Carlshorn, C., Jin, D., Wartren, F., Keck, P., and Oppermann, H., Medical applications of single-chain antibodies, *Int. Rev. Immunol.*, 10, 195, 1993.
17. Gadina, M., Newton, D. L., Rybak, S. M., Wu, Y.-N., and Youle, R. J., Humanized immunotoxins. *Ther. Immunol.*, 1, 59, 1994.
18. Pietersz, G. A. and McKenzie, I. F. C., The genetic engineering of antibody constructs for diagnosis and therapy, in *Monoclonal Antibodies: The Second Generation*, Zola, H., Ed., BIOS Scientific Publishers Ltd., Oxford, 1995, 93.
19. Haber, E., Antibody-enzyme fusion proteins and bispecific antibodies, in *The Pharmacology of Monoclonal Antibodies, Handbook of Experimental Pharmacology, Vol. 113*, Rosenberg, M. and Moore, G. P., Eds., Springer-Verlag, Berlin, 1994, 179.
20. Huennekens, F. M., Tumor targeting: activation of prodrugs by enzyme-monoclonal antibody conjugates, *Trends Biotechnol.*, 12, 234, 1994.
21. Gascoigne, N. R., Goodnow, C. C., Dudzik, K. I., Oi, V. T., and Davis, M. M., Secretion of a chimeric T-cell receptor-immunoglobulin protein, *Proc. Natl. Acad. Sci. U.S.A.*, 84, 2936, 1987
22. Chamow, S. M. and Ashkenazi, A., Immunoadhesins: principles and applications, *Trends Biotechnol.*, 14, 52, 1996

23. Bebbington, C. R., Expression of antibody genes in nonlymphoid mammalian cells, *Methods: A Companion to Methods in Enzymology,* 2, 136, 1991.
24. Horwitz, A. H., Chang, C. P., Better, M., Hellstrom, K. E., and Robinson, R. R., Secretion of functional antibody and Fab fragment from yeast cells, *Proc. Natl. Acad. Sci. U.S.A.,* 85, 8678, 1988.
25. Jones, P. T., Dear, P. H., Foote, J., Neuberger, M. S., and Winter, G., Replacing the complementarity-determining regions in a human antibody with those from a mouse, *Nature,* 321, 522, 1986.
26. LoBuglio, A. F., Wheeler, R. H., Trang, J., Haynes, A., Rogers, K., Harvey, E. B., Sun, L., Ghrayeb, J., and Khazaeli, M. B., Mouse/human chimeric monoclonal antibody in man: kinetics and immune response, *Proc. Natl. Acad. Sci. U.S.A.,* 86, 4220, 1989.
27. Hale, G., Dyer, M. J., Clark, M. R., Phillips, J. M., Marcus, R., Riechmann, L., Winter, G., and Waldmann, H., Remission induction in non-Hodgkin lymphoma with reshaped human monoclonal antibody CAMPATH-1H, *Lancet,* ii, 1394, 1988.
28. Emery, S. C. and Adair, J. R., Humanized monoclonal antibodies for therapeutic applications, *Exp. Opin. Invest. Drugs,* 3, 241, 1994.
29. Adair, J. R. and Bright, S., Progress with humanized antibodies — an update, *Exp. Opin. Invest. Drugs,* 4, 863, 1995.
30. Chin, L. T., Hinkula, J., Levi, M., Ohlin, M., Wahren, B., and Borrebaeck, C. A. K., Site directed primary *in vitro* immunization: production of HIV-neutralizing human monoclonal antibodies from lymphocytes obtained from seronegative donors, *Immunology,* 81, 428, 1994.
31. Mountain, A. and Adair, J. R., Engineering antibodies for therapy, *Biotech. Gen. Eng. Rev.,* 10, 1, 1992.
32. Zanetti, M., Rossi, F., Lanza, P., Filaci, G., Lee, R. H., and Billetta, R., Theoretical and practical aspects of antigenized antibodies, *Immunol. Rev.,* 130, 125, 1992.
33. Davies, J. and Riechmann, L., Antibody VH domains as small recognition units, *Bio/Technology,* 13, 475, 1995.
34. Martin, F., Toniatti, C., Salvati, A. L., Venturini, S., Ciliberto, G., Cortese, R., and Sollazzo, M., The affinity-selection of a minibody polypeptide inhibitor of human interleukin-6, *EMBO J.,* 13, 5303, 1994.
35. Saragovi, H. U., Greene, M. I., Chrusciel, R. A., and Kahn, M., Loops and secondary structure mimetics: development and applications in basic science and rational drug design, *Bio/Technology,* 10, 773, 1992.
36. Ward, E. S. and Bebbington, C. R., Genetic manipulation and expression of antibodies, in *Monoclonal Antibodies: Principles and Applications,* Birch, J. R. and Lennox, E. S., Eds., Wiley-Liss Inc., New York, 1995, 137.
37. Reff, M., High-level production of recombinant immunoglobulins in mammalian cells, *Curr. Opin. Biotechnol.,* 4, 573, 1993.
38. Carter, P., Kelley, R. F., Rodrigues, M. L., Snedcor, B., Covarrubias, M., Velligan, M. D., Wong, W. L. T., Rowland, A. M., Kotts, C. E., Carver, M. E., Yang, M., Bourell, J. H., Shepard, H. M., and Henner, D., High level *Escherichia coli* expression and production of a bivalent humanized antibody fragment, *Bio/Technology,* 10, 163, 1992.
39. Ma, J. K.-C. and Hein, M., Immunotherapeutic potential of antibodies produced in plants, *Trends Biotechnol.,* 13, 522, 1995.
40. Maga, E. A. and Murray, J. D., Mammary gland expression of transgenes and the potential for altering the properties of milk, *Bio/Technology,* 13, 1452, 1995.
41. Anon. *Gen. Eng. News,* 15, 12, 1995.

The Editors

William J. Harris, Ph.D., C.Biol., is Professor of Genetics at the University of Aberdeen, Scotland. He obtained a first class honors B.Sc. degree in Biochemistry in 1966 from the University of St. Andrews and Ph.D. in 1969 from the University of Dundee. He served as lecturer in Biochemistry at the University of Aberdeen from 1969 to 1978; Head of *In Vitro* Toxicology at Inveresk Research International, Edinburgh, 1978 to 1980; Head of Biotechnology at Inveresk Research International, 1980 to 1986; Research Director of Bioscot Ltd. 1986 to 1987, and assumed his present position in 1987.

He was technical advisor in Biotechnology to Cogent Investments Ltd., U.K. 1980 to 1986. In 1987 he founded Scotgen Ltd. and remained its managing director until 1993. During this time Scotgen Ltd. developed a large number of humanized antibodies against a broad range of disease targets and several of these are currently in clinical trials. He was awarded four SMART awards by the U.K. Department of Trade and Industry between 1987 and 1991.

He is a member of the Biochemical, Genetics, Immunology, and Microbiology societies of U.K., American Society of Microbiology, Institute of Biology. Since 1990 he has been the recipient of over £1 million of research grants from U.K. Biotechnology and Biologicals Sciences Research Council, U.K. Ministry of Agriculture Fisheries and Food, Scottish Hospital Endowments Research Trust, and Tenovus Charity for Cancer Research.

Professor Harris is author of over 40 papers in peer reviewed journals, 15 chapters in books, editor of two books and co-author of one book. He is a co-inventor on 15 patent applications. His current research interests relate to the development of high-affinity antibody fragments for detection and bioremediation of organic pollutants, and the molecular immunology of multiples sclerosis and posterior uveitis.

John R. Adair, Ph.D., is Product Development Manager at Axis Genetics, Plc. Between 1975 to 1981, at the University of Warwick, U.K. he obtained First Class B.Sc. (Hons.) and Ph.D. degrees in Biological Sciences.

From 1981 to 1986, as a Research Scientist at G. D. Searle & Co. Ltd., he was involved with developing novel modified human interferons using protein engineering techniques. Between 1986 and 1993 in the Molecular Immunology group at Celltech Plc. he helped establish their recombinant antibody engineering program, developing processes for engineering novel human-like antibodies and antibody fragments for own-product and contract development. Several candidates developed during this time by the research group are now in clinical studies. During this time he became Head of the Protein Engineering Department and later was Principal Scientist and Molecular Immunology Team Leader in the Oncology Biology Section.

He was appointed Research Manager at Scotgen Biopharmaceuticals in 1993. Scotgen was a leader in antibody engineering technology and developed antibody-based therapeutics and diagnostics for infectious disease, cancer, and atherosclerosis. He took up his current position in 1996.

Current interests include developing novel presentation systems for peptide therapeutics and vaccines, novel production systems for therapeutic proteins, and the continuing generation of antibody-based therapeutics and diagnostics.

Dr. Adair is a member of the U.K. Biochemical Society. He is named as co-inventor on 13 granted and pending antibody patent families and has published papers and invited reviews on antibody engineering and production.

Contributors

John R. Adair
Axis Genetics, Plc.
Babraham, Cambridge
United Kingdom

Maria-Luisa Alegre
Gwen Knapp Center
University of Chicago
Chicago, Illinois

Claudio Anasetti
University of Washington
Seattle, Washington

Itai Benhar
Department of Molecular Microbiology and Biotechnology
Tel-Aviv University
Tel-Aviv, Israel

Kate J. Bentley
Department of Biochemistry and Molecular Biology
University of Leeds
Leeds, England

Marc Better
XOMA Corporation
Santa Monica, California

Lucienne Chatenoud
Clinical Immunology
INSERM U25 — Hopital Necker
Paris, France

Mike Clark
Department of Pathology
Cambridge University
Cambridge, United Kingdom

Pauline M. Cupit
Department of Molecular and Cell Biology
University of Aberdeen
Institute of Medical Sciences
Aberdeen, Scotland

Yashwant M. Deo
Medarex, Inc.
Annandale, New Jersey

Susan B. Dillon
Molecular Virology and Host Defense
SmithKline Beecham Pharmaceuticals
King of Prussia, Pennsylvania

Patrick Gavit
XOMA Corporation
Santa Monica, California

John Hakimi
Inflammation and Autoimmune Diseases
Hoffmann-LaRoche
Nutley, New Jersey

William J. Harris
Department of Molecular and Cell Biology
University of Aberdeen
Institute of Medical Sciences
Aberdeen, Scotland

Robert J. Kreitman
Laboratory of Molecular Biology
National Cancer Institute
National Institutes of Health
Bethesda, Maryland

Kathy J. Lambert
Cantab Pharmaceuticals
Cambridge, United Kingdom

Susan E. Light
Clinical Sciences
Hoffmann-LaRoche
Nutley, New Jersey

John A. Lipani
SmithKline Beecham Pharmaceuticals
King of Prussia, Pennsylvania

Diane Mould
SmithKline Beecham Pharmaceuticals
King of Prussia, Pennsylvania

Roland A. Newman
IDEC Pharmaceutical Corporation
La Jolla, California

Ira H. Pastan
Laboratory of Molecular Biology
National Cancer Institute
National Institutes of Health
Bethesda, Maryland

Andy J.R. Porter
Department of Molecular and Cell Biology
University of Aberdeen
Institute of Medical Sciences
Aberdeen, Scotland

Terence G. Porter
Department of Protein Biochemistry
SmithKline Beecham Pharmaceuticals
King of Prussia, Pennsylvania

Cary L. Queen
Protein Design Laboratories, Inc.
Mountain View, California

David K. Robinson
Merck Research Laboratories
Rahway, New Jersey
Current address:
Schering-Plough Research Institute
Union, New Jersey

Alan M. Solinger
IDEC Pharmaceutical Corporation
San Diego, California

Mark Sopwith
Celltech Therapeutics, Ltd.
Slough, Berkshire, United Kingdom

Sue Stephens
Celltech Therapeutics, Ltd.
Slough, Berkshire, United Kingdom

Alemseged Truneh
SmithKline Beecham Pharmaceuticals
King of Prussia, Pennsylvania

Olivia Vetterlein
Celltech Therapeutics Ltd.
Slough, Berkshire, United Kingdom

Thomas A. Waldmann
National Cancer Institute
National Institutes of Health
Bethesda, Maryland

T. Paul Wallace
Peptide Therapeutics Ltd.
Cambridge, England

Vijay Yabannavar
Chiron Corporation
Emeryville, California

G. Yarranton
Celltech Therapeutics, Ltd.
Slough, Berkshire, United Kingdom

Table of Contents

PART III. DEVELOPMENT OF ANTIBODY THERAPEUTICS

PART IV. RECOMBINANT ANTIBODIES IN THE CLINIC

Part I

Antibodies as Therapeutics

Chapter 1

Unconjugated Antibodies as Therapeutics

Mike Clark

CONTENTS

0-8493-8547-4/97/$0.00+$.50

1.1 INTRODUCTION

This chapter will attempt to review the background work to the development of unconjugated antibodies for potential therapeutic uses *in vivo*. Essentially there are two key features to consider: (1) the antibody specificity and (2) its associated effector functions. From a basic knowledge of antibody structures we know that the specificity of an antibody is determined by the precise combination of heavy chain V_H domain with light chain V_L domain, while the effector functions are thought to be largely a property of the heavy chain constant region domains.

The immunoglobulin molecules and their associated humoral and cellular effector systems are broadly conserved across species.[1] Classical experiments within immunology have exploited this homology showing that in many instances the components of the antibody-mediated effector systems can be mixed and matched, e.g., human cells, mouse antibodies, and rabbit complement. However, as will be discussed in this chapter, the conservation of structure and function is not absolute and this can be exploited, or alternatively and more often, it can impose limitations on the therapeutic application of antibodies. A full knowledge of the relevant structural features of antibodies which determine biological function will allow for the development of novel therapeutic agents which are fine tuned for their required activities *in vivo*. It must also be taken into account that in addition the immune system itself, as well as providing us with the source of therapeutic antibodies can be a barrier to the proposed therapeutic strategies. The obvious example is when therapeutic antibodies are neutralized by the recipient's antiglobulin response to the therapeutic antibody which is seen as a foreign immunogenic protein.

1.2 DERIVATION OF ANTIBODIES

1.2.1 Immunization and Specificity

Conventionally antibodies are raised by immunizing animals with a chosen antigen. Those determinants of an antigen that are seen as foreign are potentially able to be recognized by surface immunoglobulin on B cells and this can then trigger the differentiation of B cells into plasma cells resulting in the secretion of the immunoglobulin molecules. Some antigens, for example, complex carbohydrate antigens (e.g., bacterial polysaccharides and antigens cross-reacting with the blood group ABO molecules), are able to trigger B cells without a requirement for any "classical" T-cell help and these are called the "thymus-independent antigens." However, for many antigens and in particular for most protein-containing antigens there is an absolute requirement for T-cell recognition and help before a B-cell response can be generated. T cells see processed peptide antigens presented in the context of major histocompatibility complex (MHC) class II. It seems that B cells can process and present antigens that have been captured by their own surface immunoglobulin very effectively to activated T cells but not to naive T cells. This T-cell activation seems to require previous exposure to antigen presented on dendritic cells along with appropriate costimulatory signals. In some circumstances following an encounter with an antigen it is possible to induce anergy and tolerance rather than activation and this is, of course, crucial in preventing autoreactive cells from causing damage.

The complex nature of this T-B cooperation therefore means that the precise nature of the B-cell response to a given antigen is difficult to predict and depends upon such variables as the route of immunization, the purity, the dose, the frequency, the use of carriers or adjuvant, and previous exposure to antigens as well as the species and strain of animal used. Initially the immune responses to thymus-dependent antigens start off as low-affinity antibodies of the IgM class, but during the course of the immune response and particularly following repeat immunizations class switching to IgG, IgA, and IgE, and affinity maturation through somatic hypermutation are usually observed.

1.2.2 Monoclonal Antibodies (MAbs)

It is now two decades since Kohler and Milstein published their original observations on the immortalization of specific antibody-producing cell lines. This was achieved through the cell fusion of a tissue culture of adapted plasmacytoma line with spleen cells from a mouse immunized with sheep red blood cells.[2] The basic method with a few minor technical changes was quickly established as a principal method of producing highly specific and clonal antibodies from immunized laboratory mice and rats. Although the method has been adapted to the production of MAbs from other species, including human, it has proven to be most effective and routinely applicable for production of mouse and rat antibodies.[3-5] A majority of MAbs which have been made and studied are of the IgM class and IgG subclasses from mice and rats.

One of the earlier observations made using somatic cell fusion was that the immunoglobulin encoding genes of both parental cells are codominantly expressed in the hybrid cells.[6] During normal B-cell development the rearrangement of immunoglobulin encoding gene segments is tightly regulated so that only one heavy chain and one light chain are successfully rearranged and expressed, giving rise to allelic and isotypic exclusion; however, hybridoma and transfected cells can be constructed to express multiple light and/or heavy chains. In such cells the chains are able to associate to give rise to mixtures of antibodies with altered valency for antigen and novel functions.[7-11] As discussed below, such novel antibodies may have unusual properties and thus confer therapeutic advantages over conventional antibodies.[12] As an alternative to codominant expression of antibody chains in the same cell line it is possible to reproduce similar monovalent or bispecific reagents through the *in vitro* covalent modification of conventional MAbs.[13-15]

1.2.3 Phage Antibodies

A more recent approach to the production of antigen-specific immunoglobulin fragments is in the use of bacteriophage vectors to clone and express genes encoding Fv or Fab structures.[16-18] Originally these vectors were used to clone V genes as libraries derived from immunized animals. Degenerate oligonucleotide primers, specific for conserved sequences at the 5′ and 3′ ends of the heavy and light chain V regions, were used in the polymerase chain reaction (PCR). Fragments of the heavy and light chains from the library were expressed in different combinations and the specific Fv or Fab encoding phage was purified by affinity selection on antigen.[19] More recently, some success has been obtained in the use of totally synthetic libraries containing randomized "hypervariable" or "complementarity determining region" (CDR) sequences within conserved "framework region" (FwR) sequences.[20] Again the libraries can be selected by affinity for antigen and subsequent rounds of mutation and affinity maturation can be introduced into the system.

Phage libraries allow for the production of new antibodies in ways that are more convenient to those research workers with expertise in molecular biology. They can be used to clone and express antibodies from species that might prove difficult to use for the conventional Kohler and Milstein methods, and they can also be used with antigens for which it might be impossible to immunize an animal, either for practical or for ethical reasons. Synthetic libraries are, of course, not constrained by the normal requirements of antigen processing and presentation and T-B cooperation described above. However, unless it is possible to use the phage-derived antibodies directly for therapy, as Fab or Fv fragments, it is most likely that the antibody V regions will need to be subcloned along with suitable constant regions into expression vectors capable of producing whole antibody molecules.

1.3 RODENT MAbs

1.3.1 Functional Properties of Rodent MAbs

As mentioned above a majority of MAbs which have been well studied are of the mouse or rat, IgM class or IgG subclasses. From the point of view of the potential of these antibodies as therapeutics it is important to consider how such antibodies are likely to mediate their functions by interacting with the host, and in the context of human therapy this requires a comparison of mouse, rat, and human immunoglobulins. From a sequence comparison it is obvious that the immunoglobulin classes IgM and IgG are homologous in the three species.[21,22] However, it is not so clearly defined for the subclasses of IgG, despite the fact that all three species have four subclasses.[23] A look at the gene organization and a comparison of the protein sequences suggest that gene duplication to give rise to four IgG subclasses took place after species diversion. For rats and mice it appears that the immediate ancestor to both species probably had three IgG subclasses and that a different gene in each species duplicated to give the fourth subclass.[22] In an ancestor of man it would appear that a gene organization of μ–δ–γ–γ–ε–α recently gave rise to a duplication creating the four isotypes as μ–δ–γ–γ–ε–α–γ–γ–ε–α. In addition in man this created two subclasses of IgA (unlike in mouse or rat), but one of the ε genes is a pseudo gene so that there is only one functional IgE.[24] There is also an additional pseudo γ sequence present in the middle of the human locus. In all three species the different subclasses do show functional differences from each other but it should not be assumed that the four subclasses have direct equivalent functional counterparts in the other species.[22,23]

In addition to the gene organizations giving rise to different classes and subclasses, there are also allelic forms of some of the genes which encode protein sequence differences and give rise to serologically recognized allotypes of the immunoglobulins.[25,26] Functional differences may be associated with these allotypic differences.[23,26,27] Early experiments demonstrated some interesting properties of antibodies in activation of the effector functions, as detailed below.

For a given antigen the observations made were that, as expected, different subclasses were found to have different abilities to activate complement as a result of differences in the affinity for the early complement component C1q.[28] When experiments were conducted with human cell-surface antigens as targets and human serum as a complement source, there were other major influences on the outcome for cell lysis. Thus there were bigger differences in lysis when comparing the results for different antigen specificities than when comparing different isotypes.[28-32] For example, the CD52 antigen and MHC class I and II antigens on lymphocytes are very good targets for complement-mediated lysis and rat antibodies of the isotypes IgM, IgG1, IgG2a, IgG2b, and IgG2c are all very effective, although IgM is usually the most effective and IgG2b is the best IgG subclass.[30-32] Other good but artificial targets studied extensively were based on the covalent linkage of small hapten groups such as DNP (dinotrophenyl),[33,34] NIP (3-iodo-4-hydroxy-5-nitrophenylacetate),[35-37] and DNS (5-dimethylamino-1-naphthalenesulfonyl dansyl chloride),[38,39] to proteins or membrane soluble lipids. Further studies indicated that the amount of observed lysis caused by a given isotype was often a result of differences in the efficiencies of activation and complexing of several stages in the complement cascade and not just the affinity of the initial components of the classical pathway C1q, C1r, and C1s for that subclass.[28,40]

In contrast to the above observations the antigens CD3 and CD45 are very poor targets (as are the vast majority of human cell-surface antigens studied), and even antibodies of the rat subclass IgG2b give next to no lysis.[31,32,40] The study of antibodies to these poor targets has, however, highlighted ways of improving lysis. Mixtures of antibodies directed to different determinants of the CD45 antigen were found to give greatly improved synergistic lysis.[32] Used separately two rat IgG2b antibodies gave next to no lysis even at saturating antibody concentrations while when mixed together the pair of antibodies produced substantial lysis even at subsaturating levels of antibodies. Clearly the local antibody density and steric arrangement is more important than the average density of antibody on the cell.[28] This is probably a clue as to why some antigens are better targets than others. The synergistic pair of rat CD45 antibodies was used in experiments to reduce the incidence of graft rejection by using them to attempt to remove "passenger leukocytes" from allo–kidneys prior to transplantation.[41] Synergistic lysis with MAbs was first described for rat monoclonal allo–antibodies to the rat MHC–class I molecule RT1.[42,43] This system has been very well studied *in vitro* and *in vivo* for different antibody isotypes and for different antigen densities and by using this system optimum depletion was shown to depend upon the antigen density as well as the rat isotypes used.[44,45] In addition, evidence was provided which suggested that optimum clearance by some antibodies might depend on complement fixation, while for other antibodies Fc receptor-mediated clearance was probably involved.

While investigating functions of MAbs *in vitro*, particularly with regard to potential therapeutic applications, it was found that antibody-dependent cellular cytotoxicity (ADCC) against human tumor cell lines and normal peripheral blood leukocytes were mediated by a lymphocyte subpopulation which seemed to express the CD16 receptor.[46] The ADCC was triggered by rat IgG2b MAbs and was mediated by peripheral blood mononuclear cell populations used as the effectors. Effector cells depleted of monocytes/macrophages were still active but ADCC was abrogated by depletion of effector cells bearing the HNK-1 marker. Alternatively, incubation of the effectors with CD16 antibody also blocked ADCC. Using matched sets of recombinant antibodies specific for the hapten NP, we confirmed the rat isotype which worked best in ADCC was rat IgG2b[47] and for human isotypes it was found that IgG1 and IgG3 were active.[37]

1.3.2 Therapeutic Use of Rodent Antibodies

The ability to make MAbs and the observations that they could bind to and cause destruction of cells *in vitro* either through complement activation or through antibody-dependent cell-mediated cytotoxicity led to their uses in patient therapy. The rat IgM antibody CAMPATH-1 M against the human CD52 antigen has been widely used *in vitro* for the removal of lymphocytes from bone marrow prior to transplantation, in order to prevent graft-versus-host disease.[48,49] The antibody was also administered *in vivo* for the attempted treatment of lymphoma and lymphocytic leukemias; however, both the IgM and a rat IgG2a antibody also specific for CD52 produced only transient cell reductions in the patients. Based on the results obtained *in vitro* with rat IgG2b antibodies in assays for ADCC a class switch variant of the rat IgG2a hybridoma to IgG2b was sought and this, when used *in vivo*, was able to induce partial and complete remissions.[50,51] This result emphasized that it was necessary for an antibody to mediate an appropriate effector function as well as to bind to the right target population.

Another antibody which has been successfully used *in vivo* is the mouse IgG2a monoclonal OKT3 specific for the T-lymphocyte CD3 antigen. This antibody is able to cause immunosuppression by blocking T-cell receptor function.[52] Interestingly CD3 turns out to be a poor target for complement-dependent lysis, however, it was discovered that antibodies could be significantly improved by rendering them univalent for antigen.[10] A monovalent version of a rat IgG2b antibody to CD3 was derived and used *in vivo* for immunosuppression of patients suffering heart organ graft rejection episodes.[53,54] Interestingly, the monovalent antibody seemed to be effective at a relatively low dose and did not seem to produce high levels of cytokine release; a complication often seen with OKT3.[54]

1.3.3 Bispecific Antibodies

The preparation of monovalent MAbs, such as the monovalent rat CD3 antibody described above, relies upon the observation that immunoglobulin genes are codominantly expressed in a cell.[6,10] Thus, the individual protein chains are able to randomly associate, within the limits of a heavy chain class, and the secreted products consist of a mixture of hybrid antibodies (see Figure 1). Normally, a process of allelic exclusion acts during the differentiation of B cells to prevent two heavy chain encoding genes or two light chain encoding genes from being functionally rearranged. This can be overcome by fusing two hybridoma cells together to make a hybrid-hybridoma (sometimes called a quadroma), or by transfecting extra immunoglobulin genes.[7-12]

Purification of different molecular species away from each other not only allows for selection of the monovalent antibodies described above but also for bispecific antibodies.[7-9,11,12] Such antibodies are capable of binding to two different antigens simultaneously and thus can have some interesting properties (see Figure 1). With regard to therapy two particular examples of bispecific antibodies have been pursued. First, MAbs specific for cell-surface antigens present on tumors have been combined with MAbs specific for cytotoxic agents, for example, toxins such as gelonin and saponin.[55,56] These bispecific antibodies are able to crosslink the toxic agent to a target cell and give rise to very potent killing. A second use of bispecific antibodies has been in the enhancement or recruitment of additional cell-mediated effector mechanisms.[11-14] Bispecific antibodies which again recognize cell-surface antigens on tumor cell targets can be combined with specificities for activation molecules on effector cells, e.g., the antigen-specific receptor complex on T lymphocytes or the Fc receptors on macrophages and other leukocytes.[11-14,57,58]

A therapeutic example of a bispecific antibody is the CD3xCD19 antibody SHR1 which was prepared by fusion of a rat IgG2b (CD3) producing hybridoma with a mouse IgG1 (CD19) hybridoma.[53] In a series of *in vitro* experiments that antibody was shown to be a potent activator of cytotoxic T cells and could be used to target them to destroy CD19-positive B-lymphoma and leukemia cells.[59-61] More recently these studies have led to phase I/II clinical trials and again the ability to activate T cells is apparent *in vivo*.[62,63] Currently the important questions

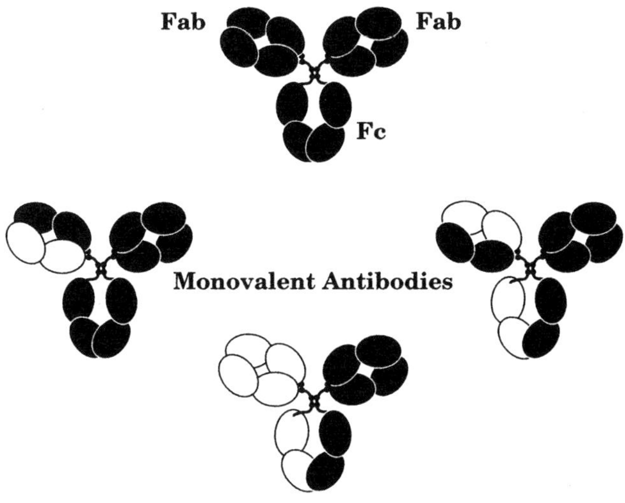

FIGURE 1
Novel MAb species. Shown are schematic representations of antibody molecules. The top represents a conventional bivalent IgG molecule with two identical heavy chains and two identical light chains. The two Fab regions and the Fc region of the molecule are labeled. Underneath are two types of monovalent IgG molecule which arise from the inappropriate pairing of heavy chains (white or black) or light chains (white or black) in cell lines which do not show allelic or isotypic exclusion. The bottom molecule represents the special case of an antibody which is monovalent for each of two different antigens giving rise to a bispecific antibody.

of such therapeutic uses concern the dose and timing of administration of antibody as well as the need to maintain activation of T cells through additional administration of cytokines.

1.4 RECOMBINANT ANTIBODIES

1.4.1 Reshaping or Humanization of Antibody V Regions

As has been described above, through careful selection of species and isotype, it has proved possible to select rodent antibodies with profound therapeutic activities *in vivo*.[23,44,45,48,51-55] The general conservation of immunoglobulin structure and function across species means that antibodies capable of activating human complement or of binding to and activating human Fcγ receptors, such as the rat IgG2b CAMPATH-1G (CD52) or the mouse IgG2a OKT3 (CD3) can be found. However, a major limitation in the long-term use of such agents in therapy has been the rapid onset after 10 to 15 days of a human antiglobulin response to the rat- or mouse-specific residues.[52,53,64,65] A partial solution to this problem was the production of recombinant chimeric antibodies in which the rodent constant regions were replaced with human constant regions.[33-39,66] This also had the advantage that it was possible to select a constant region which endowed the antibody with the appropriate biological effector functions.[37,66] A further step was the recognition that even within the variable regions there were human- and rodent-specific residues within the framework sequences which could be exchanged without altering the specificity of the antibody, while reducing further the chance of an antiglobulin response.[67-69]

The first such fully "reshaped" or "humanized" rodent MAbs were generated by grafting the rodent CDR sequences onto human framework sequences from human myeloma proteins for which crystallographic structures had been determined.[67-69] This has proved successful in a number of cases, but sometimes additional changes to the sequence of the frameworks are required for a restoration of the full binding affinity.[70,71] An alternative technique which has proven to be highly successful has been the selection of human germline V gene sequences which are most homologous to the rodent sequence, followed by mutation of the rodent frameworks to these sequences.[72,73] This closest fit strategy has an additional benefit in that the choice of myeloma-derived framework regions has the disadvantage of maybe including somatic mutations not found in the general human population, whereas germline genes can be selected that are generally represented in majority of individuals.[70]

Future development of new MAb-based therapies is likely to involve either direct selection of human-like sequences from combinatorial or synthetic phage libraries or the full reshaping ("humanization") of rodent-derived MAbs. These V regions will then be coexpressed along with appropriate constant regions, selected on the basis of the required biological functions.

1.4.2 Biological Functions of Antibody Isotypes

Based on a comparison of the amino acid sequences of IgG antibodies from several species and a knowledge of which ones were capable of activating complement or binding to Fcγ receptors, residues which might be responsible for the different functions were identified[1] (see Figure 2). This led to a series of experiments in which site-directed mutations of such residues were introduced into a mouse IgG2b antibody, with specificity for the hapten NIP. A sequence motif in the C_H2 region involving Glu 318, Lys 320, and Lys 322 was identified as being crucial for the binding of the first component of the complement cascade C1q.[74] However, this motif is present in isotypes from antibody

```
               233                                                                        296                 318      327
               | 235                                                                      |                   | 320    |  330
               | |  238                                                                   |297                | | 322  |  |331
               | |  |                                                                     ||                  | | |    |  ||
Human IgG1     APELLGGPSVFLFPPKPKDTLMISRTPEVTCVVVDVSHEDPEVKFNWYVDGVEVHNAKTKPREEQYNSTYRVVSVLTVLHQDWLNGKEYKCKVSNKALPAPIEKTISKAK
Human IgG2     APP_VAGPSVFLFPPKPKDTLMISRTPEVTCVVVDVSHEDPEVQFNWYVDGVEVHNAKTKPREEQFNSTFRVVSVLTVVHQDWLNGKEYKCKVSNKGLPAPIEKTISKTK
Human IgG3     APELLGGPSVFLFPPKPKDTLMISRTPEVTCVVVDVSHEDPEVQFKWYVDGVEVHNAKTKPREEQYNSTFRVVSVLTVLHQDWLNGKEYKCKVSNKALPAPIEKTISKTK
Human IgG4     APEFLGGPSVFLFPPKPKDTLMISRTPEVTCVVVDVSQEDPEVQFNWYVDGVEVHNAKTKPREEQFNSTYRVVSVLTVLHQDWLNGKEYKCKVSNKGLPSSIEKTISKAK

Mouse IgG1     VPEV___SSVFIFPPKPKDVLTITLTPKVTCVVVDISKDDPEVQFSWFVDDVEVHTAQTQPREEQFNSTFRSVSELPIMHQDWLNGKEFKCRVNSAAFPAPIEKTISKTK
Mouse IgG2a[b]  APDLLGGPSVFIFPPKIKDVLMISLSPMVTCVVVDVSEDDPDVQISWFVNNVEVHTAQTQTHREDYNSTLRVVSALPIQHQDWMSGKEFKCKVNNRALPSPIEKTISKPR
Mouse IgG2a[a]  APNLLGGPSVFIFPPKIKDVLMISLSPIVTCVVVDVSEDDPDVQISWFVNNVEVHTAQTQTHREDYNSTLRVVSALPIQHQDWMSGKEFKCKVNNKDLPAPIERTISKPK
Mouse IgG2b    APNLEGGPSVFIFPPNIKDVLMISLTPKVTCVVVDVSEDDPDVQISWFVNNVEVHTAQTQTHREDYNSTIRVVSTLPIQHQDWMSGKEFKCKVNNKDLPSPIERTISKIK
Mouse IgG3     AGNILGGPSVFIFPPKPKDALMISLTPKVTCVVVDVSEDDPDVHVSWFVDNKEVHTAWTQPREAQYNSTFRVVSALPIQHQDWMRGKEFKCKVNNKALPAPIERTISKPK

Rat   IgG1     GSEV___SSVFIFPPKTKDVLTITLTPKVTCVVVDISQNDPEVRFSWFIDDVEVHTAQTHAPEKQSNSTLRSVSELPIVHRDWLNGKTFKCKVNSGAFPAPIEKSISKPE
Rat   IgG2a    GSEV___SSVFIFPPKPKDVLTITLTPKVTCVVVDISQDDPEVHFSWFVDDVEVHTAQTRPPEEQFNSTFRSVSELPILHQDWLNGRTFRCKVTSAAFPSPIEKTISKPE
Rat   IgG2b    VPELLGGPSVFIFPPKPKDILLISQNAKVTCVVVDVSEEEPDVQFSWFVNNVEVHTAQTQPREEQYNSTFRVVSALPIQHQDWMSGKEFKCKVNNKALPSPIEKTISKPK
Rat   IgG2c    DDNL_GRPSVFIFPPKPKDILMITLTPKVTCVVVDVSEEEPDVQFSWFVDNVRVFTAQTQPHEEQLNGTFRVVSTLHIQHQDWMSGKEFKCKVNNKDLPSPIEKTISKPR
                      .***.***. ** * *. .. *******.*...*.*. .*....  * .* *...  . *.* * ** * . *.**..*....*.*.. ..*..**..***
```

FIGURE 2
Alignment of the CH_2 sequences of human, mouse, and rat IgG subclasses. The CH_2 domain of IgG is thought to play a crucial role in complement and Fc receptor-mediated functions. Shown are aligned sequences for the four human subclasses IgG1, IgG2, IgG3, and IgG4, together with sequences for mouse and rat subclasses. Two allotypes, a and b, of the mouse IgG2a subclass are shown. Gaps have been introduced in some of the sequences to maximize alignments ("_" character). Absolute homology is indicated by an "*" under the sequence, while conservative changes are indicated by a "." character. Residues referred to in the text as being implicated in functional differences are indicated by the residue numbers above the sequences.

subclasses such as human IgG4, so there must be other features of the sequences of the C_H2 which are crucial to function.[1,21,23,27,37] In the same system a mutation of the mouse IgG2b residue Glu 235 to Leu resulted in a dramatic increase in the affinity of the antibody for binding to the human high-affinity FcγRI (CD64).[75]

Matched sets of chimeric and humanized antibodies have been used to provide considerable information on the relative roles of different immunoglobulin isotypes in both *in vitro* and *in vivo* effector systems (reviewed in References 27 and 76–78). These studies allow completely autologous systems to be set up, for example, the killing of human cells by human complement or cellular cytotoxicity as mediated by human Ig isotypes.[27,37] Using recombinant DNA technology, rodent MAbs with suitable specificities can be reconstructed as chimeric, or fully reshaped humanized antibodies with different human constant region domains corresponding to different isotypes.[68] The advantage of matched panels of antibodies prepared in this way is that the specificities and single site affinities for antigens are the same and any functional differences are thus dependent upon the structural differences in the constant regions.[27,76-78]

A complete matched set of MAbs consisting of the human isotypes IgM, IgG1(allotype G1m[za], IgG2, IgG3 (allotypes G3m[b] and G3m[g]), IgG4, IgA2, and IgE was constructed with specificity for the hapten NP and its derivative NIP.[37] The antibodies were tested for their abilities to mediate autologous complement-dependent lysis of human red blood cells labeled with NIP, and for ADCC of a NIP conjugated human lymphoblastoid cell line by activated human mononuclear cells. The IgG1 antibody proved to be the most effective in both complement-dependent and cell-mediated cytotoxicity. The effector cells in ADCC were inhibited by a CD16 (FcγRIII) MAb and had the phenotype of killer cells (K cells). As expected, the IgM antibody proved to be good at complement activation but poor in ADCC. Surprisingly the two IgG3 antibodies were not quite as good as the IgG1 antibody in either assay. For complement, this was despite the fact that IgG3 was shown to be fixing many more molecules of C1q. Bindon et al.[40] later went on to show that although human IgG1 bound less C1 than human IgG3 there was a much more efficient deposition of C4b on the cell surface which accounted for the more effective cell lysis by IgG1. None of the other isotypes IgG2, IgG4, IgA2, and IgE, showed any significant functional activity in these assays.

Other groups making use of this set of antibodies have extended the original observations. Two groups have investigated the effect of varying the antigen density as well as the epitope patchiness for complement lysis triggered by the NIP chimeric MAbs.[79,80] The IgG1 antibody was most effective when the antigen concentration was higher, whereas the IgG3 antibody was relatively better at lower concentrations.

The IgG2 antibody gave good lysis at very high concentrations of antigen, but the IgG4 antibody did not give lysis under any conditions. It was also shown that IgG1 and IgG3, along with IgM, activated the classical pathway of complement but not the alternative pathway. At high antigen concentration the IgG2 antibody could also activate the classical pathway but the IgG4 and IgA2 antibodies could not; however, the IgA2 antibody, and to a lesser extent the IgG2 antibody, did activate the alternative pathway of complement.

The matched panel of human antibodies to the hapten NIP has also been used to look at effector functions in a different system, immunity to parasites.[81] The parasite *Schistosoma mansoni schistosomula* was incubated with NIP-kephalin, which incorporated the hapten into the parasite surface membrane. The killing of these parasites was then determined in the presence of different human isotypes by eosinophils activated in different ways. An interesting observation was that as well as the expected killing by some IgG subclasses and by IgE, the isotype IgA2 proved to be a very potent mediator of ADCC in this system. This result clearly illustrates the usefulness of these matched panels in investigating the roles of different isotypes in immunity and highlights the fact that our preoccupation with IgG subclasses and their receptors may be ignoring important mechanisms of immunity mediated by other classes such as IgA.

Other studies have been carried out with matched sets of human antibodies to conventional human cell-surface antigens such as IgG antibodies to CD52 (CAMPATH-1) antigen and to CD3 and CD4.[68,72,73] For the CD52 antibodies the IgG1 antibody was found to be the most effective antibody in both complement-mediated lysis and ADCC.[68] The IgG3 antibody was also active in both assays while the IgG2 antibody had a lower titer in complement-mediated lysis and gave very little ADCC. The IgG4 antibody did not work in either system. Comparing these results with the NIP chimeric MAbs revealed a large degree of similarity except that the IgG2 antibody to CD52 antigen was more active in complement lysis.[68] As described above, this observation may be due to different antigen densities, or clustering of antigen, with the CD52 antigen being equivalent to the NIP antigen at high concentrations.[79,80]

1.5 THE STRUCTURAL BASIS FOR IgG EFFECTOR FUNCTIONS

A striking feature of the human IgG subclasses is the very high sequence homology between them. Within the constant region domains C_H1, C_H2, and C_H3 this is greater than 90% at the amino acid level.[1,21,23] The biggest differences are within the hinge region which differs in

```
Human  IgG1    EPKSCDKTHTCPPCP
Human  IgG2    ERKCCVECPPCP
Human  IgG3    ELKTPLGDTTHTCPRCP----EPKSCDTPPPCPRCP----EPKSCDTPPPCPRCP----EPKSCDTPPPCPRCP
Human  IgG4    ESKTGPPCPSCP

Mouse  IgG1    VPRDCGCKPCICT
Mouse  IgG2a^b EPRVPITQNPCPPLKECPPCA
Mouse  IgG2a^a EPRGPTIKPCPPCKCP
Mouse  IgG2b   EPSGPISTINPCPPCKECHKCP
Mouse  IgG3    EPRIPKPSTPPGSSCP

Rat  IgG1      VPRNCGGDCKPCICT
Rat  IgG2a     VPRECNPCGCT
Rat  IgG2b     ERRNGGIGHKCPTCPTCHKCP
Rat  IgG2c     EPRRPKPRPPTDICSC
```

FIGURE 3
Hinge region sequences of human, mouse, and rat IgG subclasses. Shown are the sequences of the genetic hinge regions of human, mouse, and rat IgG subclasses. All are encoded by single exons except for the elongated hinge of human IgG3 which is encoded by four exons each of which appears to have a degree of homology with the human IgG1 hinge exon. The amino acid sequence of human IgG3 is shown punctuated to indicate which amino acids are encoded in each exon.

both sequence and length between subclasses (see Figure 3). At the genomic level it can be seen that the genetic hinge has almost certainly been duplicated along with the rest of the constant regions, but that many more mutations have been allowed to accumulate since the subclasses diverged.[21] The hinge of the subclass IgG3 is actually encoded by four repeats of an exon homologous to the hinge region of IgG1 (indicated in Figure 3). Clearly the functional differences observed in comparisons of the human IgG subclasses mentioned above must be dependent on some or all of these sequence differences. A knowledge of the crucial sequences might reveal ways in which novel effector function properties could be introduced into recombinant antibodies such that they could be exploited in therapeutic strategies.[23,27,76-78] Also it would be possible to investigate which are the crucial effector mechanisms that operate under different circumstances, for example, in the control of infections by antibody-mediated responses. Just as it is possible to prepare matched panels of recombinant antibodies of different isotypes it is also possible to prepare matched panels of antibodies in which crucial residues have been changed by site-directed mutations of the genes or in which regions of sequence from one subclass are swapped with the homologous regions from another.

1.5.1 Complement Activation

With regard to the four human IgG subclasses a logical starting place for these investigations concerned investigation of the role of the hinge region. The site of interaction of C1q with IgG was thought to be within the C_H2 domain and, as mentioned above, a C1q binding motif had been identified in mouse IgG2b.[74] However, the four human IgG subclasses are identical within the region of this motif and are very homologous for the rest of the C_H2.[1,21] It was proposed that the difference between IgG3 and IgG4 was therefore dependent upon the former having a long and very flexible hinge region while the latter has a short and more rigid hinge. Thus the greater segmental flexibility of the IgG3 might allow greater access to the Fc region of the antibody for complement binding. To answer this question, the hinges of IgG3 and IgG4 were swapped in anti-DNS antibodies, but it was found that although the upper hinge length was responsible for the big differences in segmental flexibility, this was not responsible for the differences seen in complement binding.[39] Further experiments with domain swap mutants involving IgG1, 3, and 4 with specificity for the hapten DNS[82] and then domain swaps involving IgG1 and IgG4 with specificity for the lymphocyte antigen CD52[83] confirmed that the genetic hinge region only has a marginal effect on complement activation and the crucial differences between IgG4 and IgG1 are in the COOH terminal half of the C_H2 domain (see Figure 2). There are in fact only four residues that differ in this region (IgG1:IgG4, 296 Tyr:Phe, 327 Ala:Gly, 330 Ala:Ser, 331 Pro:Ser), in the anti-DNS antibody system[84] and also repeated with an NIP hapten specific antibody[85] it was shown that a substitution of serine at position 331 in IgG4 for proline (as in IgG1, 2 and 3) endows IgG4 with the ability to activate complement. Recently, starting with a human IgG1 antibody specific for the human MHC class II, HLA-DR antigen, mutations were introduced to attempt to alter complement and FcγR binding.[86] Surprisingly, two results with this human IgG1 antibody show a big difference with earlier studies using mouse IgG2b antibodies specific for NIP. First, a change in the residue 320, previously reported from experiments with mouse IgG2b as being a crucial residue for C1q binding,[74] from Lys to Ala had no effect on complement. In contrast, a change in the residue Leu 235 to Glu, which had previously been implicated in FcγRI binding[75] but not in complement activation using the mouse IgG2b,[74] abolished complement lysis by the human IgG1.[86]

The question of the role of the hinge in IgG is still not settled completely.[87] In the experiments with anti-DNS the hinge length of the IgG3 was shortened by deleting the repeat exons (see Figure 3). While it was reported that an antibody without a hinge was inactive in complement activation, the shortened hinge versions were all apparently similarly active.[39] However, in a system using antibodies specific for the hapten NIP it was reported that shortening the hinge of IgG3 resulted in an improvement in the complement activation by this isotype.[88,89] Also in this NIP system the hinge could be completely replaced with a single disulfide bond while still retaining the ability to activate complement.[90] In human IgG1 but not IgG2, 3, or 4 the light chain is disulfide bonded to a residue within the upper hinge region of the antibody. A set of mutated chimeric antibodies specific for the GD2, melanoma surface antigen, in which the arrangement of the light-heavy chain bond in IgG1 was altered to be more like the other subclasses, was prepared and compared in complement lysis with human complement.[91] The mutated IgG1 antibodies lost their ability to activate complement indicating that residues in the Fab and upper hinge region are critical.

Further evidence for an involvement of residues in the Fab comes from recent studies on mutated human IgG1 antibodies to the CD52 antigen. In human IgG1 there are several naturally occurring allotypes of the heavy chain in the human population which vary in frequency in different racial groups.[25] Alternative allotypic residues are recognized at positions 214 in the C_H1 (proximal to the hinge) and at positions in the C_H3. A gene encoding the wild-type allotype G1m(1,17) was mutated to give either the alternative natural allotype G1m(3), or artificial allotypes G1m(1,3) or G1m(17). Surprisingly it was found that the ability of the antibodies to cause complement-mediated lysis was quantitatively dependent on the residue found at position 214 in the Fab.[27,92]

1.5.2 Fcγ Receptors

The interaction of human IgG antibodies with Fc receptors needs to take into account the different classes of receptor. In humans there are three identified classes of Fc receptors for human IgG (FcγR). Much is known about the gene organization and the structure and function of these receptors (reviewed by van de Winkel and Capel[93]) and they can be readily detected on the cell surface using specific MAbs. Human FcγRI (CD64) can bind monomeric IgG with high affinity and is expressed constitutively on macrophages and monocytes and can be induced on neutrophils and eosinophils. Human FcγRII (CD32) binds IgG only in complexed or polymeric forms and is widely expressed on a range of cell types including monocytes, macrophages, basophils, eosinophils, Langerhans cells, B cells, and platelets. Human FcγRIII (CD16) is also a medium-to-low-affinity receptor and is expressed on macrophages, large granular lymphocytes (LGL; K cells, and NK cells), and neutrophils and can be induced on eosinophils and monocytes. The expression of these three receptor classes on cell types is, however, quite complex for several reasons. First, each of these three classes of receptors is encoded by several closely related genes; thus there are FcγRIA, B and C, FcγRIIA, B and C, and FcγRIIIA and B. The FcγRIIIa form which is a transmembrane receptor, expressed in conjunction with γ, ζ, and β chains, is found on K/NK cells, monocytes, and macrophages while FcγRIIIB is a GPI anchored receptor found on neutrophils and eosinophils. Second, some of these genes then give rise to multiple transcripts, e.g., FcγRIIb1, b2, and b3. (3) Finally, some of these genes exist within the population in different polymorphic forms, e.g., FcγRIIa-R131/FcγRIIa-H131 and $Fc\gamma RIIIb^{NA1}$/$Fc\gamma RIIIb^{NA2}$.

Of particular interest and significance, the polymorphism in FcγRIIa leads to a functional difference in the ability of the receptor to discriminate between different IgG isotypes. This was originally identified for mitogenic responses with murine CD3 antibodies but has been found to affect binding of rat and human isotypes.[94,95] Thus FcγRIIa–R131 binds mouse IgG1 but not human IgG2 while FcγRIIa–H131 does not bind mouse IgG1 but does bind human IgG2. Both forms of the receptor bind human IgG1 but do not bind human IgG4. Only a single amino acid change in the receptor (R → H131) is responsible for this remarkable ability to discriminate between the different isotypes.[93] Further studies have also indicated that the polymorphism affects binding of rat IgG2b.[95] Rat IgG2b behaves in a similar way to human IgG2 and opposite to mouse IgG1; however, unlike human IgG2 the rat IgG2b also binds to the high-affinity FcγRI receptor.[95] Recent results suggest that functionally the FcγRIIa polymorphism may have important consequences regarding resistance to certain infections as mediated by IgG2 and the racial differences in the allele frequencies may in part explain the observed geographical and racial differences in disease incidences such as *Haemophilus influenzae* infections.[93,96] In another clinical situation, this polymorphism in the binding of human IgG2 by FcγRIIa has been implicated as a risk factor in the development of heparin-induced thrombocytopenia.[97]

1.5.3 High-Affinity FcγRI (CD64) Binding

Just as it has proved possible to exploit the homology of the four human IgG subclasses to investigate which residues are involved in complement binding and activation, the same strategies outlined above can be used to determine residues critical for Fcγ receptor binding and activation. The high-affinity binding of monomeric IgG to the FcγRI receptor allowed this interaction to be studied. Human IgG1 and IgG3 bind FcγRI with the highest affinity (K_d 10^{-8} to 10^{-9} M) followed by IgG4 which is about tenfold weaker in its interaction while IgG2 does not readily bind to the receptor.[93] Rat IgG2b and mouse IgG2a also bind human FcγRI readily while mouse IgG2b antibodies were found to be poor at binding.[23,93] A sequence comparison of IgG classes indicated that residues in the IgG lower hinge region (encoded by the 5′ end of the C_H2 exon) might be crucial[1] (see Figure 2). Using site-directed mutagenesis it was shown that by changing the residue Glu 235 to Leu improved the affinity of mouse IgG2b for FcγRI by 100-fold.[75] Using reciprocal domain swap mutants between TNP-specific IgG1 and IgG2 antibodies it was shown that a region spanning 233–238 (Glu Leu Leu Gly Gly Pro in IgG1) was critical for binding, and the introduction of this sequence into IgG2 produced an antibody that bound with higher affinity than IgG1.[98] This result would indicate that there are, of course, other critical residues, probably in the C terminal half of the C_H2 region which are critical. Domain swap mutants between DNS-specific IgG2 and IgG3 antibodies also support the critical role of these residues encoded in the C_H2 regions.[99] Investigation of the residues responsible for the lower binding affinity of IgG4 compared to IgG1 and 3 showed that a change of Phe 234 in IgG4 to Leu improved the affinity.[99] However, it was also found that in IgG3 the change of Pro 331 for Ser as found in IgG4 decreased the affinity of IgG3 for FcγRI.[99] In addition to these domain swap experiments, the introduction of point mutations into NIP-specific IgG3 antibodies in which individual residues were changed to alanine indicated the critical role of the residues Leu 234, Leu 235, and Gly 237.[100]

1.5.4 Low-Affinity FcγRII (CD32) Binding

Studies of the direct binding of IgG to the low-affinity FcγRII are more difficult and so most experimental systems employ some form of complexed or aggregated IgG. One system involves the rosetting of IgG sensitized red cells by FcγRII-bearing leukocytes.[100] Alternatively, IgG can be aggregated into small multimeric complexes using antigen or $F(ab)_2$ fragments of anti-light chain specific antibodies mixed in a 1:1 ratio with the IgG.[101] A different assay exploits the ability of CD3-specific antibodies to trigger a mitogenic response from T cells if the antibody Fc aggregates upon binding to Fc receptors on accessory cells.[95] Generally the observations that IgG1 and IgG3 bound well to FcγRII but IgG4 and IgG2 did not again suggest that the sequence differences in the hinge and lower hinge regions might be critical (see Figure 2). Using rosette formation between red cells sensitized by point mutated IgG3 antibodies with the cell lines Daudi and K562 has indicated that some of the crucial residues for binding are Leu 234 and Leu 237.[100] However, as mentioned above, the more recent observation that two alternative alleles of human FcγRIIa exist and that one can bind human IgG2 and rat IgG2b while the other cannot would suggest that the lower hinge region is not the only critical set of residues and that further studies are required.[95]

1.5.5 ADCC via FcγRIII (CD16)

Most studies of IgG interactions with the low-affinity IgG receptor FcγRIII have concentrated on functional assays of ADCC using effector cells expressing the transmembrane FcγRIIIa form of the receptor. As mentioned above, the rat IgG2b and the human IgG1 antibodies to NIP and to CD52 were particularly potent at triggering ADCC with human peripheral blood mononuclear cells and activated lymphocytes as the effectors.[37,47,68] A series of domain swap mutants between IgG1 and IgG4 were constructed to identify residues responsible for the observed functional differences.[83] First, it was verified that all of the critical differences between these two isotypes lie in the C_H2 domain and secondly, that they were in the COOH terminal end of the C_H2 domain, a result similar to complement activation as described above and involving four possible amino acid changes (IgG1:IgG4, 296 Tyr:Phe,

327 Ala:Gly, 330 Ala:Ser, 331 Pro:Ser) with in particular the residue change Pro 331 in IgG1 for Ser in IgG4 prominent (see Figure 2). However, in a different set of experiments using point mutations of residues in the lower hinge region of IgG3, the residues 235 and 237 were identified as critical for ADCC.[102] The importance of this region for ADCC through FcγRIIIa was confirmed with the anti-HLA DR IgG1 antibody, where changing the Gly at 237 to Ala or exchanging the whole region 233 to 236 for the sequence found in IgG2 reduced activity. As mentioned above, in this same system a change of Leu 235 to Glu not only abolished binding for FcγRI and also complement activation, but had no affect on ADCC through FcγRIIIa.

The results obtained with the domain swap mutants of IgG1 and IgG4 antibodies were, however, further complicated. It was found that the results obtained in this system were dependent upon the donor of the lymphocyte effectors.[83] With some donors IgG1 was effective while IgG4 was ineffective, and in this case the domain swap mutants implicated the residues in the COOH half of the C_H2 as critical. For some donors it was surprisingly found that IgG1 and IgG4 were both effective in ADCC and all of the domain swap mutants were indistinguishable. With such donors of effectors it was found that the four isotypes IgG1, IgG2, IgG3, and IgG4 gave very similar levels of activity. Several genetic polymorphisms of the FcγRIIIa gene have recently been described, but it remains to be demonstrated which if any of these might be responsible for the functional polymorphism seen with the CD52 antibodies.[103]

1.5.6 Glycosylation and Effector Functions

One feature of the IgG antibodies that has been found to be critical for complement-mediated lysis as well as binding to and activation of all three FcγR classes of receptor is the conserved N linked glycosylation site within the C_H2 domain at Asp 297[1,21] (see Figure 2). Antibodies produced without carbohydrate, either through use of metabolic inhibitors, endoglycosidases by site-directed mutation of the attachment site, or produced in bacterial expression systems all show greatly reduced biological functions.[1,27,74-78,104,105] It is not yet clear what is the precise role of the carbohydrate. While glycosylation of antibody is important for function, the precise structures attached to the IgG are complex and can vary from one cell line to another depending upon the glycosyltransferases present.[105] There is some suggestion that the precise carbohydrate structure present on an antibody might have some influence over the biological activity of the antibody in complement activation and FcγR binding, although further investigation is required for a definitive answer.[76,105]

Indeed, an aglycosylated human IgG antibody with specificity for the mouse CD8 antigen was found not to deplete mouse CD8 lymphocytes *in vivo* whereas the glycosylated human IgG subclasses were very effective at depleting cells.[106] This property has been exploited in the production of an aglycosylated form of a humanized IgG1 CD3 antibody which can block T-cell functions without depleting the cells or triggering cytokine release, thus eliminating some of the severe side effects of CD3 antibody therapy.[107]

1.5.7 Acquisition of Maternal IgG by the Neonate

For some considerable time there has been a debate as to the nature of the receptor responsible for transport of human IgG across the placenta. Some have argued for evidence in favor of all three of the receptors described above (CD64, CD32, CD16), however, it has always been a distinct possibility that a previously undescribed receptor was involved. In the rat an Fc receptor was described, FcRn, which was responsible for the neonatal transport of IgG across the intestinal epithelium. This receptor does not show homology to the other FcγR but instead is an MHC class I like molecule with a heavy chain associated with a β_2 microglobulin light chain. Recently a crystal structure of the rat FcRn has been published along with a second crystal structure of the receptor complexed with rat IgG.[108,109] The receptor appears to interact with the IgG forming important contacts with the C_H2 and C_H3 interface. A number of histidine residues are involved and these are likely to be responsible for the observed pH dependence of the transport of IgG by this receptor. In another recent development, the cloning and expression of a human homolog of the rat FcRn from a placental cDNA library has been reported.[110] This receptor shows a similar pH dependency for binding of IgG and the evidence is compelling that this receptor termed hFcRn represents the receptor responsible for placental transport of IgG in the human. From the high homology of this human receptor to the rat FcRn it seems reasonable that it interacts with IgG in a similar structural way as determined for the crystal structure. This should facilitate the modeling of the sites of interaction of human IgG with hFcRn and the present data would indicate that this interaction is likely to involve different sites to the residues identified as important in the association with the three FcγR as detailed above. There are a number of diseases which involve maternal IgG specific for paternal alloantigens, for example, hemolytic disease of the newborn (HDN). The IgG is transported across the placenta where it causes damage in the fetus or newborn through activation of effector mechanisms as described above. It is interesting to speculate whether novel future therapeutic strategies could be developed based on a detailed knowledge of all of the interactions with FcγR and complement discussed above.

1.5.8 Properties of Rat IgG2b vs. Human IgG1/IgG3

Despite the apparent homology of the IgG classes across species, there is in fact no absolute conservation of the number or functional properties of the different IgG subclasses. This is of particular importance when comparing properties of rodent MAbs with their humanized forms in an attempt to derive the best isotype for therapy. As an example of this, during the humanization of the rat IgG2b antibody CAMPATH-1G the original rat antibody was compared to the four human IgG isotypes in various *in vitro* assays.[68] The human IgG1 isotype appeared to be a close match for the rat IgG2b in complement-mediated lysis and antibody-dependent-cell mediated cytotoxicity.[68] The CAMPATH-1 antigen CD52 is a very good target for lysis and the humanized IgG1 antibody CAMPATH-1H proved to work both *in vitro* and *in vivo*.[111] However, recent data suggest that the rat IgG2b might interact with human effector mechanisms in a way which is unique and not directly comparable to any of the four human IgG subclasses. During the humanization of a rat IgG2b CD3 antibody it was noticed that while the rat antibody gave some measurable complement-mediated lysis, a human IgG1 version gave no significant lysis.[73] Also, while a monovalent version of the rat IgG2b antibody proved to be potently lytic a monovalent version of the human IgG1 showed only a small improvement.[53,54,73] Following up these observations we have recently measured the activation of complement by several versions of the CD3 antibody. Three different allotypes of the human IgG1 failed to show detectable lysis or binding of the early complement components C1q, C1s, C4, and C3 while the original rat IgG2b showed significant binding of all four components (Clark et al., unpublished). Interestingly, a human IgG3 version of the CD3 antibody and a second version in which the longer hinge of the IgG3 antibody had been truncated to the same length as IgG1 both showed complement activation, but were not as good as the rat IgG2b (Clark et al., unpublished). The rat IgG2b also shows a different pattern of binding to human FcγR. Rat IgG2b behaves like human IgG1 and IgG3 in binding to FcγRI and also mediating ADCC through FcγRIII, however, it behaves like human IgG2 in that it binds to only the H-131 allelic form of the FcγRIIa receptor.[95] These observations do raise interesting questions regarding whether it can be expected that humanized forms of rat IgG2b antibodies such as the CD52 antibody CAMPATH-1H or the human IgG1 CD3 antibody will behave the same *in vivo* or whether they might give different therapeutic results.

1.6 CONCLUSION

It is clear from the above that conventional rodent MAbs are able to interact with human effector systems although they may not do so in an entirely predictable fashion. These antibodies can also be used to derive therapeutic reagents with novel properties, such as monovalent and bispecific binding properties. Problems with antiglobulin responses and a requirement to carry out precise manipulation of the structure and function of antibodies has led to the use of recombinant techniques for the manipulation and expression of immunoglobulin genes. Recombinant antibodies allow for the investigation of the structural basis for the observed functions, such as antigen binding, complement binding, and activation, and also Fc receptor binding and activation. Investigation of how antibodies interact with cells expressing these Fc receptors in assisting in particular types of cell-mediated responses is also possible. At present, many of these studies have yielded interesting observations but the results are not definitive. It remains to be seen how many of these observations can be put into successful clinical practice. One encouraging observation is that many of the amino acid changes which might be introduced into antibodies to alter effector functions may still retain the long biological half-lives seen with conventional antibodies.[112]

REFERENCES

1. Burton, D. R., Immunoglobulin G: functional sites, *Mol. Immunol.*, 22, 161, 1985.
2. Kohler, G. and Milstein, C., Continuous cultures of fused cells secreting antibody of predefined specificity, *Nature*, 256, 495, 1975.
3. Clark, M. R. and Milstein, C., Expression of spleen cell immunoglobulin phenotype in hybrids with myeloma cell lines, *Som. Cell Genet.*, 7, 657, 1981.
4. Galfre, G. and Milstein, C., Preparation of monoclonal antibodies: strategies and procedures, *Methods Enzymol.*, 73, 3, 1981.
5. Clark, M. and Waldmann, H., Production of murine monoclonal antibodies, *Methods Hematol.*, 13, 1, 1986.
6. Cotton, R. G. H. and Milstein, C., Fusion of two immunoglobulin producing cell lines, *Nature*, 244, 42, 1973.
7. Staerz, U. D. and Bevan, M. J., Hybrid hybridoma producing a bispecific monoclonal antibody that can focus effector T-cell activity, *Proc. Natl. Acad. Sci. U.S.A.*, 83, 1453, 1986.
8. Suresh, M. R., Cuello, A. C., and Milstein, C., Advantages of bispecific hybridomas in one-step immunocytochemistry and immunoassays, *Proc. Natl. Acad. Sci. U.S.A.*, 83, 789, 1986.
9. Suresh, M. R., Cuello, A. C., and Milstein, C., Bispecific monoclonal antibodies from hybrid hybridomas, *Methods Enzymol.*, 121, 210, 1986.
10. Cobbold, S. P. and Waldmann, H., Therapeutic potential of monovalent monoclonal antibodies, *Nature*, 308, 460, 1984.

11. Clark, M. R. and Waldmann, H., T-cell killing of target cells induced by hybrid antibodies: comparison of two bispecific monoclonal antibodies, *J. Natl. Cancer Inst.*, 79, 1393, 1987.
12. Clark, M., Gilliland, L., and Waldmann, H., Hybrid antibodies for therapy, *Prog. Allergy*, 45, 31, 1988.
13. Liu, M. A., Kranz, D. M., Kurnick, J. T., Boyle, L. A., Levy, R., and Eisen, H. N., Heteroantibody duplexes target cells for lysis by cytotoxic T lymphocytes, *Proc. Natl. Acad. Sci. U.S.A.*, 82, 8648, 1985.
14. Perez, P., Hoffman, R. W., Shaw, S., Bluestone, J. A., and Segal, D. M., Specific targeting of cytotoxic T cells by anti-T3 linked to anti-target cell antibody, *Nature*, 316, 354, 1985.
15. Stevenson, G. T., Glennie, M. J., and Kan, K. S., Chemically engineered chimaeric and multi-Fab antibodies, in *Protein Engineering of Antibody Molecules for Prophylactic and Therapeutic Applications in Man*, Clark, M., Ed., Academic Titles, Nottingham, UK, 1993, 127.
16. Huse, W. D., Sastry, S., Iverson, S. A., Kang, A. S., Alting-Mees, M., Burton, D. R., Benkovic, S. J., and Lerner, R. A., Generation of a large combinatorial library of the immunoglobulin repertoire in phage lambda, *Science*, 246, 1275, 1989.
17. Ward, E. S., Gussow, D., Griffiths, A. D., Jones, P. T., and Winter, G., Binding activities of a repertoire of single immunoglobulin variable domains secreted from *Escherichia coli*, *Nature*, 341, 544, 1989.
18. McCafferty, J., Griffiths, A. D., Winter, G., and Chiswell, D. J., Phage antibodies-filamentous phage displaying antibody variable domains, *Nature*, 348, 552, 1990.
19. Griffiths, A. D. and Hoogenboom, H. R., Building an *in vitro* immune system: human antibodies from phage display libraries, in *Protein Engineering of Antibody Molecules for Prophylactic and Therapeutic Applications in Man*, Clark, M., Ed., Academic Titles, Nottingham, UK, 1993, 45.
20. Burton, D. R. and Barbas III, C. F., Human antibodies from combinatorial libraries, in *Protein Engineering of Antibody Molecules for Prophylactic and Therapeutic Applications in Man*, Clark, M., Ed., Academic Titles, Nottingham, UK, 1993, 65.
21. Kabat, E. A., Wu, T. T., Reid-Miller, M., Perry, H. M., and Gottesman, K. S., *Sequences of Proteins of Immunological Interest*, U.S. Department of Health and Human Services, U.S. Government Printing Office, 1987.
22. Bruggemann, M., Evolution of the rat immunoglobulin gamma heavy chain gene family, *Gene*, 74, 473, 1988.
23. Clark, M., General Introduction, in *Monoclonal Antibodies: Principles and Applications*, Birch, J. S. and Lennox, E., Eds., John Wiley & Sons, New York, 1995, 1.
24. Esser, C. and Radbruch, A., Immunoglobulin class switching: Molecular and cellular analysis, *Annu. Rev. Immunol.*, 8, 717, 1990.
25. WHO, Review of the notation for the allotypic and related markers of human immunoglobulins, *J. Immunogenetics*, 3, 357, 1976.
26. Loghem, E. van, Allotypic markers, *Monogr. Allergy*, 19, 40, 1986.
27. Greenwood, J. and Clark, M., Effector functions of matched sets of recombinant human IgG subclass antibodies, in *Protein Engineering of Antibody Molecules for Prophylactic and Therapeutic Applications in Man*, Clark, M., Ed., Academic Titles, Nottingham, UK, 1993, 85.
28. Howard, J. and Hughes-Jones, N., Complement-mediated lysis with monoclonal antibodies, *Prog. Allergy*, 45, 1, 1988.
29. Hale, G., Bright, S., Chumbley, G., Hoang, T., Metcalf, D., Munro, A. J., and Waldmann, H., Removal of T cells from bone marrow for transplantation: a monoclonal antilymphocyte antibody that fixes human complement, *Blood*, 62, 873, 1983.
30. Hale, G., Hoang, T., Prospero, T., Watt, S. M., and Waldmann, H., Removal of T cells from bone marrow for transplantation: comparison of rat monoclonal antilymphocyte antibodies of different isotypes, *Mol. Biol. Med.*, 1, 305, 1983.

31. Bindon, C. I., Hale, G., and Waldmann, H., Importance of antigen specificity for complement-mediated lysis by monoclonal antibodies, *Eur. J. Immunol.*, 18, 1507, 1988.
32. Bindon, C. I., Hale, G., Clark, M. R., and Waldmann, H., Therapeutic potential of monoclonal antibodies to the leukocyte common antigen: synergy and interference in complement-mediated lysis, *Transplantation*, 40, 538, 1985.
33. Boulianne, G. L., Hozumi, N., and Schulman, M. J., Production of functional chimaeric mouse/human antibody, *Nature*, 312, 643, 1984.
34. Boulianne, G. L., Isenman, D. E., Hozumi, N., and Shulman, M. J., Biological properties of chimeric antibodies: interaction with complement, *Mol. Biol. Med.*, 4, 37, 1987.
35. Neuberger, M. S., Williams, G. T., and Fox, R. O., Recombinant antibodies possessing novel effector functions, *Nature*, 312, 604, 1984.
36. Neuberger, M. S., Williams, G. T., Mitchell, E. B., Jouhal, S. S., Flanagan, J. G., and Rabbitts, T. H., A hapten-specific chimeric immunoglobulin E antibody which exhibits human physiological effector function, *Nature*, 314, 268, 1985.
37. Bruggemann, M., Williams, G. T., Bindon, C. I., Clark, M. R., Walker, M. R., Jefferis, R., Waldmann, H., and Neuberger, M. S., Comparison of the effector functions of human immunoglobulins using a matched set of chimeric antibodies, *J. Exp. Med.*, 166, 1351, 1987.
38. Schneider, W. P., Wensel, T. G., Stryer, L., and Oi, V. T., Genetically engineered immunoglobulins reveal structural features controlling segmental flexibility, *Proc. Natl. Acad. Sci. U.S.A.*, 85, 2509, 1988.
39. Tan, L. K., Shopes, R. J., Oi, V. T., and Morrison, S. L., Influence of the hinge region on complement activation, C1q binding, and segmental flexibility in chimeric human immunoglobulins, *Proc. Natl. Acad. Sci. U.S.A.*, 87, 162, 1990.
40. Bindon, C. I., Hale, G., Bruggemann, M., and Waldmann, H., Human monoclonal IgG antibodies differ in complement activating function at the level of C4 as well as C1q, *J. Exp. Med.*, 166, 351, 1988.
41. Brewer, Y., Palmer, A., Taube, D., Welsh, K., Bewick, M., Hale, G., Waldmann, H., Dische, F., Parsons, V., and Snowden, S., Randomised control trial of the pretreatment of human renal allografts with a synergistic pair of monoclonal antibodies against the leucocyte common antigen for the prevention of rejection, *Lancet*, 2, 935, 1989.
42. Hughes-Jones, N. C., Gorick, B. D., and Howard, J. C., The mechanism of synergistic complement-mediated lysis of rat red cells by monoclonal IgG antibodies, *Eur. J. Immunol.*, 13, 635, 1983.
43. Hughes-Jones, N. C., Gorick, B. D., Miller, N. G. A., and Howard, J. C., IgG pair formation on one antigenic molecule is the main mechanism of synergy between antibodies in complement-mediated lysis, *Eur. J. Immunol.*, 14, 974, 1984.
44. Yousaf, N., Howard, J. C., and Williams, B. D., Targeting behaviour of rat monoclonal IgG antibodies *in vivo* — role of antibody isotype, specificity and the target-cell antigen density, *Eur. J. Immunol.*, 21, 943, 1991.
45. Yousaf, N., Howard, J. C., and Williams, B. D., Complement-dependent synergistic effects of rat monoclonal IgG antibodies *in vivo*, *Eur. J. Immunol.*, 23, 369, 1993.
46. Hale, G., Clark, M., and Waldmann, H., Therapeutic potential of rat monoclonal antibodies: isotype specificity of antibody-dependant cell-mediated cytotoxicity with human lymphocytes, *J. Immunol.*, 134, 3056, 1985.
47. Bruggemann, M., Teale, C., Clark, M., Bindon, C., and Waldmann, H., A matched set of rat/mouse chimeric antibodies. Identification and biological properties of rat H chain constant regions μ, $\gamma 1$, $\gamma 2a$, $\gamma 2b$, $\gamma 2c$, ε, and α, *J. Immunol.*, 142, 3145, 1989.
48. Hale, G., Swirsky, D. M., Hayhoe, F. G. J., and Waldmann, H., Effects of monoclonal anti-lymphocyte antibodies *in vivo* in monkeys and humans, *Mol. Biol. Med.*, 1, 321, 1983.

49. Hale, G., Cobbold, S., and Waldmann, H., T cell depletion with CAMPATH-1 in allogeneic bone marrow transplantation, *Transplantation*, 45, 753, 1988.
50. Hale, G., Cobbold, S. P., Waldmann, H., Easter, G., Matejtschuk, P., and Coombs, R. A., Isolation of low-frequency class-switch variants from rat hybrid myelomas, *J. Immunol. Methods*, 103, 59, 1987.
51. Ortho Multicentre Transplant Study Group, A randomized clinical trial of OKT3 monoclonal antibody for acute rejection of cadaveric renal transplants, *N. Engl. J. Med.*, 313, 337, 1985.
52. Cobbold, S. P. and Waldmann, H., Therapeutic potential of monovalent monoclonal antibodies, *Nature*, 308, 460, 1984.
53. Clark, M., Bindon, C., Dyer, M., Friend, P., Hale, G., Cobbold, S., Calne, R., and Waldmann, H., The improved lytic function and *in-vivo* efficacy of monovalent monoclonal CD3 antibodies, *Eur. J. Immunol.*, 19, 381, 1989.
54. Abbs, I. C., Clark, M., Waldmann, H., Chatenoud, L., Koffman, C. G., and Sacks, S. H., Sparing of the first dose effect of monovalent anti-CD3 antibody used in allograft rejection is associated with diminished release of pro-inflammatory cytokines, *Ther. Immunol.*, 1, 325, 1994.
55. French, R. R., Hamblin, T. J., Bell, A. J., Tutt, A. L., and Glennie, M. J., Treatment of B-cell lymphomas with combination of bispecific antibodies and saporin, *Lancet*, 346, 223, 1995.
56. French, R. R., Penney, C. A., Browning, A. C., Stirpe, F., George, A. J. T., and Glennie, M. J., Delivery of the ribosome-inactivating protein, gelonin, to lymphoma cells via CD22 and CD38 using bispecific antibodies, *Br. J. Cancer*, 71, 986, 1995.
57. Shen, L., Guyre, P. M., Anderson, C. L., and Fanger, M. W., Heteroantibody-mediated cytotoxicity: antibody to the high affinity Fc receptor for IgG mediates cytotoxicity by human monocytes that is enhanced by interferon-gamma and is not blocked by human IgG, *J. Immunol.*, 137, 3378, 1986.
58. Clark, M., Bolt, S., Tunnacliffe, A., and Waldmann, H., Use of bispecific monoclonal antibodies to treat hematological malignancies: a model system using CD3 transgenic mice in *Bispecific Antibodies and Targeted Cellular Cytotoxicity: Second International Conference*, Romet-Lemonne, J. L., Fanger, M. W., and Segal, D. M., Eds., 1990, 243.
59. Haagen, I. A., van de Griend, R., Clark, M., Geerars, A., Bast, B., and de Gast, B., Killing of human leukemia lymphoma B-cells by activated cytotoxic T-lymphocytes in the presence of a bispecific monoclonal-antibody (CD3/CD19), *Clin. Exp. Immunol.*, 90, 368, 1992.
60. Haagen, I.-A., de Lau, W. B. M., Bast, B. J. E. G., Geerars, A. J. G., Clark, M. R., and de Gast, B. C., Unprimed CD4+ and CD8+ T cells can be rapidly activated by a CD3xCD19 bispecific antibody to proliferate and become cytotoxic, *Cancer Immunol. Immunother.*, 39, 391, 1994.
61. Haagen, I.-A., Geerars, A., de Lau, W., Clark, M., van de Griend, R., Bast, B., and de Gast, B., Killing of autologous B-lineage malignancy using CD3xCD19 bispecific monoclonal antibody in end stage leukemia and lymphoma, *Blood*, 84, 556, 1994.
62. de Gast, G. C., Haagen, I.-A., van Houten, A. A., Klein, S. C., Duits, A. J., de Weger, R. A., Vroom, T. M., Clark, M. R., Phillips, J., van Dijk, A. J. G., de Lau, W. B. M., and Bast, B. J. E. G., CD8 T cell activation after intravenous administration of CD3xCD19 bispecific antibody in patients with non-Hodgkin lymphoma, *Cancer Immunol. Immunother.*, 40, 390, 1995.
63. de Gast, G. C., van Houten, A. A., Haagen, I.-A., Klein, S. C., de Weger, R. A., van Dijk, A. J. G., Phillips, J., Clark, M. R., and Bast, B. J. E. G., Clinical Experience with CD3xCD19 Bispecific Antibodies in patients with B-cell malignancies, *J. Hematother.*, 1995.
64. Chatenoud, L., Baudrihaye, M. F., Chkoff, N., Kreis, H., Goldstein, G., and Bach, J. F., Restriction of the human *in vivo* immune response against the mouse monoclonal antibody OKT3, *J. Immunol.*, 137, 830, 1986.

65. Cobbold, S. P., Rebello, P. R. U. B., Davies, H. ff. S., Friend, P. J., and Clark, M. R., A simple method for measuring patient antiglobulin responses against isotypic or idiotypic determinants, *J. Immunol Methods*, 127, 19, 1990.
66. Steplewski, Z., Sun, L. K., Shearman, C. W., Ghrayeb, J., Daddona, P., and Koprowski, H., Biological activity of human-mouse IgG1, IgG2, IgG3, and IgG4 chimeric monoclonal antibodies with antitumor specificity, *Proc. Natl. Acad. Sci. U.S.A.*, 85, 4852, 1988.
67. Jones, P. T., Dear, P. H., Foote, J., Neuberger, M. S., and Winter, G., Replacing the complementarity-determining regions in a human antibody with those from a mouse, *Nature*, 321, 522, 1986.
68. Riechmann, L., Clark, M. R., Waldmann, H., and Winter, G., Reshaping human antibodies for therapy, *Nature*, 332, 323, 1988.
69. Verhoeyen, M., Milstein, C., and Winter, G., Reshaping human antibodies: grafting an antilysozyme activity, *Science*, 239, 1534, 1988.
70. Routledge, E. G., Gorman, S. D., and Clark, M., Reshaping antibodies for therapy, in *Protein Engineering of Antibody Molecules for Prophylactic and Therapeutic Applications in Man*, Clark, M., Ed., Academic Titles, Nottingham, UK, 1993, 13.
71. Queen, C., Schneider, W. P., Selick, H. E., Payne, P. W., Landolfi, N. F., Duncan, J. F., Avdalovic, N. M., Levitt, M., Junghans, R. P., and Waldmann, T. A., A humanized antibody that binds to the interleukin 2 receptor, *Proc. Natl. Acad. Sci. U.S.A.*, 86, 10029, 1989.
72. Gorman, S. D., Clark, M. R., Routledge, E. G., Cobbold, S. P., and Waldmann, H., Reshaping a therapeutic CD4 antibody, *Proc. Natl. Acad. Sci. U.S.A.*, 88, 4181, 1991.
73. Routledge, E. G., Lloyd, I., Gorman, S., Clark, M., and Waldmann, H., A humanized monovalent CD3 antibody which can activate homologous complement, *Eur. J. Immunol.*, 21, 2717, 1991.
74. Duncan, A. R. and Winter, G., The binding site for C1q on antibodies, *Nature*, 332, 738, 1988.
75. Duncan, A. R., Woof, J. M., Partridge, L. J., Burton, D. R., and Winter, G., Localization of the binding site for the human high-affinity Fc receptor on IgG, *Nature*, 332, 563, 1988.
76. Shin, S., Wright, A., Bonagura, V., and Morrison, S. L., Genetically-engineered antibodies: tools for the study of diverse properties of the antibody molecule, *Immunol. Rev.*, 130, 8, 1992.
77. Jefferis, R. and Lund, J., Molecular characterisation of IgG antibody effector sites, in *Protein Engineering of Antibody Molecules for Prophylactic and Therapeutic Applications in Man*, Clark, M., Ed., Academic Titles, Nottingham, UK, 1993, 115.
78. Morrison, S. L., Canfield, S. M., and Tao, M., Complement activation and Fc receptor binding by IgG, in *Protein Engineering of Antibody Molecules for Prophylactic and Therapeutic Applications in Man*, Clark, M., Ed., Academic Titles, Nottingham, UK, 1993, 101.
79. Valim, Y. M. L. and Lachmann., P. J., The effect of antibody isotype and antigenic epitope density on the complement-fixing activity of immune complexes, *Clin. Exp. Immunol.*, 84, 1, 1991.
80. Michaelsen, T. E., Garred, P., and Aase, A., Human IgG subclass pattern of inducing complement-mediated cytolysis depends on antigen concentration and to a lesser extent on epitope patchiness, antibody affinity and complement concentration, *Eur. J. Immunol.*, 21, 11, 1991.
81. Dunne, D. W., Richardson, B. A., Jones, F. M., Clark, M., Thorne, K. J. I., and Butterworth, A. E., The use of mouse/human chimaeric antibodies to investigate the roles of different antibody isotypes, including IgA2, in the killing of *Schistosoma mansoni schistosomula* by eosinophils, *Parasite Immunol.*, 15, 181, 1993.

82. Tao, M., Canfield, S. M., and Morrison, S. L., The differential ability of human IgG1 and IgG4 to activate complement is determined by the COOH-terminal sequence of the CH2 domain, *J. Exp. Med.*, 173, 1025, 1991.
83. Greenwood, J., Clark, M., and Waldmann, H., Structural motifs involved in human IgG antibody effector functions, *Eur. J. Immunol.*, 23, 1098, 1993.
84. Tao, M. H., Smith, R. I., and Morrison, S. L., Structural features of human immunoglobulin G that determine isotype specific differences in complement activation, *J. Exp. Med.*, 178, 661, 1993.
85. Brekke, O. H., Michaelsen, T. E., Aase, A., Sandin, R. H., and Sandlie, I., Human IgG isotype-specific amino acid residues affecting complement-mediated cell lysis and phagocytosis, *Eur. J. Immunol.*, 24, 2542, 1994.
86. Morgan, A., Jones, N. D., Nesbitt, A. M., Chaplin, L., Bodmer, M. W., and Emtage, J. S., The N-terminal end of the CH2 domain of chimeric human IgG1 anti-HLA DR is necessary for C1q, FcγRI and FcγRIII binding, *Immunology*, 86, 319, 1995.
87. Brekke, O. H., Michaelsen, T. E., and Sandlie, I., The structural requirements for complement activation by IgG: does it hinge on the hinge? *Immunol. Today*, 16, 85, 1995.
88. Michaelsen, T. E., Aase, A., Westby, C., and Sandlie, I., Enhancement of complement activation and cytolysis of human IgG3 by deletion of hinge exons, *Scan. J. Immunol.*, 32, 517, 1990.
89. Michaelsen, T. E., Aase, A., Norderhaug, L., and Sandlie, I., Antibody dependent cell-mediated cytotoxicity induced by chimeric mouse-human IgG subclasses and IgG3 antibodies with altered hinge regions, *Mol. Immunol.*, 29, 319, 1992.
90. Brekke, O. L., Michaelsen, T. E., Sandin, R., and Sandlie, I., Activation of complement by an IgG molecule without a genetic hinge, *Nature*, 363, 628, 1993.
91. Dorai, H., Wesolowski, J. S., and Gillies, S. D., Role of inter-heavy and light chain disulphide bonds in the effector functions of human immunoglobulin IgG1, *Mol. Immunol.*, 29, 1487, 1992.
92. Gorman, S. D. and Clark, M. R., Humanization of monoclonal antibodies for therapy, *Semin. Immunol.*, 2, 457, 1990.
93. van de Winkel, J. G. J. and Capel, P. J. A., Human IgG Fc receptor heterogeneity: molecular aspects and clinical implications, *Immunol. Today*, 14, 215, 1993.
94. Tax, W. J. M., Hermes, F. F. M., Willems, R. W., Capel, P. J. A., and Koene, R. A. P., Fc receptors for mouse IgG1 on human monocytes: polymorphism and role in antibody-induced T cell proliferation, *J. Immunol.*, 133, 1185, 1984.
95. Haagen, I.-A., Geerars, A. J. G., Clark, M. R., and van de Winkel, J. G. J., Interaction of human monocyte Fcγ receptors with rat IgG2b: a new indicator for the FcRγIIA (R-H131) polymorphism, *J. Immunol.*, 154, 1852, 1995.
96. Bredius, R. G. M., de Vries, C. E. E., Troelstra, A., van Alphen, L., Weening, R. S., van der Winkel, J. G. J., and Out, T. A., Phagocytosis of *Staphylococcus aureus* and *Haemophilus influenzae* type B opsonised by polyclonal human IgG1 and IgG2 antibodies: functional hFcγRIIa polymorphism to IgG2, *J. Immunol.*, 151, 1463, 1993.
97. Burgess, J. K., Lindeman, R., Chesterman, C. N., and Chong, B. H., Single amino acid mutation of Fcγ receptor is associated with the development of heparin-induced thrombocytopenia, *Br. J. Haematol.*, 91, 761, 1995.
98. Chappel, M. S., Isenman, D. E., Everett, M., Xu, Y., Dorrington, K. J., and Klein, M. H., Identification of the Fcγ receptor class I binding site in human IgG through the use of recombinant IgG1/IgG2 hybrid and point-mutated antibodies, *Proc. Natl. Acad. Sci. U.S.A.*, 88, 9036, 1991.
99. Canfield, S. M. and Morrison, S. L., The binding affinity of human IgG for its high affinity Fc receptor is determined by multiple amino acids in the CH2 domain and is modulated by the hinge region, *J. Exp. Med.*, 173, 1483, 1991.

100. Jefferis, R., Lund, J., and Pound, J., Molecular definition of interaction sites on human IgG for Fc receptors (huFcγR), *Mol. Immunol.*, 27, 1237, 1990.
101. Huizinga, T. W. J., Kerst, M., Nuyens, J. H., Vlug, A., von dem Borne, A. E. G. K., Roos, D., and Tetteroo, P. A. T., Binding characteristics of dimeric IgG subclass complexes to human-neutrophils, *J. Immunol.* 142, 2359, 1989.
102. Sarmay, G., Lund, J., Rozsnyay, Z., Gergely, J., and Jefferis, R., Mapping and comparison of the interaction sites on the Fc region of the IgG responsible for the triggering antibody dependent cellular cytotoxicity (ADCC) through different types of human Fcγ receptor, *Mol. Immunol.*, 29, 633, 1992.
103. de Haas, M., Koene, H. R., Kleijer, M., de Vries, E., Simsek, S., van Tol, M. J. D., Roos, D., and von dem Borne, A. E. G., A triallelic FcγRIIIA polymorphism influences the binding of human IgG by NK cell FcγRIIIA, *J. Immunol.*, 156, 2948, 1996.
104. Nose, M., Takano, R., Nakamura, S., Arata, Y., and Kyoguku, M., Recombinant Fc of human IgG1 prepared in *Escherichia coli* system escapes recognition by macrophages, *Int. Immunol.*, 2, 1109, 1990.
105. Lund, J., Takahashi, N., Pound, J. D., Goodall, M., Nakagawa, H., and Jefferis, R., Oligosaccharide-protein interactions in IgG can modulate recognition by Fcγ receptors, *FASEB J.*, 9, 115, 1994.
106. Isaacs, J. D., Clark, M. R., Greenwood, J., and Waldmann, H., Therapy with monoclonal antibodies — an *in vivo* model for the assessment of therapeutic potential, *J. Immunol.*, 148, 3062, 1992.
107. Bolt, S., Routledge, E., Lloyd, I., Chatenoud, L., Pope, H., Gorman, S. D., Clark, M., and Waldmann, H., The generation of a humanized, non-mitogenic CD3 monoclonal antibody which retains *in vitro* immunosuppressive properties, *Eur. J. Immunol.*, 23, 403, 1993.
108. Burmeister, W. H., Gastinel, L. N., Simister, N. E., Blum, M. L., and Bjorkman, P. J., Crystal structure at 2.2 Å resolution of the MHC-related neonatal Fc receptor, *Nature*, 372, 336, 1994.
109. Burmeister, W. P., Huber, A. H., and Bjorkman, P. J., Crystal structure of the complex of rat neonatal Fc receptor with Fc, *Nature*, 372, 379, 1994.
110. Story, C. M., Mikulska, J. E., and Simister, N. E., A major histocompatibility complex class I-like Fc receptor cloned from human placenta: possible role in transfer of immunoglobulin G from mother to fetus, *J. Exp. Med.*, 180, 2377, 1994.
111. Hale, G. and Waldmann, H., CAMPATH-1 monoclonal antibodies in bone marrow transplantation, *J. Haematother.*, 3, 15, 1994.
112. Wawrzynczak, E. J., Denham, S., Parnell, G. D., Cumber, A. J., Jones, P. T., and Winter, G., Recombinant mouse monoclonal antibodies with single amino acid substitutions affecting C1q and high affinity Fc receptor binding have identical serum half-lives in the BALB/c mouse, *Mol. Immunol.*, 29, 221, 1992.

Chapter 2

Immunotoxins for Treating Cancer and Autoimmune Disease

Robert J. Kreitman and Ira Pastan

CONTENTS

0-8493-8547-4/97/$0.00+$.50

2.1 INTRODUCTION

At the present time nearly half of all human malignancies remain incurable, primarily due to the ineffectiveness of therapy for systemic cancer. Often, the metastatic cells that are least amenable to cytotoxic chemotherapy are composed of relatively differentiated malignant cells, which are biochemically similar to their nonmalignant cell of origin. Hence, the cytotoxic agents in current use have insufficient specificity in killing the target cells. These relatively differentiated malignant cells often display, as part of their malignant phenotype, various receptors or antigens on their cell surface in numbers much higher than normal cells. The same high levels of specific receptors are also present on the activated T lymphocytes which mediate autoimmune disorders. To target cells mediating malignant and autoimmune disease, immunotoxins are being developed which bind with high specificity to specific receptors or antigens, are internalized into the cells, and kill cells by inhibition of protein synthesis. This review will highlight the current development of immunotoxins for treatment of cancer and autoimmune disease, and will focus on the development of *Pseudomonas* exotoxin-containing immunotoxins for hematologic malignancies.

2.1.1 Introduction to Protein Toxins

Plants and bacteria produce protein toxins which interfere with protein synthesis in animal cells. Plant toxins, such as ricin, gelonin, pokeweed antiviral protein (PAP), and saporin inhibit protein synthesis by inactivating ribosomes,[1] while bacterial toxins including *Pseudomonas* exotoxin (PE) and diphtheria toxin (DT), inactivate elongation factor 2 (EF-2).[2,3] Toxins are active in minute quantities because they function enzymatically and only one or a few molecules need to reach the cytosol to kill a cell.[1,4] This extremely high potency is necessary when targeting cells by their surface receptors, since such cells may only have hundreds or thousands of receptors per cell, and only a minority of toxin molecules that are internalized may reach the cytosol.

Plant toxins are either holotoxins, like ricin, abrin, and modeccin, which exist in nature as a cell-binding domain disulfide-bonded to an enzymatic domain, or hemitoxins, like PAP, saporin, and gelonin, which are composed of only the enzymatic domain. Immunotoxins can be made by chemically coupling the enzymatic domain to the antibody. Once internalized into a target cell, the enzymatic domain inactivates ribosomes. Many plant toxins, including ricin, abrin, modeccin, saporin, gelonin, and PAP have been shown to inactivate the elongation factor-1 (EF-1) and EF-2 associated functions of the 60 S ribosomal subunit by removing the base of $A^{3,4}$ in 28 S rRNA.[5,6] Bacterial toxins, such as PE and DT also kill cells by inhibition of protein synthesis. By ADP ribosylation they inactivate EF-2 directly without affecting ribosomes.[2,3,7]

2.1.1.1 *Structure and Function of PE and DT*

The full-length 613 amino acid PE contains three functional domains which are necessary for cellular intoxication.[8,9] Domain Ia (amino acids 1-252) is the binding domain, domain II (amino acids 253-364) is responsible for translocating the toxin to the cytosol, and domain III (amino acids 400-613) contains the ADP-ribosylating enzyme which inactivates EF-2 in the cytosol and results in cell death. The function of domain Ib (amino acids 365–399) is unknown. A current model of how PE kills cells contains the following steps: (1) the C terminal residue (lysine-613) is removed by a carboxypeptidase in the plasma or culture medium; (2) domain Ia binds to the $\alpha 2$ macroglobulin receptor present on animal cells and is internalized via endosomes to the transreticular Golgi;[10] (3) after internalization, domain II is proteolytically cleaved between amino acids 279 and 280 by Furin;[11-13] (4) the disulfide bond between cysteines 265 and 287, which joins the two fragments generated by proteolysis, is reduced; (5) amino acids 609-612 (REDL) bind to an intracellular sorting receptor which transports the 37-kDa carboxy terminal fragment from the transreticular Golgi apparatus to the endoplasmic reticulum;[14,15] (6) amino acids 280–313 mediate translocation of the toxin to the cytosol;[16,17] and (7) the ADP-ribosylating enzyme within amino acids 400–602 inactivates EF-2.[2]

DT, like PE, is composed of a single polypeptide chain which after cleavage translocates an ADP-ribosylating fragment to the cytosol. However, in contrast to PE, the 535 amino acid DT protein, traditionally divided into A and B domains, contains the enzymatic domain (A domain) at the amino terminus (amino acids 1-193) and the binding domain at the carboxyl terminus (amino acids 482–535).[3,7,18] The crystal structure of DT shows a third domain, which is the translocation or transmembrane (T) domain, and it is located in the center of the molecule.[19] After proteolytic cleavage of DT near amino acid 193, the T domain promotes the formation of a channel, and after reduction of the disulfide bond linking amino acids 186 and 201 the amino terminal fragment is released into the cytoplasm.[20,21]

2.1.2 Mutated Bacterial Toxins for Attaching to Ligands

To connect PE or DT to ligands, mutants are created in which the binding domain of the toxin is deleted or nonfunctional. Full-length toxins with mutated binding domains include PE^{4E} containing glutamate replacing basic residues at positions 57, 246, 247, and 249 of PE, and CRM107, containing phenylalanines replacing a leucine at position 390 and serine at position 525 of DT.[22,23] Deletion mutants include PE40, amino acids 253–613 of PE, and DAB_{486}, the first 485 amino acids of DT.[8,24,25] Shorter and more desirable versions recently constructed include PE38, composed of amino acids 253–364 and 381–613 of PE, and DT388 or DAB_{389}, containing the first 388 amino acids of DT.[26-29] Because these mutants of PE and DT are proteolytically cleaved prior to delivery of the catalytic domain to the cytosol, they may be fused in single-chain form to ligands to create recombinant toxins. This is difficult to accomplish with plant toxins. To allow the ADP-ribosylating domain to enter the cytosol without the ligand, the ligand is placed at the amino terminus of PE and at the carboxyl terminus of DT. Growth factors can be used instead of antibodies to make chimeric toxins, but these molecules will not be reviewed here.

2.2 TARGET CELLS FOR IMMUNOTOXINS

During the early development of immunotoxins, exciting advances were also being made in characterizing the interleukin-2 receptor (IL-2R), and thus IL-2R-bearing cells became early targets for immunotoxins. The IL-2R binds IL-2 with high, intermediate, or low affinity depending on which receptor subunits are present (α-β-γ_c, Kd = 10^{-11} M; β-γ_c, Kd = 10^{-9} M; α alone, Kd = 10^{-8} M).[30] IL-2Rα is overexpressed on the malignant cells in adult T-cell leukemia (ATL), peripheral T-cell leukemia/lymphomas, cutaneous T-cell lymphoma, B-cell non-Hodgkin's lymphomas, Hodgkin's disease, hairy cell leukemia, chronic lymphocytic leukemia (CLL), and acute myeloblastic leukemia, as well as on activated T cells.[31-35] The IL-2Rβ subunit is expressed without detectable IL-2Rα in large granular lymphocytic leukemia (LGLL), childhood acute lymphoblastic leukemia, and in many cases of chronic myelogenous leukemia and acute myelogenous leukemia.[36] We will review the development of immunotoxins targeting the IL-2R, as well as parallel studies performed with other immunotoxins.

2.3 IMMUNOTOXINS TARGETING IL-2R-BEARING CELLS

In 1981, anti-Tac, a murine monoclonal antibody (MAb) binding to human IL-2Rα, was isolated.[37] The first attempt to target interleukin-2 receptor (IL-2Rα)-bearing cells with an immunotoxin employed a chemical conjugate of murine anti-Tac and whole PE. The PE portion was treated with iminothiolane which modifies lysine residues in domain Ia and thereby decreases the binding of PE to its receptor[38] and facilitates conjugation of the toxin to anti-Tac. Anti-Tac-PE inhibited protein synthesis in an HTLV-I positive T-cell line HUT-102 by 50% (IC_{50}) at 1.2 ng/ml (5 pM), compared to 90–880 ng/ml for IL-2Rα negative cells.[24] The nonspecific toxicity of the toxin was dramatically reduced by using PE40 instead of PE.[24] The chemical conjugate (anti-Tac-Lys-PE40) was less cytotoxic than anti-Tac-PE toward HUT-102 cells, with an IC_{50} of 13 pM compared to 5 pM, but the non-specific cytotoxicity toward non-IL-2Rα-bearing cells improved 6- to 100-fold.[24,39]

In the next several years, PE, PE40, and PE38 were conjugated to a variety of other MAbs. These included: (1) OVB3, recognizing an ovarian cancer antigen,[40] (2) HB21, recognizing the human transferrin receptor,[39,41] (3) B1, B3, and BR96, recognizing Lewis-y (Le^y) antigens on breast and gastrointestinal carcinomas,[42-44] (4) MRK16, recognizing P-glycoprotein on multiply drug resistant cells,[45,46] (5) C242, recognizing human colon cancer,[47] and (6) LL2, recognizing CD22 on B-cell lymphoma.[48] All of these immunotoxins showed *in vivo* activity in mice bearing human target antigens. Immunotoxins have also been made using CRM107 and other derivatives of DT and MAbs such as (1) T101 and UCHT1, recognizing the respective T-cell antigens CD5 and CD3,[49] (2) 9.2.27, recognizing human melanoma,[50] (3) D3, recognizing hepatocarcinoma,[51] and (4) 454A12, recognizing the human transferrin receptor.[52]

Immunotoxins containing plant toxins have a potential advantage over chemical conjugates containing PE40, PE38, or CRM107, in that these PE or DT derivatives require proteolysis prior to translocation of the active toxin fragment to the cytosol. Indeed, it has been found that some tumor cells lack Furin, the protease needed to produce the active fragment of PE. To address this problem, PE35, the processed translocated portion of PE38 was expressed and purified from *E. coli*. PE35 contains amino acids 281–364 and 381–613 of PE. It has only one cysteine residue at position 287, so like ricin A chain it can be conjugated to antibodies through a disulfide bond and does not require proteolytic processing for activity. It was found that immunotoxins made from MAbs HB21 and B3 were more active if conjugated to PE35 compared to PE38.[53] Anti-Tac-PE35 was found to have an IC_{50} on HUT-102 cells of ~20 pM, which was not improved over that of anti-Tac-PE40.[24,39,53]

2.4 THE NEXT GENERATION: RECOMBINANT TOXINS

Immunotoxins containing an antibody or antibody fragment like a Fab′ chemically conjugated to a toxin have several disadvantages. First, their large size (100–200 kDa), often results in reduced tumor penetration. Second, for conjugation to antibodies, toxins such as PE40 and PE38 must be derivatized with reagents which modify the lysine residues, many of which are near the carboxyl terminus. Similarly, the antibody may require derivatization of lysine residues within the antigen-binding domains. The resulting immunotoxins are therefore a heterogeneous mixture with respect to sites of attachment of the antibody and toxin, as well as the number of toxin and antibody components per immunotoxin molecule. Finally, chemical conjugates are difficult to produce, because the toxin and antibody must be purified separately, conjugated, and then the product repurified.

2.4.1 Recombinant Immunotoxins

To more effectively target IL-2R-bearing cells, our goal was to use a high-affinity ligand which could be fused in single-chain form to PE. The anti-Tac MAb has a very high affinity for IL-2Rα (Kd ~ 10^{-10} M), almost 100-fold over IL-2.[54] The smallest fragment of an antibody that will still bind effectively to antigen is the Fv, composed of one variable heavy (V_H) and one variable light (V_L) domain.[55,56] A single-chain Fv molecule composed of one variable domain connected to the next through a peptide linker is only 26 kDa in size, less than 20% of the size of an IgG. Anti-Tac(Fv) was constructed by fusing V_H to V_L via the 15 amino acid linker $(Gly_4Ser)_3$ and the resulting Fv fragment of anti-Tac was fused to PE40.[57] Anti-Tac(Fv)-PE40 retained one third of the binding affinity of the dimeric anti-Tac IgG. This recombinant immunotoxin was extremely cytotoxic with an IC_{50} of 0.15 ng/ml (~2 pM) toward HUT-102 cells[57] and 0.05–0.1 ng/ml toward activated human T cells.[27,58] Anti-Tac(Fv)-PE40 and its slightly smaller version anti-Tac(Fv)-PE38 were very cytotoxic toward fresh malignant cells from 46 of 46 patients with ATL,[27,59-61] showed antitumor activity against IL-2Rα-expressing human tumors in mice,[62] and is being prepared for a phase I clinical trial for patients with IL-2Rα-expressing malignancies.

2.4.2 Recombinant Immunotoxins Made from Other Antibodies

Since the development of anti-Tac(Fv)-PE40 began, a large number of other recombinant immunotoxins have been reported. Table 1 lists 14 examples of antigen-binding domains fused to derivatives of PE. DT388 has also been fused to anti-Tac(Fv) and HB21(Fv).[60,63,64] In these two cases the cytotoxic activity of the DT388- and PE40-containing immunotoxins were comparable. Thus far, recombinant single-chain immunotoxins binding to IL-2Rα, Le^y, and erbB2 have been reported to display excellent antitumor activity against human tumors in nude

TABLE 1

Active Recombinant Single-Chain Fv Immunotoxins

Binding Domain	Toxin(s)	Antigen	Cell Type	Cell Line	Cytotoxicity IC_{50} (ng/ml)	Ref.
Anti-Tac(Fv)	PE40,PE38, PE38XXXL	IL-2Rα	Leukemias, lymphomas	HUT-102	0.15	57
					0.035–0.08	15
	DT388				0.37	60, 63, 64
B1(Fv)	PE38	Le^y	Breast, GI CA	A431	0.25	69, 78
B3(Fv)	PE38, PE38KDEL	Le^y	Breast, GI CA	A431	2	78-80
B3(hFv)	PE38	Le^y	Breast, GI CA	A431	2.2	81
B5(Fv)	PE38	Le^y	Breast, GI CA	A431	20	78
BR96(Fv)	PE40	Le^y	Breast, GI CA	MCF7	0.3	82
e6(Fv)	PE40	TrR	Human cells	K562	7	83
e23(Fv)	PE40,PE38	erbB2	Solid tumors	SK-OV-3	62–80	84
	PE38KDEL				5	
	PE40KDEL				22	
FRP5(Fv)	PE40	erbB2	Solid tumors	SK-OV-3	195	85
G28-5(Fv)	PE40	CD40	Lymphoma, myeloma, leukemia	BJAB	2.5	86
HB21(Fv)	PE40	TrR	Human cells	HUT-102	2.4	64
	DT388				0.7	
Mik-b1(Fv)	PE40,	IL-2Rβ	NK leukemia	YT-S	6.5	87
	PE40KDEL				2.5	
OVB3(Fv)	PE	NR	Ovarian CA	Ovcar-3	4	88
PR1(Fv)	PE38KDEL	NR	Prostate CA	LNCaP	0.8	89

Note: In the toxin PE38XXXL fused to anti-Tac(Fv), XXX denotes either the amino acids KDD, KDE, KED, KEE, RDD, RDE, RED, or REE. B3(hFv) denotes a humanized form of B3(Fv). Other abbreviations: IL-2Rα, (subunit of the interleukin-2 receptor; GI, gastrointestinal; CA, carcinoma; Le^y, Lewis y; TrR, transferrin receptor; IC_{50}, concentration necessary for 50% inhibition of protein synthesis; and NR, not reported.

mice. B3(Fv)-PE38 (LMB-7) which targets Le^y is now being tested in a phase I trial against epithelial tumors at the National Cancer Institute and a similar immunotoxin (BR96(Fv)-PE40) has been developed using MAb BR96 (Table 3). Anti-Tac (Fv)-PE38 (LMB-2) is also now undergoing Phase I testing.

2.4.3 Production of Recombinant Toxins

The protocol used in our laboratory for the production of recombinant toxins has been adapted from procedures used to renature and purify recombinant Fab molecules.[65] The goal is to produce in high yield recombinant protein which is fully active, homogeneous with respect to tertiary structure, and free of contaminants such as bacterial proteins and endotoxin. A plasmid encoding the recombinant toxin under control of the T7 promoter is used to transform *E. coli* BL21/λDE3.[66] The culture is grown and induced with the lactose analog IPTG, after which the recombinant protein accumulates in insoluble inclusion bodies. The inclusion bodies are washed in detergent, which extracts many bacterial proteins and endotoxin. The resulting inclusion body protein on an SDS-PAGE reducing gel contains >90% recombinant protein, but it is aggregated and improperly folded. After dissolving, denaturing, and reducing in a guanidine-dithioerythritol solution, the protein is then refolded in a redox buffer. The renatured protein is then purified by anion exchange and sizing chromatography. For anti-Tac(Fv)-PE38, 1 l of culture induced in a fermentor at OD_{650} around 8 yields approximately 1 g of inclusion body protein, which after purification yields approximately 50 mg of pure immunotoxin.

2.4.4 Disulfide-Stabilized Fv-Immunotoxins

One disadvantage of recombinant immunotoxins is that in many cases the single-chain (Fv) does not fold correctly and hence does not bind to the antigen with the same affinity as would the corresponding Fab molecule. For example, e23(Fv)-PE38KDEL was found to bind to receptor-bearing cells with 20% of the affinity of e23(Fab), and only 7.5% of the affinity of e23(IgG).[67] One hypothesis to explain poor binding is that V_H and V_L have low affinity for each other. Thus, when the two variable domains dissociate to the distance allowed by the peptide linker, the molecules could aggregate or adopt a less appropriate monomeric structure. To improve the stability and hence binding of single-chain recombinant immunotoxins, the two variable domains were attached with a disulfide bond, instead of a peptide linker. To engineer a disulfide bond between the two variable domains, the structures of several antibodies were evaluated and a pair of conserved amino acids were found, one on V_H and the other on V_L, which in the antibody were the appropriate distance apart. These two residues were converted to cysteines, and when a denatured inclusion body mixture of V_L + V_H-toxin (or V_H + V_L-toxin) were mixed in refolding buffer, disulfide-stabilized Fv (dsFv) immunotoxins were formed.[68] Disulfide-stabilized immunotoxins were produced with the Fv domains for anti-Tac, e23, B3, and B1.[69,70] Anti-Tac(dsFv)-PE38KDEL, B3(dsFv)-PE38KDEL, and e23(dsFv)-PE38KDEL each proved to be more stable than their respective single-chain recombinant immunotoxins, and in the case of e23(dsFv)-PE38KDEL the binding improved so that is was indistinguishable from that of the Fab fragment.[67,70]

2.4.4.1 *Recombinant Immunotoxin Anti-Tac-(dsFv)-PE38KDEL*

Anti-Tac(dsFv)-PE38KDEL is composed of V_H disulfide-bonded to a fusion protein composed of V_L and PE38KDEL. The disulfide bond was created by converting G44 of V_H and S99 of V_L to cysteines. Inclusion bodies are prepared from V_H and (V_L)-PE38KDEL separately, mixed at a 2:1 ratio, and during refolding the disulfide bond forms to make the dsFv. There was no difference in the receptor binding or cytotoxic activity of anti-Tac(Fv)-PE38KDEL and anti-Tac(dsFv)-PE38KDEL toward target cells. This is probably because anti-Tac(Fv)-PE38KDEL is already tightly folded to a relatively stable structure. However, anti-Tac(dsFv)-PE38KDEL retained full activity in human serum after 3 days at 37°C, while anti-Tac(Fv)-PE38KDEL was stable for only 2 h.[71] Nevertheless, both recombinant immunotoxins displayed the same pharmacokinetics in mice, indicating that disappearance of immunotoxin in the serum of animals is due to distribution into the extracellular space and renal excretion, and not due to breakdown by plasma. One advantage of an agent having better stability in the serum is that it would be more stable in the extravascular space within a tumor.

2.4.4.2 *A Recombinant Immunotoxin with Increased Plasma Lifetime*

While it is expected that the smaller recombinant immunotoxins will penetrate tumors better than the larger IgG-toxin conjugates, the trade off is that their lifetime in the plasma would be shorter. Clearly, the goal is optimal tumor penetration, but penetration is a product of the rate of permeation and the time that the drug is in the plasma. Thus it is not clear what is the optimum immunotoxin size which allows good tumor penetration and sufficient plasma lifetime. To determine whether a recombinant immunotoxin having an improved plasma lifetime could be made and would be useful, anti-Tac(Fab)-PE40 was produced. This completely recombinant immunotoxin is composed of the Fd (V_H + C_H1) domain of anti-Tac disulfide-bonded to a fusion of the anti-Tac light chain (V_L + C_κ). Each of these two polypeptide chains were encoded on a single plasmid, under control of the phoA promoter.[72] The active recombinant immunotoxin could be purified equally well from denatured and renatured inclusion bodies, or from secreted protein in the periplasm. The binding and cytotoxic activity of anti-Tac(Fab)-PE40 and anti-Tac(Fv)-PE40 did not differ, but in mice the $t_{1/2}\beta$ was 430 min for anti-Tac(Fab)-PE40, compared to 57 min for anti-Tac(Fv)-PE40. The antitumor activity of anti-Tac(Fv)-PE40 and anti-Tac(Fab)-PE40 in the ATAC-4 model was similar, but both were more active than a chemical conjugate of anti-Tac(IgG) with toxin.[72] Thus, the optimal size of a targeting protein may be close to 66 or 100 kDa, but further experiments and perhaps clinical trials will be needed to establish this.

More recently, fully recombinant Fab-immunotoxins have also been reported for MAbs B3 and C242.[73,74] In the latter case, it was found again that the 86-kDa recombinant immunotoxin produced much better regression of tumors than the IgG chemical conjugate.[74]

2.5 CLINICAL TRIALS OF OTHER IMMUNOTOXINS

Tables 2 and 3 list clinical trials performed and ongoing for several immunotoxins. Most of the reported clinical trials have treated patients with hematologic tumors, including both direct targeting of hematopoietic antigens CD5, CD19, CD22, and CD30, as well as targeting of activated T cells to treat graft-versus-host disease (GVHD). Many of the ricin-based conjugates cause vascular leak syndrome (VLS), manifested by decreased albumin concentration and third-spacing of fluid. Blocked ricin as well as saporin causes transaminase elevations and thrombocytopenia.

Similar toxicities for toxins with different binding domains indicate that the toxicity is due to binding of the toxin itself to the normal tissues. Indeed, it has been found that ricin A chain binds to and kills human endothelial cells, possibly leading to VLS.[75] The Le^y immunotoxins B3-LysPE38 and B3(Fv)-PE38 also bind to endothelial cells, and the larger IgG conjugate has been found to cause VLS clinically. The binding to endothelial cells is mediated by the antibody (B3) and not by PE38, since other immunotoxins including anti-Tac(Fv)-PE38 did not bind to endothelial cells.[76] BR96(Fv)-PE40 was found to cause VLS in rats, but only when very high doses were administered.[77]

In general, hematologic tumors respond more frequently to immunotoxins than solid tumors. One reason is that antibodies to hematopoietic tumors are more specific than antibodies to solid tumors and produce fewer side effects on essential normal cells. Another reason is that in hematologic malignancies, particularly leukemias, the immunotoxins have a better chance of reaching the tumor. Small recombinant immunotoxins are now entering clinical trials and it will be interesting to see if they have an advantage over the larger IgG chemical conjugates for both hematologic and solid tumors.

TABLE 2

Clinical Trials of Immunotoxins

Name	Antigen	Diseases	PT	Toxicity	Response	Ref.
T,p67-RTA	CD5	GVHD	1	None	1 CR	90
T101-RTA	CD5	CLL	4	Mild fever	0	91
T101-RTA	CD5	CLL	2	None	40% reduction	92
H65-RTA	CD5	GVHD	8	Infections	6 prevented	93
H65-RTA	CD5	RA	12	NR	T-cell changes	94
H65-RTA	CD5	SLE	6	Mild fever, VLS	2 improved	95
Xomazyme-Mel	Melanoma	Melanoma	22	VLS	1 CR	96
260F9-RTA	Breast CA	Breast CA	4	VLS, neuropathy	0	97, 98
791T/36-RTA	Colon CA	Colon CA	17	Fever, VLS	5 mixed	99
454A12-rRTA	TrR	IP CA	20	VLS, cerebral edema	0	100
RFB4-dgA	CD22	B-cell	26	VLS	5 PR, 1 CR	101
RFB4-Fab′-dgA	CD22	B-cell	15	VLS, rhabdomyolysis	6 PR	102
Anti-B4-bR	CD19	B-cell	25	Liver	1 CR, 2 PR	103
Anti-B4-bR	CD19	B-cell	34	Liver, thrombocytopenia	2 CR, 3 PR (CI)	104
Anti-B4-bR	CD19	B-cell	12	Liver, thrombocytopenia	11 still CR (Adj)	105
N901-bR	SCLC	SCLC	19	VLS	1 PR	106
B43-PAP	CD19	B-ALL	17	VLS	4 CR, 1 PR	107
Ber-H2-Saporin	CD30	Hodgkin's	4	Liver, thrombocytopenia	3 transient	108
Anti-Tac-PE	IL-2Rα	ATL	5	Liver	0	
OVB3-PE	Ovarian	Ovarian	16	Encephalopathy	0	109

Note: Abbreviations: Adj, adjuvant setting; ALL, acute lymphoblastic leukemia; ATL, adult T-cell leukemia; B-cell, B-cell malignancies; bR, blocked whole ricin; CA, carcinoma; CLL, chronic lymphocytic leukemia; CI, continuous infusion; CIS, carcinoma *in situ;* CTCL, cutaneous T-cell lymphoma; CR, complete response; dgA, deglycosylated ricin A chain; EGFR, epidermal growth factor receptor; GVHD, graft versus host disease; HIV, human immunodeficiency virus; IL-2R, interleukin-2 receptor; IL-2Rα, α (p55) subunit of the IL-2R; IP, intraperitoneal; NR, not reported; PAP, pokeweed antiviral protein; PE, *Pseudomonas* exotoxin; PR, partial response; PT, number of patients in the study; RA, rheumatoid arthritis; RTA, ricin A chain; rRTA, recombinant ricin A chain; SCLC, small cell lung cancer; SLE, systemic lupus erythematosis; TrR, transferrin receptor; VLS, vascular leak syndrome. This review does not include chimeric toxins containing growth factors instead of antibodies.

TABLE 3

Unpublished or Ongoing Clinical Trials on Other Immunotoxins

Name	Antigen	Diseases	Ref.
RFT5-dgA	IL-2Rα	Hodgkin's disease	110
Anti-CD7-dgA	CD7	T-ALL	
Anti-CD33-bR	CD33	Transplanted AML	
IgG-HD37-dgA	CD19	B-cell lymphoma	111
B3-LysPE38	Le^y	Breast, GI CA	79
B3(Fv)-PE38	Le^y	Breast, GI CA	79
Anti-Tac(Fv)-PE38	IL2Rα	Hematologic tumors	

Note: Many immunotoxins listed in Table 2 are also in ongoing clinical trials testing different dosing schemes or combination therapy. Abbreviations not listed in Table 2: AML, acute myelogenous leukemia and GI, gastrointestinal.

REFERENCES

1. Eiklid, K., Olsnes, S., and Pihl, A., Entry of lethal doses of abrin, ricin and modeccin into the cytosol of HeLa cells, *Exp. Cell Res.*, 126, 321, 1980.
2. Carroll, S. F. and Collier, R. J., Active site of *Pseudomonas aeruginosa* exotoxin A. Glutamic acid 553 is photolabeled by NAD and shows functional homology with glutamic acid 148 of diphtheria toxin, *J. Biol. Chem.*, 262, 8707, 1987.
3. Uchida, T., Pappenheimer, A. M., Jr., and Harper, A. A., Reconstitution of diphtheria toxin from two nontoxic cross-reacting mutant proteins, *Science*, 175, 901, 1972.
4. Yamaizumi, M., Mekada, E., Uchida, T., and Okada, Y., One molecule of diphtheria toxin fragment A introduced into a cell can kill the cell, *Cell*, 15, 245, 1978.
5. Endo, Y., Mitsui, K., Motizuki, M., and Tsurugi, K., The mechanism of action of ricin and related toxic lectins on eukaryotic ribosomes, *J. Biol. Chem.*, 262, 5908, 1987.
6. Zamboni, M., Brigotti, M., Rambelli, F., Montanaro, L., and Sperti, S., High pressure liquid chromatographic and fluorimetric methods for the determination of adenine released from ribosomes by ricin and gelonin, *Biochem. J.*, 259, 639, 1989.
7. Uchida, T., Pappenheimer, A. M., Jr., and Greany, R., Diphtheria toxin and related proteins I. Isolation and properties of mutant proteins serologically related to diphtheria toxin, *J. Biol. Chem.*, 248, 3838, 1973.
8. Hwang, J., FitzGerald, D. J., Adhya, S., and Pastan, I., Functional domains of *Pseudomonas* exotoxin identified by deletion analysis of the gene expressed in *E. coli*, *Cell*, 48, 129, 1987.
9. Allured, V. S., Collier, R. J., Carroll, S. F., and McKay, D. B., Structure of exotoxin A of *Pseudomonas aeruginosa* at 3.0 Angstrom resolution, *Proc. Natl. Acad. Sci. U.S.A.*, 83, 1320, 1986.
10. Kounnas, M. Z., Morris, R. E., Thompson, M. R., FitzGerald, D. J., Strickland, D. K., and Saelinger, C. B., The a2-macroglobulin receptor/low density lipoprotein receptor-related protein binds and internalizes *Pseudomonas* exotoxin A, *J. Biol. Chem.*, 267, 12420, 1992.
11. Chiron, M. F., Fryling, C. M., and FitzGerald, D. J., Cleavage of *Pseudomonas* exotoxin and diphtheria toxin by a furin-like enzyme prepared from beef liver, *J. Biol. Chem.*, 269, 18167, 1994.

12. Fryling, C., Ogata, M., and FitzGerald, D., Characterization of a cellular protease that cleaves *Pseudomonas* exotoxin, *Infect. and Immun.*, 60, 497, 1992.
13. Ogata, M., Fryling, C. M., Pastan, I., and FitzGerald, D. J., Cell-mediated cleavage of *Pseudomonas* exotoxin between Arg^{279} and Gly^{280} generates the enzymatically active fragment which translocates to the cytosol, *J. Biol. Chem.*, 267, 25396, 1992.
14. Chaudhary, V. K., Jinno, Y., FitzGerald, D., and Pastan, I., *Pseudomonas* exotoxin contains a specific sequence at the carboxyl terminus that is required for cytotoxicity, *Proc. Natl. Acad. Sci. U.S.A.*, 87, 308, 1990.
15. Kreitman, R. J. and Pastan, I., Importance of the glutamate residue of KDEL in increasing the cytotoxicity of *Pseudomonas* exotoxin derivatives and for increased binding to the KDEL receptor, *Biochem. J.*, 307, 29, 1995.
16. Theuer, C., Kasturi, S., and Pastan, I., Domain II of *Pseudomonas* exotoxin A arrests the transfer of translocating nascent chains into mammalian microsomes, *Biochemistry*, 33, 5894, 1994.
17. Theuer, C. P., Buchner, J., FitzGerald, D., and Pastan, I., The N-terminal region of the 37-kDa translocated fragment of *Pseudomonas* exotoxin A aborts translocation by promoting its own export after microsomal membrane insertion, *Proc. Natl. Acad. Sci. U.S.A.*, 90, 7774, 1993.
18. Rolf, J. M., Gaudin, H. M., and Eidels, L., Localization of the diphtheria toxin receptor-binding domain to the carboxyl-terminal M_r ~6000 region of the toxin, *J. Biol. Chem.*, 265, 7331, 1990.
19. Choe, S., Bennett, M. J., Fujii, G., Curmi, P. M. G., Kantardjieff, K. A., Collier, R. J., and Eisenberg, D., The crystal structure of diphtheria toxin, *Science*, 357, 216, 1992.
20. Papini, E., Schiavo, G., Tomasi, M., Colombatti, M., Rappuoli, R., and Montecucco, C., Lipid interaction of diphtheria toxin and mutants with altered fragment B. 2. Hydrophobic photolabelling and cell intoxication, *Eur. J. Biochem.*, 169, 637, 1987.
21. Moskaug, J. O., Stenmark, H., and Olsnes, S., Insertion of diphtheria toxin B-fragment into the plasma membrane at low pH. Characterization and topology of inserted regions, *J. Biol. Chem.*, 266, 2652, 1991.
22. Greenfield, L., Johnson, V. G., and Youle, R. J., Mutations in diphtheria toxin separate binding from entry and amplify immunotoxin selectivity, *Science*, 238, 536, 1987.
23. Chaudhary, V. K., Jinno, Y., Gallo, M. G., FitzGerald, D., and Pastan, I., Mutagenesis of *Pseudomonas* exotoxin in identification of sequences responsible for the animal toxicity, *J. Biol. Chem.*, 265, 16306, 1990.
24. Kondo, T., FitzGerald, D., Chaudhary, V. K., Adhya, S., and Pastan, I., Activity of immunotoxins constructed with modified *Pseudomonas* exotoxin A lacking the cell recognition domain, *J. Biol. Chem.*, 263, 9470, 1988.
25. Williams, D. P., Parker, K., Bacha, P., Bishai, W., Borowski, M., Genbauffe, F., Strom, T. B., and Murphy, J. R., Diphtheria toxin receptor binding domain substitution with interleukin-2: genetic construction and properties of a diphtheria toxin-related interleukin-2 fusion protein, *Prot. Eng.*, 1, 493, 1987.
26. Siegall, C. B., Chaudhary, V. K., FitzGerald, D. J., and Pastan, I., Functional analysis of domains II, Ib, and III of *Pseudomonas* exotoxin, *J. Biol. Chem.*, 264, 14256, 1989.
27. Kreitman, R. J., Batra, J. K., Seetharam, S., Chaudhary, V. K., FitzGerald, D. J., and Pastan, I., Single-chain immunotoxin fusions between anti-Tac and *Pseudomonas* exotoxin: relative importance of the two toxin disulfide bonds, *Bioconj. Chem.*, 4, 112, 1993.
28. Williams, D. P., Snider, C. E., Strom, T. B., and Murphy, J. R., Structure/function analysis of interleukin-2-toxin (DAB_{486}-IL-2). Fragment B sequences required for the delivery of fragment A to the cytosol of target cells, *J. Biol. Chem.*, 265, 11885, 1990.
29. Chaudhary, V. K., FitzGerald, D. J., and Pastan, I., A proper amino terminus of diphtheria toxin is important for cytotoxicity, *Biochem. Biophys. Res. Commun.*, 180, 545, 1991.

30. Taniguchi, T. and Minami, Y., The IL2/IL-2 receptor system: a current overview, *Cell*, 73, 5, 1993.
31. Kodaka, T., Uchiyama, T., Ishikawa, T., Kamio, M., Onishi, R., Itoh, K., Hori, T., Uchino, H., Tsudo, M., and Araki, K., Interleukin-2 receptor β-chain (p70-75) expressed on leukemic cells from adult T cell leukemia patients, *Jpn. J. Cancer Res.*, 81, 902, 1990.
32. Yagura, H., Tamaki, T., Furitsu, T., Tomiyama, Y., Nishiura, T., Tominaga, N., Katagiri, S., Yonezawa, T., and Tarui, S., Demonstration of high-affinity interleukin-2 receptors on B-chronic lymphocytic leukemia cells: functional and structural characterization, *Blut*, 60, 181, 1990.
33. Kreitman, R. J. and Pastan, I., Recombinant single-chain immunotoxins against T and B cell leukemias, *Leuk. Lymphoma*, 13, 1, 1994.
34. Robb, R. J., Greene, W. C., and Rusk, C. M., Low and high-affinity cellular receptors for interleukin 2, *J. Exp. Med.*, 160, 1126, 1984.
35. Gazzola, M., Collins, N. H., Tafuri, A., and Keever, C. A., Recombinant interleukin 3 induces interleukin 2 receptor expression on early myeloid cells in normal human bone marrow, *Exp. Hematol.*, 20, 201, 1992.
36. Hoshino, S., Oshimi, K., and Mizoguchi, H., Interleukin-2 receptor β chain in leukemias and lymphomas, *Leuk. Lymphoma*, 1992, 107, 1992.
37. Uchiyama, T. A., Broder, S., and Waldmann, T. A., A monoclonal antibody (anti-Tac) reactive with activated and functionally mature human T cells. I. Production of anti-Tac monoclonal antibody and distribution of Tac (+) cells, *J. Immunol.*, 126, 1393, 1981.
38. FitzGerald, D. J. P., Waldmann, T. A., Willingham, M. C., and Pastan, I., *Pseudomonas* exotoxin-Anti-Tac: cell specific immunotoxin active against cells expressing the human T cell growth factor receptor, *J. Clin. Invest.*, 74, 966, 1984.
39. Batra, J. K., Jinno, Y., Chaudhary, V. K., Kondo, T., Willingham, M. C., FitzGerald, D. J., and Pastan, I., Antitumor activity in mice of an immunotoxin made with anti-transferrin receptor and a recombinant form of *Pseudomonas* exotoxin, *Proc. Natl. Acad. Sci. U.S.A.*, 86, 8545, 1989.
40. Willingham, M. C., FitzGerald, D. J., and Pastan, I., *Pseudomonas* exotoxin coupled to a monoclonal antibody against ovarian cancer inhibits the growth of human ovarian cancer cells in a mouse model, *Proc. Natl. Acad. Sci. U.S.A.*, 84, 474, 1987.
41. FitzGerald, D. J., Willingham, M. C., and Pastan, I., Antitumor effects of an immunotoxin made with *Pseudomonas* exotoxin in a nude mouse model of human ovarian cancer, *Proc. Natl. Acad. Sci. U.S.A.*, 83, 6627, 1986.
42. Pastan, I., Lovelace, E. T., Gallo, M. G., Rutherford, A. V., Magnani, J. L., and Willingham, M. C., Characterization of monoclonal antibodies B1 and B3 that react with mucinous adenocarcinomas, *Cancer Res.*, 51, 3781, 1991.
43. Pai, L. H., Batra, J. K., FitzGerald, D. J., Willingham, M. C., and Pastan, I., Antitumor effects of B3-PE and B3-LysPE40 in a nude mouse model of human breast cancer and the evaluation of B3-PE toxicity in monkeys, *Cancer Res.*, 52, 3189, 1992.
44. Siegall, C. B., Gawlak, S. L., Chin, J. J., Zoeckler, M. E., Kadow, K. F., Brown, J. P., and Braslawsky, G. R., Cytotoxicity of chimeric (human-murine) monoclonal antibody BR96 IgG, $F(ab')_2$, and Fab′ conjugated to *Pseudomonas* exotoxin, *Bioconj. Chem.*, 3, 302, 1992.
45. FitzGerald, D. J., Willingham, M. C., Cardarelli, C. O., Hamada, H., Tsuruo, T., Gottesman, M. M., and Pastan, I., A monoclonal antibody-*Pseudomonas* toxin conjugate that specifically kills multidrug-resistant cells, *Proc. Natl. Acad. Sci. U.S.A.*, 84, 4288, 1987.
46. Mickisch, G. H., Pai, L. H., Siegsmund, M., Campain, J., Gottesman, M. M., and Pastan, I., *Pseudomonas* exotoxin conjugated to monoclonal antibody MRK16 specifically kills multidrug resistant cells in cultured renal carcinomas and in MDR-transgenic mice, *J. Urol.*, 149, 174, 1993.

47. Debinski, W., Karlsson, B., Lindholm, L., Siegall, C. B., Willingham, M. C., FitzGerald, D., and Pastan, I., Monoclonal antibody C242-*Pseudomonas* exotoxin A. A specific and potent immunotoxin with antitumor activity on a human colon cancer xenograft in nude mice, *J. Clin. Invest.*, 90, 405, 1992.
48. Kreitman, R. J., Hansen, H. J., Jones, A. L., FitzGerald, D. J. P., Goldenberg, D. M., and Pastan, I., *Pseudomonas* exotoxin-based immunotoxins containing the antibody LL2 or LL2-Fab′ induce regression of subcutaneous human B-cell lymphoma in mice, *Cancer Res.*, 53, 819, 1993.
49. Youle, R. J., Uckun, F. M., Vallera, D. A., and Colombatti, M., Immunotoxins show rapid entry of diphtheria toxin but not ricin via the T3 antigen, *J. Immunol.*, 136, 93, 1986.
50. Bumol, T. F., Wang, Q. C., Reisfeld, R. A., and Kaplan, N. O., Monoclonal antibody and an antibody-toxin conjugate to a cell surface proteoglycan of melanoma cells suppress *in vivo* tumor growth, *Proc. Natl. Acad. Sci. U.S.A.*, 80, 529, 1983.
51. Bernhard, M. I., Foon, K. A., Oeltmann, T. N., Key, M. E., Hwang, K. M., Clarke, G. C., Christensen, W. L., Hoyer, L. C., Hanna, M. G., Jr., and Oldham, R. K., Guinea pig line 10 hepatocarcinoma model: characterization of monoclonal antibody and *in vivo* effect of unconjugated antibody and antibody conjugated to diphtheria toxin A chain, *Cancer Res.*, 43, 4420, 1983.
52. Sung, C., Youle, R. J., and Dedrick, R. L., Pharmacokinetic analysis of immunotoxin uptake in solid tumors: role of plasma kinetics, capillary permeability, and binding, *Cancer Res.*, 50, 7382, 1990.
53. Theuer, C. P., Kreitman, R. J., FitzGerald, D. J., and Pastan, I., Immunotoxins made with a recombinant form of *Pseudomonas* exotoxin A that do not require proteolysis for activity, *Cancer Res.*, 53, 340, 1993.
54. Waldmann, T. A., Goldman, C. K., Robb, R. J., Depper, J. M., Leonard, W. J., Sharrow, S. O., Bongiovanni, K. F., Korsmeyer, S. J., and Greene, W. C., Expression of interleukin 2 receptors on activated human B cells, *J. Exp. Med.*, 160, 1450, 1984.
55. Huston, J. S., Levinson, D., Mudgett-Hunter, M., Tai, M.-S., Novotny, J., Margolies, M. N., Ridge, R. J., Bruccoleri, R. E., Haber, E., Crea, R., and Oppermann, H., Protein engineering of antibody binding sites: Recovery of specific activity in an antidigoxin single-chain Fv analogue produced in *Escherichia coli*, *Proc. Natl. Acad. Sci. U.S.A.*, 85, 5879, 1988.
56. Bird, R. E., Hardman, K. D., Jacobson, J. W., Johnson, S., Kaufman, B. M., Lee, S. M., Lee, T., Pope, S. H., Riordan, G. S., and Whitlow, M., Single-chain antigen-binding proteins, *Science*, 242, 423, 1988.
57. Chaudhary, V. K., Queen, C., Junghans, R. P., Waldmann, T. A., FitzGerald, D. J., and Pastan, I., A recombinant immunotoxin consisting of two antibody variable domains fused to *Pseuodomonas* exotoxin, *Nature*, 339, 394, 1989.
58. Batra, J. K., FitzGerald, D., Gately, M., Chaudhary, V. K., and Pastan, I., Anti-Tac(Fv)-PE40: a single chain antibody *Pseudomonas* fusion protein directed at interleukin 2 receptor bearing cells, *J. Biol. Chem.*, 265, 15198, 1990.
59. Kreitman, R. J., Chaudhary, V. K., Waldmann, T., Willingham, M. C., FitzGerald, D. J., and Pastan, I., The recombinant immunotoxin anti-Tac(Fv)-*Pseuodomonas* exotoxin 40 is cytotoxic toward peripheral blood malignant cells from patients with adult T-cell leukemia, *Proc. Natl. Acad. Sci. U.S.A.*, 87, 8291, 1990.
60. Kreitman, R. J., Chaudhary, V. K., Waldmann, T. A., Hanchard, B., Cranston, B., FitzGerald, D. J. P., and Pastan, I., Cytotoxic activities of recombinant immunotoxins composed of *Pseudomonas* toxin or diphtheria toxin toward lymphocytes from patients with adult T-cell leukemia, *Leukemia*, 7, 553, 1993.
61. Saito, T., Kreitman, R. J., Hanada, S.-I., Makino, T., Utsunomiya, A., Sumizawa, T., Arima, T., Chang, C. N., Hudson, D., Pastan, I., and Akiyama, S.-I., Cytotoxicity of recombinant Fab and Fv immunotoxins on adult T-cell leukemia lymph node and blood cells in the presence of soluble interleukin-2 receptor, *Cancer Res.*, 54, 1059, 1994.

62. Kreitman, R. J., Bailon, P., Chaudhary, V. K., FitzGerald, D. J. P., and Pastan, I., Recombinant immunotoxins containing anti-Tac(Fv) and derivatives of *Pseudomonas* exotoxin produce complete regression in mice of an interleukin-2 receptor-expressing human carcinoma, *Blood*, 83, 426, 1994.
63. Chaudhary, V. K., Gallo, M. G., FitzGerald, D. J., and Pastan, I., A recombinant single-chain immunotoxin composed of anti-Tac variable regions and a truncated diphtheria toxin, *Proc. Natl. Acad. Sci. U.S.A.*, 87, 9491, 1990.
64. Batra, J. K., FitzGerald, D. J., Chaudhary, V. K., and Pastan, I., Single-chain immunotoxins directed at the human transferrin receptor containing *Pseudomonas* exotoxin A or diphtheria toxin: Anti-TFR(Fv)-PE40 and DT388-Anti-TFR(Fv), *Mol. Cell. Biol.*, 11, 2200, 1991.
65. Buchner, J., Pastan, I., and Brinkmann, U., A method for increasing the yield of properly folded recombinant fusion proteins: single-chain immunotoxins from renaturation of bacterial inclusion bodies, *Anal. Biochem.*, 205, 263, 1992.
66. Studier, F. W. and Moffatt, B. A., Use of bacteriophage T7 polymerase to direct selective expression of cloned genes, *J. Mol. Biol.*, 189, 113, 1986.
67. Reiter, Y., Brinkmann, U., Jung, S., Lee, B., Kasprzyk, P. G., King, C. R., and Pastan, I., Improved binding and antitumor activity of a recombinant anti-erbB2 immunotoxin by disulfide stabilization of the Fv fragment, *J. Biol. Chem.*, 269, 18327, 1994.
68. Brinkmann, U., Reiter, Y., Jung, S., Lee, B., and Pastan, I., A recombinant immunotoxin containing a disulfide-stabilized Fv fragment, *Proc. Natl. Acad. Sci. U.S.A.*, 90, 7538, 1993.
69. Benhar, I. and Pastan, I., Characterization of B1(Fv)PE38 and B1(dsFv)PE38: single-chain and disulfide-stabilized Fv Immunotoxins with increased activity that cause complete remissions of established human carcinoma xenografts in nude mice, *Clin. Cancer Res.*, 1, 1023, 1995.
70. Reiter, Y., Brinkmann, U., Kreitman, R. J., Jung, S.-H., Lee, B., and Pastan, I., Stabilization of the Fv fragments in recombinant immunotoxins by disulfide bonds engineered into conserved framework regions, *Biochemistry*, 33, 5451, 1994.
71. Reiter, Y., Kreitman, R. J., Brinkmann, U., and Pastan, I., Cytotoxic and antitumor activity of a recombinant immunotoxin composed of disulfide-stablized anti-Tac Fv fragment and truncated *Pseudomonas* exotoxin, *Int. J. Cancer*, 58, 142, 1994.
72. Kreitman, R. J., Chang, C. N., Hudson, D. V., Queen, C., Bailon, P., and Pastan, I., Anti-Tac(Fab)-PE40, a recombinant double-chain immunotoxin which kills interleukin-2-receptor-bearing cells and induces complete remission in an *in vivo* tumor model, *Int. J. Cancer*, 57, 856, 1994.
73. Choe, M., Webber, K. O., and Pastan, I., B3(Fab)-PE38 M: a recombinant immunotoxin in which a mutant form of *Pseudomonas* exotoxin is fused to the Fab fragment of monoclonal antibody B3, *Cancer Res.*, 54, 3460, 1994.
74. Debinski, W. and Pastan, I., Recombinant F(ab′) C242-*Pseudomonas* exotoxin, but not the whole antibody-based immunotoxin, causes regression of a human colorectal tumor xenograft, *Clin. Cancer Res.*, 1, 1015, 1995.
75. Soler-Rodriguez, A.-M., Ghetie, M.-A., Oppenheimer-Marks, N., Uhr, J. W., and Vitetta, E. S., Ricin A-chain and ricin A-chain immunotoxins rapidly damage human endothelial cells: Implications for vascular leak syndrome, *Exp. Cell Res.*, 206, 227, 1993.
76. Kuan, C., Pai, L. H., and Pastan, I., Immunotoxins containing *Pseudomonas* exotoxin targeting Le^Y damage human endothelial cells in an antibody-specific mode: relevance to vascular leak syndrome, *Clin. Cancer Res.*, 1, 1589, 1995.
77. Siegall, C. B., Liggitt, D., Chace, D., Tepper, M. A., and Fell, H. P., Prevention of immunotoxin-mediated vascular leak syndrome in rats with retention of antitumor activity, *Proc. Natl. Acad. Sci. U.S.A.*, 91, 9514, 1994.

78. Benhar, I. and Pastan, I., Cloning, expression and characterization of the Fv fragments of the anti-carbohydrate mAbs B1 and B5 as single-chain immunotoxins, *Prot. Eng.*, 7, 1509, 1994.
79. Pai, L. H. and Pastan, I., Immunotoxin therapy for cancer, *JAMA*, 269, 78, 1993.
80. Brinkmann, U., Pai, L. H., FitzGerald, D. J., Willingham, M., and Pastan, I., B3(Fv)-PE38KDEL, a single-chain immunotoxin that causes complete regression of a human carinoma in mice, *Proc. Natl. Acad. Sci. U.S.A.*, 88, 8616, 1991.
81. Benhar, I., Padlan, E. A., Jung, S., Lee, B., and Pastan, I., Rapid humanization of the Fv of monoclonal antibody B3 by using framework exchange of the recombinant immunotoxin B3(Fv)-PE38, *Proc. Natl. Acad. Sci. U.S.A.*, 91, 12051, 1994.
82. Friedman, P. N., McAndrew, S. J., Gawlak, S. L., Chace, D., Trail, P. A., Brown, J. P., and Siegall, C. B., BR96 sFv-PE40, a potent single-chain immunotoxin that selectively kills carcinoma cells, *Cancer Res.*, 53, 334, 1993.
83. Nicholls, P. J., Johnson, V. G., Andrew, S. M., Hoogenboom, H. R., Raus, J. C. M., and Youle, R. J., Characterization of single-chain antibody (sFv)-toxin fusion proteins produced *in vitro* in rabbit reticulocyte lysate, *J. Biol. Chem.*, 268, 5302, 1993.
84. Batra, J. K., Kasprzyk, P. G., Bird, R. E., Pastan, I., and King, C. R., Recombinant anti-erbB2 immunotoxins containing *Pseudomonas* exotoxin, *Proc. Natl. Acad. Sci. U.S.A.*, 89, 5867, 1992.
85. Wels, W., Harwerth, I.-M., Mueller, M., Groner, B., and Hynes, N. E., Selective inhibition of tumor cell growth by a recombinant single-chain antibody-toxin specific for the erbB-2 receptor, *Cancer Res.*, 52, 6310, 1992.
86. Francisco, J. A., Gilliland, L. K., Stebbins, M. R., Norris, N. A., Ledbetter, J. A., and Siegall, C. B., Activity of a single-chain immunotoxin that selectively kills lymphoma and other B-lineage cells expressing the CD40 antigen, *Cancer Res.*, 55, 3099, 1995.
87. Kreitman, R. J., Schneider, W. P., Queen, C., Tsudo, M., FitzGerald, D. J. P., Waldmann, T. A., and Pastan, I., Mik-b1(Fv)-PE40, a recombinant immunotoxin cytotoxic toward cells bearing the β-chain of the IL-2 receptor, *J. Immunol.*, 149, 2810, 1992.
88. Chaudhary, V. K., Batra, J. K., Gallo, M. G., Willingham, M. C., FitzGerald, D. J., and Pastan, I., A rapid method of cloning functional variable-region antibody genes in *Escherichia coli* as single-chain immunotoxins, *Proc. Natl. Acad. Sci. U.S.A.*, 87, 1066, 1990.
89. Brinkmann, U., Gallo, M., Brinkmann, E., Kunwar, S., and Pastan, I., A recombinant immunotoxin that is active on prostate cancer cells and that is composed of the Fv region of monoclonal antibody PR1 and a truncated form of *Pseudomonas* exotoxin, *Proc. Natl. Acad. Sci. U.S.A.*, 90, 547, 1993.
90. Kernan, N. A., Byers, V., Scannon, P. J., Mischak, R. P., Brochstein, J., Flomenberg, N., Dupont, B., and O'Reilly, R. J., Treatment of steroid resistant acute graft-vs-host disease by *in vivo* administration of an anti-T-cell ricin A chain immunotoxin, *JAMA*, 259, 3154, 1988.
91. Hertler, A. A., Schlossman, D. M., Borowitz, M. J., Laurent, G., Jansen, F. K., Schmidt, C., and Frankel, A. E., A phase I study of T101-ricin A chain immunotoxin in refractory chronic lymphocytic leukemia, *J. Biol. Response Mod.*, 7, 97, 1988.
92. Laurent, G., Pris, J., Farcet, J.-P., Carayon, P., Blythman, H., Casellas, P., Poncelet, P., and Jansen, F. K., Effects of therapy with T101 ricin A-chain immunotoxin in two leukemia patients, *Blood*, 67, 1680, 1986.
93. Koehler, M., Hurwitz, C. A., Krance, R. A., Coustan-Smith, E., Williams, L. L., Santana, V., Ribeiro, R. C., Brenner, M. K., and Heslop, H. E., XomaZyme-CD5 immunotoxin in conjunction with partial T cell depletion for prevention of graft rejection and graft-versus-host disease after bone marrow transplantation from matched unrelated donors, *Bone Marrow Transplant.*, 13, 571, 1994.

94. Fishwild, D. M. and Strand, V., Administration of an anti-CD5 immunoconjugate to patients with rheumatoid arthritis: Effect on peripheral blood mononuclear cells and *in vitro* immune function, *J. Rheumatol.*, 21, 596-604, 1994.
95. Stafford, F. J., Fleisher, T. A., Lee, G., Brown, M., Strand, V., Austin, H. A., III, Balow, J. E., and Klippel, J. H., A pilot study of anti-CD5 ricin A chain immunoconjugate in systemic lupus erythematosus, *J. Rheumatol.*, 21, 2068, 1994.
96. Spitler, L. E., Rio, M. D., Khentigan, A., Wedel, N. I., Brophy, N. A., Miller, L. L., Harkonen, W. S., Rosendorf, L. L., Lee, H. M., Mischak, R. P., Kawahata, R. T., Stoudemire, J. B., Fradkin, L. B., Bautista, E. E., and Scannon, P. J., Therapy of patients with malignant melanoma using a monoclonal antimelanoma antibody-ricin A chain immunotoxin, *Cancer Res.*, 47, 1717, 1987.
97. Weiner, L. M., O'Dwyer, J., Kitson, J., Comis, R. L., Frankel, A. E., Bauer, R. J., Konrad, M. S., and Groves, E. S., Phase I evaluation of an anti-breast carcinoma monoclonal antibody 260F9-recombinant ricin A chain immunoconjugate, *Cancer Res.*, 49, 4062, 1989.
98. Gould, B. J., Borowitz, M. J., Groves, E. S., Carter, P. W., Anthony, D., Weiner, L. M., and Frankel, A. E., Phase I study of an anti-breast cancer immunotoxin by continuous infusion: report of a targeted toxic effect not predicted by animal studies, *J. Natl. Cancer Inst.*, 81, 775, 1989.
99. Byers, V. S., Rodvien, R., Grant, K., Durrant, L. G., Hudson, K. H., Baldwin, R. W., and Scannon, P. J., Phase I study of monoclonal antibody-ricin A chain immunotoxin XomaZyme-791 in patients with metastatic colon cancer, *Cancer Res.*, 49, 6153, 1989.
100. Byers, V. S. and Baldwin, R. W., Rationale for clinical use of immunotoxins in cancer and autoimmune disease, *Semin. Cell Biol.*, 2, 59, 1991.
101. Amlot, P. L., Stone, M. J., Cunningham, D., Fay, J., Newman, J., Collins, R., May, R., McCarthy, M., Richardson, J., Ghetie, V., Ramilo, O., Thorpe, P. E., Uhr, J. W., and Vitetta, E. S., A phase I study of an anti-CD22-deglycosylated ricin A chain immunotoxin in the treatment of B-cell lymphomas resistant to conventional therapy, *Blood*, 82, 2624, 1993.
102. Vitetta, E. S., Stone, M., Amlot, P., Fay, J., May, R., Till, M., Newman, J., Clark, P., Collins, R., Cunningham, D., Ghetie, V., Uhr, J., and Thorpe, P. E., Phase I immunotoxin trial in patients with B-cell lymphoma, *Cancer Res.*, 51, 4052, 1991.
103. Grossbard, M. L., Freedman, A. S., Ritz, J., Coral, F., Goldmacher, V. S., Eliseo, L., Spector, N., Dear, K., Lambert, J. M., Blattler, W. A., Taylor, J. A., and Nadler, L. M., Serotherapy of B-cell neoplasms with anti-B4-blocked ricin: a phase I trial of daily bolus infusion, *Blood*, 79, 576, 1992.
104. Grossbard, M. L., Lambert, J. M., Goldmacher, V. S., Spector, N. L., Kinsella, J., Eliseo, L., Coral, F., Taylor, J. A., Blattler, W. A., Epstein, C. L., and Nadler, L. M., Anti-B4-blocked ricin: a Phase I trial of 7-day continuous infusion in patients with B-cell neoplasms, *J. Clin. Oncol.*, 11, 726, 1993.
105. Grossbard, M. L., Gribben, J. G., Freedman, A. S., Lambert, J. M., Kinsella, J., Rabinowe, S. N., Eliseo, L., Taylor, J. A., Blattler, W. A., Epstein, C. L., and Nadler, L. M., Adjuvant immunotoxin therapy with anti-B4-blocked ricin after autologous bone marrow transplantation for patients with B-cell non-Hodgkin's lymphoma, *Blood*, 81, 2263, 1993.
106. Lynch, T. J., Immunotoxin therapy of small-cell lung cancer. N901-blocked ricin for relapsed small-cell lung cancer, *Chest*, 103, 436s, 1993.
107. Uckun, F., Immunotoxins for the treatment of leukaemia, *Br. J. Haematol.*, *85*, 435, 1993.
108. Falini, B., Bolognesi, A., Flenghi, L., Tazzari, P. L., Broe, M. K., Stein, H., Durkop, H., Aversa, F., Corneli, P., Pizzolo, G., Barbabietola, G., Sabattini, E., Pileri, S., Martelli, M. F., and Stirpe, F., Response of refractory Hodgkin's disease to monoclonal anti-CD30 immunotoxin, *Lancet*, 339, 1195, 1992.

109. Pai, L. H., Bookman, M. A., Ozols, R. F., Young, R. C., Smith, J. W., II, Longo, D. L., B., G., Frankel, A., McClay, E. F., Howell, S., Reed, E., Willingham, M. C., FitzGerald, D. J., and Pastan, I., Clinical evaluation of intraperitoneal *Pseudomonas* exotoxin immunoconjugate OVB3-PE in patients with ovarian cancer, *J. Clin. Oncol.*, 9, 2095, 1991.
110. Engert, A., Gottstein, C., Winkler, U., Amlot, P., Pileri, S., Diehl, V., and Thorpe, P., Experimental treatment of human Hodgkin's disease with ricin A-chain immunotoxins, *Leuk. Lymphoma*, 13, 441, 1994.
111. Ghetie, V. and Vitetta, E., Immunotoxins in the therapy of cancer: From bench to clinic, *Pharmacol. Ther.*, 63, 209, 1994.

Chapter **3**

ANTIBODIES AS CARRIERS FOR DRUGS AND RADIOISOTOPES

G. Yarranton

CONTENTS

0-8493-8547-4/97/$0.00+$.50

3.1 INTRODUCTION

Since the development of hybridoma technology in 1975, there has been much effort expended on attempts to conjugate monoclonal antibodies (MAbs) for the *in vivo* diagnosis and treatment of disease. Currently, two antibody radioisotope conjugates have been approved for clinical use: MyoScint®, a ^{111}In-labeled murine anti-myosin agent for imaging myocardial damage,[1] and OncoScint CR/OV, a murine antibody linked to ^{111}In for γ-camera imaging of colorectal and ovarian cancers.[2] These products demonstrate the utility of antibody conjugates for *in vivo* diagnosis, but do not establish antibody conjugates as successful therapies for human disease. Currently, a number of antibody conjugates are in clinical development for the treatment of cancer (Table 1), and there is a renewed optimism that some of those entities will become products.

TABLE 1

Immunoconjugates in Clinical Evaluation

Antibody	Antigen	Killing Agent	Phase	Target	Ref.
CTM01	PEM	Calicheamicin	I/II	Ovarian/lung	3
P67.6	CD33	Calicheamicin	I/II	AML	3
B1	CD20	Radioiodine	II/III	B-cell lymphoma	4
BR96	Lewis ^{y}	Doxorubicin	I/II	Epithelial tumors	5
A7	?	Neocarzinostatin	I/II	Colon	6
Lym-1	MHC-Class II	Radioiodine	III	B-cell lymphoma	7

Several reasons can be cited for this renewed optimism for antibody conjugates. First, the ability to engineer nonhuman MAbs such that they are no longer recognized by the human immune system,[8,9] means that effective repeat dosing is now a reality. Data on antibodies such as CDP571[10] (anti-TNF) and 4D5[11] (anti-HER2) in patients have clearly demonstrated this effect. Second, unconjugated antibodies, e.g., 17-1A appear to have some anti-tumor activity.[12] Clinical results with 17-1A, an anti-40-kDa epithelial cell-surface protein MAb, given repeatedly to colorectal cancer patients, are encouraging. A 30% reduction in overall death rate was observed in Dukes' C patients. These data have resulted in product approval in Germany. Although the mechanism by which this effect is achieved is not known, it seems likely that more potent antibody conjugates might improve efficacy. Third, early clinical results with the iodinated antibody B1 in the treatment of non-Hodgkin's lymphoma are impressive.[4,13] This antibody recognizes CD20, a cell-surface marker on B cells. Treatment of patients with ^{131}I-labeled antibody resulted in significant long-term remissions in over one third of the patients. Finally, the combination of MAb treatment and conventional chemotherapy appears to be generating interesting clinical data.

The IDEC Corporation antibody C2B8 (anti-CD20),[14] has been used in combination with CHOP chemotherapy for the treatment of low grade B-cell lymphoma. The overall response rate was 100% with 5–19 months' duration. In other studies, the anti-HER2 antibody of Genentech has demonstrated efficacy in breast cancer when used in combination with Adriamycin. These data are encouraging and may be improved upon if more effective antibody conjugates can be produced.

In this chapter some of the problems and possible solutions to the problems associated with the development of improved antibody conjugates will be discussed. Since cancer therapy is currently the major therapeutic focus of these efforts, I will focus the discussion around this objective.

3.2 ANTIBODY SPECIFICITY

The basic concept of antibody-targeted therapy, particularly for cancer, is that the antibody binds selectively to the target cell and delivers a cytotoxic agent (drug or isotope) in a directed manner, thereby sparing normal tissue. For this approach to be successful, target antigens should be tumor cell specific and the cytotoxic agent should only be active at the tumor site. Although many attempts have been made to reach this ideal, none has yet managed.

In many cases, tumor-associated antigens (TAAs) are used as immunogens for raising tumor-targeting antibodies. Although these antigens are expressed on tumors, their expression is rarely restricted to tumor cells (Table 2). Attention has been focused on epithelial-associated mucins because many antibodies developed against epithelial tumors react with these complex molecules. Human polymorphic epithelial mucin (PEM), the product of the MUC1 gene is one such antigen. This antigen is expressed on most of the epithelial tumor types, and antibodies recognizing PEM have been widely used in the clinic (Table 2). Although expressed on normal epithelia,[28] expression tends to be on the apical side of the cells and is hence inaccessible to circulating antibody. *In vivo* targeting of tumor sites without binding to normal epithelium therefore can be achieved. With hCTM01,[3] a human form of the murine MAb CTM01, tumor/normal tissue ratios of >10 have been observed using ^{111}In-labeled conjugates in ovarian cancer patients. This antibody binds to human PEM.

Carcinoembryonic antigen (CEA)[19-22] is another TAA that has been widely evaluated as a target for antibody-directed therapy. Localization of intravenously administered antibody has been observed clinically, although uptake in individual tumors is variable and the factors influencing this are poorly understood.[29]

TABLE 2

Commonly Targeted Solid Tumor Epithelial Antigens

Antigen	Antibody	Tumor Type	Ref.
PEM	CTM01	Ovarian	15–18
	BRE3	Breast	
	HMFG	Lung	
	SM3	Head and neck	
CEA	A5B7	Colorectal	19–22
	PRIA3	Lung	
	COL-1		
	IMMUN-14		
EpCAM	17-1A	Colorectal	23-25
	KS1-4	Lung	
		Breast	
Tag 72	B72.3	Colorectal	26, 27
	CC49	Ovarian	

The epithelial glycoprotein 40 (EGP40) encoded by the GA-733-2 gene has also been targeted by MAbs for cancer therapy.[23-25] EGP40 is expressed on the basolateral cell surface rather than apically and this has generated concern that normal epithelia will be targeted *in vivo*. This may explain some of the toxicities observed with KS1/4-vinca conjugates in phase I study in patients with adenocarcinoma.[24] Interestingly, EGP40 is the antigen recognized by the MAb 17-1A,[23] that is currently marketed in Germany for the treatment of colorectal cancer.[12]

Selectivity for tumor cell binding may be achieved with antibodies that recognize neoepitopes created on epithelial antigens as a result of alterations in tumor cell glycosylation. SM3, an antibody which recognizes human PEM, shows surprisingly weak reactivity with normal tissues. *In vivo* tumor imaging with SM3 produced results that were similar to those with other anti-PEM MAbs.[30] This antibody may be a good vehicle for toxic drug delivery. PRIA3,[22] an antibody that recognizes CEA, appears to bind to an epitope close to the cell surface, giving this antibody the property of recognizing cell-associated antigen but not shed antigen. This property may also be advantageous for drug delivery and targeting, since circulating immune complexes are often rapidly cleared to the liver and spleen.

In vivo targeting of tumor sites rather than tumor cells may have some advantages. Targeting of tumor sites has been achieved with a MAb that recognizes an antigen that is upregulated on normal tissue close to the tumor. F19,[31] an antibody that binds to an unknown antigen that is upregulated in the tumor stroma, has been used to target solid tumors (colorectal tumors) *in vivo*.[32] The antigen is found on activated fibroblasts, but the only other site showing uptake other than the tumor, is scar tissue. This represents an interesting approach to tumor therapy,

TABLE 3

Commonly-Targeted Leukemia and Lymphoma Antigens

Antigen	Antibody	Disease	Ref.
CD33	P67.6 M195	AML	35, 36
CD19	cCD19 Bu12	Lymphoma	37, 38
CD20	B1 C2B8	Lymphoma	4, 13, 14
CD37	MB1	Lymphoma	34
CD38	OKT10	Lymphoma	38
CD45	BC8	Lymphoma	38, 39

since these normal cells are unlikely to change their phenotype/genotype in the way that tumor cells do, and hence may provide a more stable target for radioimmunotherapy.

Another attractive approach to anti-tumor therapy is to target normal cells that are essential for tumor growth. There is considerable interest in the identification and targeting of novel antigens upregulated on tumor endothelium.[33] The expectation in this case is that targeting a toxin/drug to the blood vessels supplying the tumor will result in death of the tumor. The attractiveness of this approach for antibody-based therapies is that the endothelium is readily accessible.

For some cancer therapeutic approaches, it is not necessary to have complete selectivity for the tumor over normal tissue. This is particularly the case where leukemias and lymphomas are targeted (Table 3). The use of antibodies to CD20, a cell-surface marker on B cells, and B-cell progenitors to treat B-cell lymphoma, illustrates this point. The destruction of some normal cells of the hematopoietic system, in addition to the tumor cells, can be tolerated, particularly if those cells are not the pluripotent stem cells. Another example of this approach is the targeting of CD33 for the treatment of acute myeloid leukemia (AML).[35,36] CD33 is expressed on myeloid progenitor cells and some mature monocytes, but not on CD34 stem cells. This antigen is also expressed on myeloid leukemia cells. Currently, antibodies to this marker are being developed for the treatment of AML (see below).

Other antigens that are commonly used as targets for the delivery of immunoconjugates to solid tumors are growth factor receptors. In particular antibodies to the epidermal growth factor receptor (EGF)[40] and the HER2/neu[41] oncogene have been widely used. These antigens are expressed on normal tissues, particularly the liver. However, the use of these antibodies in combination with standard chemotherapy suggests that a selective anti-tumor effect may be achieved.

In summary, the selection of "antigen target" when considering antibody-conjugate therapies for cancer is not a simple choice. Antigen expression on normal tissues need not preclude effective *in vivo* targeting of tumor cells. High level, homogeneous expression of the target antigen on tumor cells is probably the most important consideration. Antigens that internalize into the target cell once the antibody conjugate is bound are preferred for both drugs and isotopes (see below).

3.3 SELECTING ANTIBODY FORM

Antibodies are very versatile carriers of either drugs or isotopes, since the biodistribution and pharmacokinetics can be varied almost at will by varying the size of the molecule. In addition, the immunogenicity of rodent antibodies can now be reduced by protein engineering, thereby enabling proper evaluation of these entities in the clinic.

It is now possible to replace most of the rodent-derived sequences of an antibody with sequences derived from human antibodies, without losing antigen-binding activity.[8] The first generation of engineered antibodies were chimeric molecules comprising the V regions of the rodent antibody and the constant regions of a human antibody.[42,43] Several antibodies of this type with reactivity against tumor antigens have been administered to patients. In most cases immune responses to the rodent variable regions have been detected, thereby rendering these agents unsuitable for repeated therapy. Further engineering of the rodent variable regions by integrating the antigen-binding determinants into human antibody framework regions has resulted in a number of engineered human antibodies.[8] Early clinical results on these fully engineered human antibodies suggest that these have low or no immunogenicity, and that they are suitable for repeated therapy.[10,11,36] Engineered human antibodies are now the antibody form of choice as a delivery vehicle for drugs or isotopes.

The size of antibody molecules can now be varied at will due to the use of genetic engineering techniques. Interestingly, the size, avidity, shape, and charge of the antibody may affect its pharmacokinetics (PK), biodistribution, and route of clearance. Selection of the "right" form of the antibody may be crucial for obtaining a "therapeutic window" with cytotoxic conjugates. In Figure 1, a number of different forms of MAbs are shown. Intact IgG tends to clear from the bloodstream very slowly. Engineered human antibodies in humans have a $t_{1/2}\beta$ of 7–14 days.[10] This type of PK profile may be advantageous for antibody-drug conjugates which are stable in the circulation, since accretion of antibodies into tumors is relatively slow and a long circulation time may lead to optimum tumor uptake. For radioisotope delivery, e.g., ^{90}Y, where the isotope has a $t_{1/2}\beta$ of 2.7 days, and the most

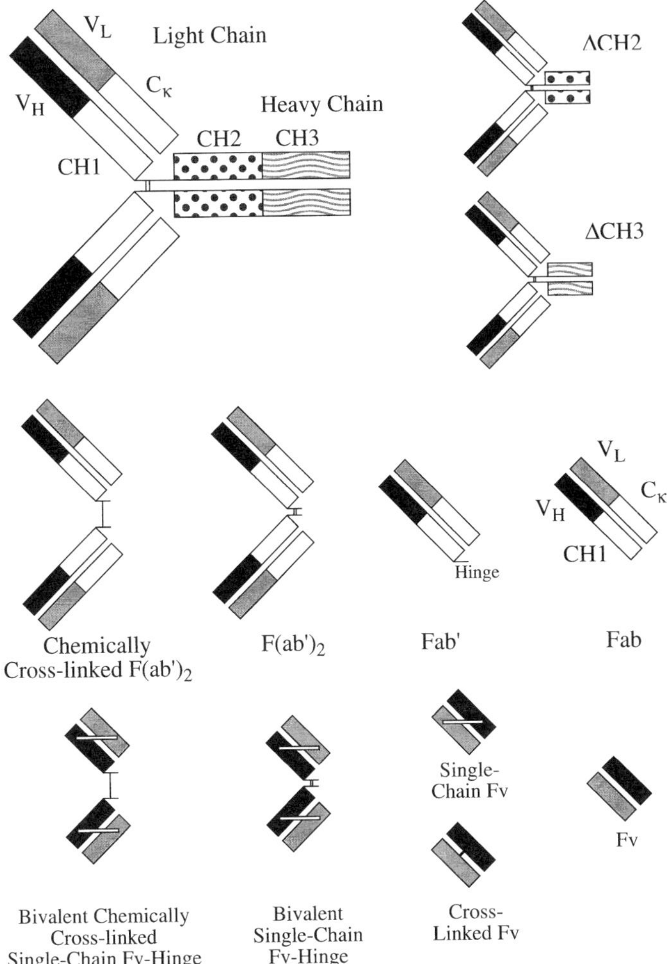

FIGURE 1
Antibody variants that have been made and evaluated as carriers of drugs or isotopes.

sensitive normal tissue is the bone marrow, the intact antibody with a $t_{1/2}\beta$ of 14 days is unlikely to produce a therapeutic benefit, unless stem cell ablation followed by transplanting is considered.

Antibody fragments are more promising carriers for radioisotope than intact IgG since they: (1) have shorter $t_{1/2}\beta$ values[44] and hence lower radiation dose exposure to the bone marrow and (2) they penetrate solid tumors faster than intact IgG, thereby generating a higher maximum dose rate to tumors at early time points.[21] Fv fragments (minimal antigen-binding regions) as non-covalently or covalently joined fragments have been evaluated as radioisotope carriers.[45] The β half-life of Fvs is very short, in the order of <1 h, suggesting that these fragments are unlikely to load sufficient radioactivity onto tumors to achieve a therapeutic effect. Fv fragments do offer an interesting option for *in vivo* diagnosis, where absolute levels retained on the tumor are less important.

$F(ab)_2$ fragments are approximately half the size of an intact antibody. The $t_{1/2}\beta$ of $F(ab)_2$ fragments is approximately 24–48 h. In terms of achieving tumor loading with relatively rapid plasma clearance, $F(ab)_2$ fragments are interesting molecules. A study of the biodistribution of $F(ab)_2$ fragments, however, using radiometals rather than radioiodine, demonstrates that the major clearance organ is the kidney.[46] Indeed up to 20% injected dose per gram of tissue (ID/g) can accumulate within the kidney, which would result in a massive radiation dose to this organ. Chemically crosslinked $F(ab')_2$ forms of antibodies have been prepared in order to prevent *in vivo* formation of Fab' forms, but have not significantly reduced rates of plasma clearance and kidney accumulation.[47]

Recently the biodistribution of a divalent (DFM) and trivalent Fab form (TFM) of the anti-tumor antibody A33[48] has been compared in guinea pigs. These chemically crosslinked, recombinant molecules were site specifically labeled in the chemical cross-linker. While the divalent form accumulated in the kidney to 9% ID/g, the trivalent form accumulated to only 1% ID/g in the kidney. This is particularly interesting because the TFM cleared only marginally slower than the DFM, hence preserving the reduced radiation exposure to the bone marrow without accumulation in the kidney. These relative rates of clearance were reproduced in the cynomolgus monkey.[49] These data suggest that the TFM may be an ideal carrier for ^{90}Y isotope, if the biodistribution and clearance observed in experimental animals is reproduced in man.

Other approaches have been used to try and optimize antibody biodistribution. In order to reduce kidney uptake of radiometal-labeled fragments, mice have been treated with basic amino acids or a range of different basic amino acid derivatives and amino sugars as well as cation peptides.[50] For Fab' and $F(ab)_2$ fragments renal uptake was reduced five- to sixfold, without reducing tumor uptake. D- and L-isomers of lysine were equally effective. D-glucosamine was effective but *N*-acetylglucosamine was not. Basic polypeptides were also effective, with their potency increasing with molecular weight. Interestingly, intact Fab' is found in the urine when the animals are treated with the basic amino acids, while in the untreated animals the radiolabel is found in low molecular weight metabolites. These data suggest that the mechanism by which these agents reduce renal uptake competes for tubular reabsorption of peptides and proteins, and that positively charged amino acids or peptides may be beneficial in reducing kidney exposure to radioactively labeled antibody fragments.

Several groups have attempted to modify Fab′ and $F(ab)_2$ PKs and renal uptake by chemical modification. PEGylation[51] and addition of oxidized dextran[52] are two such methods. Both approaches appear to reduce kidney uptake and extend the plasma half-life of the antibody. Although modification of the antibody does lead to some loss in activity, tumor uptake does not seem to be compromised. An additional advantage of such modifications may be a reduction in immunogenicity. Future advances are likely to involve the development of site-specific modification, such that antibody binding is not compromised.

In summary, antibodies have proved to be useful tools for exploring how differences in PK properties may be exploited for the targeted delivery of isotopes or cytotoxic drugs. Intact IgG has a relatively long half-life (approximately 7–14 days) and clears from the body slowly through the liver and kidney. In general, major accumulation in these organs is not observed. Antibody fragments clear rapidly by comparison, with half-life values of <1 h for Fvs and 24–48 h for Fab′. This clearance is by a large part through the kidney, where the fragments are absorbed and metabolized. Basic polypeptides or amino acids may compete out by renal absorption and this leads to fragment accumulation in the urine. Chemically cross-linked, trivalent Fab fragments may also reduce kidney accumulation.

3.4 DELIVERY OF RADIOISOTOPES

Recent clinical trials with radiolabeled antibodies directed against tumor-associated antigens have demonstrated some promise as discussed above; however, it is clear that optimization of this modality and careful selection of therapeutic targets are both key issues. Some tumors, e.g., lymphomas, are relatively radiosensitive and represent tractable targets without further optimization of current methodologies. Other tumor types, e.g., major epithelial tumors are relatively radioresistant, and isotope delivery may need to be optimized. The important question, therefore, is what are the prospects of significant improvements in delivery technology to enable solid tumors to be tractable targets?

One of the most contentious issues remains the choice of radionuclide for clinical trials. Some of the isotopes considered for radioimmunotherapy and their properties are listed in Table 4. I-131 remains the most frequently employed isotope to date because of its availability, low cost, and relatively simple radiochemistry. In addition, significant response rates have been observed in the clinic with radioimmunoconjugates of I-131.[13]

TABLE 4

Isotopes Considered for Immunotherapy

Isotope	Emission	Half-Life	Photons
^{131}I	0.34 MeV β (13%)	8.1 d	364 keV (82%)
	0.61 MeV β (86%)		
^{90}Y	2.29 MeV β (100%)	2.5 d	None
^{186}Re	0.93 MeV β (22%)	3.5 d	137 keV (9.2%)
	1.07 MeV β (70%)		
^{67}Cu	0.4 MeV β (56%)	2.5 d	91 keV (7%)
	0.48 MeV β (23%)		93 keV (17%)
	0.58 MeV β (20%)		184 keV (47%)
^{211}At	5.87 MeV α (42%)	7.2 h	None
	7.45 MeV α (58%)		

Despite its wide use, I-131 has a number of limitations. Its high-energy γ emissions cause myelosuppression which is often the dose-limiting toxicity of such conjugates. In addition, the γ emissions pose a risk to healthcare personnel and the relatively long half-life (8 days) means that hospital stays are lengthened. From an efficacy point of view, I-131-labeled antibodies prepared by the chloramine T or IodoGen methods are rapidly degraded after endocytosis by target cells, with rapid release of the isotope. This is a problem if the conjugate is metabolized by tumor cells, since retention of isotope at the tumor site is poor.[53] The development of a metabolically stable radioiodination reagent for coupling to MAbs has been a goal of several groups. Using a method that generates a stable thiourea linkage,[54] reduction of thyroid uptake of radioiodine, without reducing tumor uptake, was observed. A second approach, using a "residualizing" iodine label, dilactitol-iodotyramine, which is lysosomally trapped after catabolism of the antibody, resulted in an eightfold increase in absorbed dose to the tumor, compared to conventionally labeled I-131 antibody.[55]

Improving the metabolic stability of radioiodine conjugates is only meaningful if the targeting antibody is internalized at the tumor site, since internalization is presumably the mechanism by which conjugates are metabolized. Retention of radiolabel in the clearance organs is also predicted for these conjugates; however, the damage to these organs is not likely to be dose limiting. It does seem, therefore, based on animal data, that by using a non-metabolized iodine label and an internalizing antibody, a higher absorbed radiation dose to the tumor can be achieved, than has been achieved thus far using conventional labeling approaches for radioiodine.

Several other radionuclides may prove to be superior to I-131 for radioimmunotherapy, including the β emitters: Yttrium-90, Rhenium-186, and Copper-67, or the α emitters: Astatine-211 and Bismuth-212. β emitters may be most appropriate for radioimmunotherapy because the emissions have a long path length in tissue. This is an important consideration in the effective treatment of solid tumors. The longer path length of the β particle should ensure a more homogeneous dose distribution than the antibody distribution, therefore overcoming some of the perceived problems of poor tumor penetration and heterogeneous antigen expression.

The radioisotope ^{90}Y has been used in several radioimmunotherapy studies and is an attractive isotope for this application since: (1) it is a pure β emitter; (2) it has a half-life of 2.7 days; (3) it can be stably chelated and conjugated; and (4) internalized chelates are retained within tumor cells.

Early studies with ^{90}Y immunoconjugates were limited by the use of poor acyclic chelators, e.g., DTPA, which allow leakage of ^{90}Y with subsequent bone accumulation and bone marrow "toxicity." Co-administration of free chelator (e.g., EDTA) failed to solve this problem.[56] Stable macrocyclic chelators, e.g., DOTA, have now been developed, and these prevent the loss of ^{90}Y from immunoconjugates, under physiological conditions.[57] These conjugates perform well in mouse xenograft studies. Complete eradication of established tumors of the human colorectal cell line SW1222 in nude mice has been demonstrated using the antibody A33[49] without significant bone marrow toxicity.

Optimizing the pharmacokinetic profile and biodistribution of the antibody carrier is a key activity for radioimmunotherapy as described above. The generation of Y90-labeled TFM molecules is an interesting development that may be an optimal vehicle for the delivery of ^{90}Y. Studies using a TFM version of the antibody A33 labeled with ^{90}Y, demonstrate a clear anti-tumor effect on human xenografts in nude mice (P. Antoniw et al., in preparation). In these experiments, complete eradication of SW1222 tumors was observed at ^{90}Y doses that would have been lethal when given conjugated to intact antibody.

Although these new developments may allow the delivery of ^{90}Y-labeled antibodies to tumors, it remains unproven whether or not such conjugates will compensate for the problems of variable tumor uptake of antibody conjugates that have been reported from clinical studies.[29]

Antibody access to tumor cells is one reason for variable uptake and may be limited by the nature of the tumor vasculature. Solid tumors tend to have abnormal vessels and poor blood flow, and the lack of a lymphatic system may result in regions of high interstitial pressure.[58] Recently a number of groups have studied the ability of cytokines to increase antibody uptake by tumors. The cytokine interleukin-2 (IL-2) has been shown to increase vascular permeability and to enhance the delivery of radionuclides to tumor sites. Using an anti-CEA antibody, uptake by human CEA-positive tumors in nude mice was slightly increased (1.4–1.8 fold).[59] Tumor necrosis factor (TNF) has also been shown to produce a similar increase in tumor uptake of radioimmunoconjugates.[60] Although these results are encouraging, the improvements in uptake are modest and their significance in terms of therapy has yet to be demonstrated. Exposure of normal tissues to the injected antibody is also increased, since the increased permeability is not limited to the tumor vasculature.

3.5 DELIVERY OF CYTOTOXIC DRUGS

Early work with antibody cytotoxic drug conjugates involved attempts to evaluate conjugates of standard chemotherapeutic agents, e.g., methotrexate, Adriamycin, and vinblastine.[61-63] Although these studies were limited by the immunogenicity of the mouse antibody, the results were not encouraging as the conjugates lacked potency. A severe limitation to the generation of potent conjugates is the linking technology and the number of drug molecules per antibody molecule that are needed. Increasing the number of drug molecules above approximately 5 mol/mol antibody results in loss of antigen-binding and also antibody aggregation.

Despite these problems one antibody conjugate of a conventional chemotherapeutic drug has been developed to phase I/II clinical studies. Immunoconjugates (BR96-DOX) have been prepared between the chimeric monoclonal antibody BR96 and the anti-cancer drug doxorubicin. The antibody binds to an antigen related to Lewis Y that is abundantly expressed on the surface of a number of different tumor types. BR96 is rapidly internalized into lysosomes and endosomes after binding to tumor cells,[5] and conjugates have been designed that release drug after internalization. The DOX derivative maleimidocaproyl doxorubicin hydrazone is linked to the antibody through the maleimide. The resulting thioether linkage is stable in plasma, while the hydrazone bond is acid-labile and allows release of free drug within the endosome. BR96-DOX induced complete regressions and cures of xenografted human, lung, breast, and colon carcinomas grown subcutaneously in nude mice. This was true even when treatment was delayed until the mice displayed extensive disseminated disease.

Although these results are impressive the doses of antibody required are very high. BR96-DOX at a cumulative dose of 15 mg of DOX/kg of body weight and 700 mg of antibody/kg of body weight resulted in a 75% cure rate of established lung tumors. This dose in mice is approximately equivalent to a cumulative dose in humans of 3 g of antibody.

An alternative approach to tumor killing with cytotoxic drug antibody conjugates is to select a more potent drug molecule. One such drug is calicheamicin,[64] which is a member of the enediyne family.

Other members of this family[3,65] are: neocarzinostatin (NCS), esperamicin, and dynemicin. These potent microbial products contain a unique bicyclic ring structure that is triggered by reduction to generate a biradical which causes double-strand DNA cleavage.

The calicheamicins are small molecule enediynes with a molecular weight of approximately 1300 Da. Unlike NCS, the calicheamicins have no protein component. Calicheamicin γ is more than 1000-fold more potent than doxorubicin in murine tumor models, and is probably too toxic to be used as an unconjugated drug for cancer therapy. However, studies indicate that some derivatives of the calicheamicins, when conjugated to internalizing antibodies, show excellent anti-tumor activity.

A disulfide analog of the calicheamicin derivative, *N*-acetyl-calicheamicin γ, has been conjugated to a number of MAbs. Linkage to the antibody has been either on the carbohydrate or on lysine residues. One MAb, CTM01, which targets PEM antigen found on most of the solid tumors of epithelial origin, has shown excellent activity against human breast, ovarian, and lung tumors xenografted into nude mice.[15] Eradication of tumors was obtained at doses below the maximum tolerated dose. An engineered human form of this antibody conjugate is currently in development for the treatment of ovarian cancer.

Comparison with the BR96-DOX dosimetry calculations highlights the greater potency of the calicheamicin conjugates. Complete cure with the CTM01 conjugates is achieved at 0.45 mg calicheamicin/kg of body weight and 30 mg/kg of antibody in a mouse. Based on surface-area calculations for humans, this would approximate to a cumulative dose of 120 mg antibody dose. Hence, with the more potent conjugates a total dose reduction of greater than 20-fold is achieved.

These two examples of complete tumor eradication using antibody drug conjugates are very exciting. Since there is little scope for bystander killing of non-targeted tumor cells and it is unlikely that all the tumor cells are targeted by the conjugates, the mechanism by which complete cures are obtained remains unclear.

In addition to CTM01 conjugates of calicheamicin, a second antibody conjugate is in clinical development. An engineered human form of the anti-CD33 MAb, P67.6, is being developed for the treatment of AML.[3] Preclinical studies have shown that calicheamicin conjugates of P67.6 are potent and selective for CD33-expressing cells and that tumor eradication can be achieved in xenografted mice (unpublished data). Clinical evaluation of these conjugates will be particularly interesting, since the leukemia cells are readily accessible to the antibody conjugate and greater than 80% of the injected antibody targets to the tumor site.

Other members of the enediyene family have also been evaluated as antibody conjugates. NCS, which is not a simple, small molecule, but a complex one comprised of an acidic polypeptide chain of 11 kDa, which protects a highly labile bicyclic chromophore,[65] has been studied as a conjugate to the murine antibody A7.[66] This antibody recognizes human colon cancer cells and is internalized. Antibody conjugates show excellent activity in xenografted nude mice, and significant antitumor responses were reported in phase I human studies.[6] In the human study, dosing was limited by human anti-mouse antibodies (HAMA) responses to the murine A7 antibody. Recently, a chimeric A7 Fab conjugate has been reported.[67]

NCS has been linked by either disulfide or thioether linkages to Fab fragments of the antibody GA-17 that binds to an antigen on the surface of human astrocytomas.[68] This conjugate is active in xenograft models and could be delivered directly into tumors or into the cerebral fluid for the treatment of malignant gliomas.

Other highly potent cytotoxic agents linked to antibodies are also being developed as cancer therapies. CC-1065 (an antibiotic from *S. zelensis*) analogs attached to antibodies via a cleavable disulfide linkage have been reported. Conjugates of murine antibodies against tumor-associated antigens CD19 (B-cell lymphoma) and CD56 (melanoma and small cell lung cancer) show good *in vitro* potency and selectivity.[69] Complete cures were reported for anti-CD19 conjugates in an aggressive, metastatic human B-cell lymphoma model in SCID mice.

Maytansinoids[70] are another family of highly potent drugs that are showing promise as immunoconjugates. These compounds are ansa macrolides that are ~100-fold more potent than standard chemotherapy drugs. Derivatives of maytansinoids have been linked via disulfide bonds to a number of different antibodies, including antibodies to CD19, transferrin-receptor, and HER2/neu. These conjugates are selectively cytotoxic *in vitro* with IC_{50} values of 10^{-10} to 10^{-11} M. *In vivo* activity against A375 human melanoma cells grown intraperitoneally in SCID mice has been reported for the anti-transferrin receptor antibody conjugate.

In summary, antibody drug conjugates show surprising activity in preclinical models of cancer, despite their apparent lack of bystander killing activity. Although conjugates of conventional chemotherapeutics show activity, the more potent drugs, e.g., calicheamicins, offer more promise as viable cancer treatments.

3.6 SUMMARY

For many years the development of new cancer therapies based on MAb targeting has moved slowly. Initially, HAMA responses to murine antibody limited the ability to treat patients more than once. This problem has now been overcome. New technologies and novel killing agents now promise to finally deliver efficacious antibody therapies for cancer.

AML treatment with calicheamicin linked to an anti-CD33 antibody is an exciting prospect, since targeting (80% of the injected dose) can be readily achieved. The clinical results with anti-CD20 antibodies radiolabeled with I-131 for the treatment of B-cell lymphoma are also exciting. These two examples represent tractable cancer targets with real prospects of success.

The major solid tumors remain a difficult target for MAb therapy. Currently <1% of the injected dose of the antibody conjugate reaches the tumor site. The consequence of this poor accumulation at the tumor site is that there is a significant radiation dose to normal tissues (for radiolabeled antibody conjugates), as well as a relatively low dose to the tumor. Better chelators, use of antibody fragments, and improving tumor penetration may bring therapeutic benefits in solid tumor therapy. Currently, the use of radioimmunoconjugates in combination with bone marrow stem cell replacement may offer the best way forward for the treatment of disseminated disease. The treatment of solid tumors with conjugates of highly potent drugs may prove efficacious, since their long circulation time and stability may improve tumor uptake without resulting in non-specific toxicities. Clinical studies with these agents are awaited.

Finally, novel tumor targets, particularly the tumor endothelium, may provide the solution to the problem of solid tumor access. If tumor-specific endothelial cell markers can be found, then the application of current technology should generate some very interesting antibody-based therapeutics.

REFERENCES

1. Maguire, R. T., OncoScint image atlas, *Targeted Diagn. Ther.*, 6, 141, 1992.
2. Azrin, M. A., The uses of antibodies in clinical cardiology, *Am. Heart J.*,124, 753, 1992.
3. Hinman, L. M. and Yarranton, G. T., New approaches to non-immunogenic monoclonal antibody cancer therapies, *Annu. Rep. Med. Chem.*, 28, 237, 1993.
4. Press, O. W., Eary, J. F., Applebaum, F. R., Martin, P. J., Nelp, W. B., Glenn, S., Fisher, D. R., Porter, B., Matthews, D. C., Gooley, T., and Bernstein, I. D., Phase II trial of ^{131}I-B1 (anti-CD20) antibody therapy with autologous stem cell transplantation for relapsed B-cell lymphoma, *Lancet*, 346, 336, 1995.
5. Trail, P. A., Willner, D., Lasch, S. J., Henderson, A. J., Hofstead, S., Casazza, A. M., Firestone, R. A., Hellström, I., and Hellström, K. E., Cure of xenografted human carcinomas by BR96-Doxorubicin immunoconjugates, *Science*, 261, 212, 1993.
6. Takahashi, T., Yamaguchi, T., Kitamura, K., Noguchi, A., Honda, M., and Otsuji, E., Follow-up study of patients treated with monoclonal antibody-drug conjugate: report of 77 cases with colorectal cancer, *Jpn. J. Cancer Res.*, 84, 976, 1993.
7. DeNardo, G. L., Lewis, J. P., DeNardo, S. J., and O'Grady, L. F., Effect of Lym-1 radioimmunoconjugate on refractory chronic lymphocytic leukemia, *Cancer*, 73, 1425, 1994.

8. Adair, J. R., Athwal, D. S., and Emtage, J. S., *Humanised Antibodies*, WO91/09967.
9. Reichmann, L., Clark, M., Waldmann, H., and Winter, G., Reshaping human antibodies for therapy, *Nature*, 332, 323, 1988.
10. Stephens, S., Vetterlein, O., and Sopwith, M. CDP571, an engineered antibody to human tumor necrosis factor, in *Antibody Therapeutics*, Harris, W. J. and Adair J. R., Eds., CRC Press, Boca Raton, FL, 1997, chap. 14.
11. Shephard, H. M., Lewis, G. D., Sarup, J. C., Fendly, B. M., Maneval, D., Mordenti, J., Figari, I., Kotts, C. E., Palladino, M. A., Jr., Ullrich, A., and Slamon, D., Monoclonal antibody therapy of human cancer: taking the HER2 proto-oncogene to the clinic, *J. Clin. Immunol.*, 11, 117, 1991.
12. Riethmuller, G., Schneider-Gadicke, E., Schlimok, G., Schmiegel, W., Raab, R., Hoffken, K., Gruber, R., Pichlmaier, H., Hirche, H., Pichlmayr, R., Buggish, P., Witte, J., and the German Cancer Aid 17-1A Study Group, Randomised trial of monoclonal antibody for adjuvant therapy of resected Dukes' C colorectal carcinoma, *Lancet*, 343, 1177, 1994.
13. Press, O. W., Eary, J. F, Applebaum, F. R., Martin, P. J., Badger, C. C., Nelp, W. B., Glenn, S., Butchko, G., Fisher, D., Porter, B., Porter, B., Matthews, D. C., Fisher, L. D., and Bernstein, I. D., Radiolabelled-antibody therapy of B-cell lymphoma with autologous bone marrow support, *N. Engl. J. Med.*, 329, 1219, 1993.
14. Maloney, D. G., Liles, T. M., Czerwinski, D. K., Waldichuk, C., Rosenberg, J., Grillo-Lopez, A., and Levy, R., Phase I clinical trials escalating single-dose infusion of chimeric anti-CD20 monoclonal antibody (IDEC-C2B8) in patients with recurrent B-cell lymphoma, *Blood*, 84, 2457, 1994.
15. Hinman, L. M., Hamann, P. R., Wallace, R., Menendez, A. T., Durr, F. E., and Upeslacis, J., Preparation and characterization of monoclonal antibody conjugates of the calicheamicins; a novel and potent family of anti-tumour antibiotics, *J. Cancer Res.*, 53, 3336, 1993.
16. Couto, J. R., Blank, E. W., Peterson, J. A., Kiwan, R., Padlan, E. A., and Ceriani, R. L., Engineering of antibodies for breast cancer therapy: construction of chimeric and humanized versions of the murine monoclonal antibody BrE-3, *Adv. Exp. Med. Biol.*, 353, 55, 1994.
17. Burchell, J. and Taylor-Papadimitrou, J., Effect of modification of carbohydrate side chains on the reactivity of antibodies with core-protein epitopes of the MUC-1 gene product, *Epithelial Cell Biol.*, 2, 155, 1993.
18. Maraveyas, A., Stafford, N., Rowlinson-Busza, G., Stewart, J. S., and Epenetos, A. A., Pharmacokinetics, biodistribution and dosimetry of specific and control radiolabelled monoclonal antibodies in patients with primary head and neck squamous cell carcinoma, *Cancer. Res.*, 55, 1060, 1995.
19. Siler, K., Eggensperger, D., Hand, P. H., Milenic, D. E., Miller, L. S., Houchens, D. P., Hinkle, G., and Schlom, J., Therapeutic efficacy of a high-affinity anti-carcinoembryonic antigen monoclonal antibody (COL-1), *Biotechnol. Ther.*, 4, 163, 1993.
20. Goldenberg, D. M., Carcinoembryonic antigen as a target cancer antigen for radiolabelled antibodies: prospects for cancer imaging and therapy, *Tumour Biol.*, 16, 62, 1995.
21. Lane, D. M., Eagle, K. F., Begent, R. H. J., Hope-Stone, L. D., Green, A. J., Casey, J. L., Keep, P. A., Kelly, A. M. B., Ledermann, J. A., Glaser, M. G., and Hilson, A. J. W., Radioimmunotherapy of metastatic colorectal tumours with iodine-131-labelled antibody to CEA: phase I/II study with comparative biodistribution of intact and $F(ab')_2$ antibodies, *Br. J. Cancer*, 70, 521, 1994.
22. Durbin, H., Young, S., Stewart, L. M., Wrba, F., Rowan, A. J., Snary, D., and Bodmer, W. F., An epitope on carcinoembryonic antigen defined by clinically relevant antibody PRIA3, *Proc. Natl. Acad. Sci. U.S.A.*, 91, 4313, 1994.

23. Meredith, R. F., LoBuglio, A. L., Plott, W. E., Orr, R. A., Brezovich, I. A., Russell, C. D., Harvey, E. B., Yester, M. V., Wagner, A. J., Spencer, S. A., Wheeler, R. H., Saleh, M. N., Rogers, K. J., Polansky, A., Salter, M. M., and Khazaeli, M. B., Pharmacokinetics, immune response and biodistribution of iodine-131-labelled chimeric mouse/human IgG1,κ17-1A monoclonal antibody, *J. Nuclear Med.*, 32, 1162, 1991.
24. Petersen, B. H., Barrett, P., Lubus, J., Woodworth, J., Zimmermann, J., Bulter, F., Dugan, W., and Schneck, D. W., Murine monoclonal antibody-vinca conjugate KS1/4DAVLB hydrazide: Phase I studies in patients with adenocarcinoma, *Antibod. Immuncon. Radiopharm.*, 6, 127, 1993.
25. Velders, M. P., Litvinov, S. V., Warnaar, S. O., Gorter, A., Fleuren, G. J., Zurawski, V. R., Jr., and Coney, L. R., New chimeric anti-pan carcinoma monoclonal antibody with superior cytotoxicity-mediating potency, *Cancer Res.*, 54, 1753, 1994.
26. Khazaeli, M. B., Saleh, M. N., Liu, T. P., Meredith, R. F., Wheeler, R. H., Baker, T. S., King, D., Secher, D., Allen, L., Rogers, K., Colcher, D., Schlom, J., Shochat, D., and LoBuglio, A. F., Pharmacokinetics and immune response of 131I-chimeric mouse/human B72.3 (human γ4) monoclonal antibody in man, *Cancer Res.*, 51, 5461, 1991.
27. Divgi, C. R., Scott, A. M., Dantis, L., Capitelli, P., Siler, K., Hilton, S., Finn, R. D., Kelson, D., Kostakoglu, L., Schlom, J., and Larson, S. M., Phase I radioimmunotherapy trial with iodine-131-CC49 in metastatic colon carcinoma, *J. Nuclear Med.*, 36, 586, 1995.
28. Peat, N., Gendler, S. J., Lalani, E.-N., Duhig, T., and Taylor-Papadimitriou, J., Tissue-specific expression of a human polymorphic epithelial mucin (MUC1) in transgenic mice, *Cancer Res.*, 52, 1954, 1992.
29. Boxer, G. M., Begent, R. H. J., Kelly, A. M. B., Southall, P. J., Blair, S. B., Theodorou, N. A., Dawson, P. M., and Ledermann, J. A., Factors influencing variability of localisation of antibodies to CEA in patients with colorectal carcinoma — implications for radioimmunotherapy, *Br. J. Cancer*, 65, 825, 1992.
30. Jobling, T. W., Granowska, M., Britton, K. F., Lowe, D. G., Mather, S. J., Burchell, J., Nueem, M., and Shepherd, J. H., Radioimmunoscintigraphy of ovarian tumours using a new monoclonal antibody SM-3, *Gynecol. Oncol.*, 38, 468, 1990.
31. Rettig, W. J., Chesa-Garin, P., Beresford, H. R., Oeltgen, H. F., Melamed, M. R., and Old, L. J., Cell surface glycoproteins of human sarcomas: differential expression in normal and malignant tissues and cultured cells, *Proc. Natl. Acad. Sci. U.S.A.*, 85, 3110, 1988.
32. Welt, S., Divgi, C. R., Scott, A. M., Garin-Chesa, P., Finn, R. D., Graham, M., Carswell, E. A., Cohen, A., Larson, S. M., Old, L. J., and Rettig, W. J., Antibody targeting in metastatic colon cancer: a phase I study of monoclonal antibody F19 against a cell-surface protein of reactive tumour stromal fibroblasts, *J. Clin. Oncol.*, 12, 1193, 1994.
33. Rettig, W. J., Garin-Chesa, P., Healey, J. H., Su, S. L., Jaffe, E. A., and Old, L. J., Identification of endosialin, a cell surface glycoprotein of vascular endothelial cells in human cancer, *Proc. Natl. Acad. Sci. U.S.A.*, 89, 10832, 1992.
34. Kuminski, M. S., Fig, L. M., Zasadng, K. R., Koral, K. F., Del Rosario, R. B., Francis, I. R., Hunson, C. A., Normolle, D. P., Madgett, E., Liu, C. P., Moon, S., Scott, P., Miller, R. A., and Wahl, R. L., Imaging, dosimetry and radioimmunotherapy with iodine 131-labelled anti-CD37 antibody in B-cell lymphoma, *J. Clin. Oncol.*, 10, 1696, 1992.
35. Van der Jagt, R. H., Badger, C. C., Appelbaum, F. R., Press, O. W., Matthews, D. C., Eary, J. F., Krohn, K. A., and Bernstein, I. D., Localization of radiolabelled antimyeloid antibodies in a human acute leukemia xenograft tumour model, *Cancer Res.*, 52, 89, 1992.

36. Caron, P. C., Juricic, J. G., Scott, A. M., Finn, R. D., Divgi, C. R., Graham, M. C., Jureldini, I. M., Sgouros, G., Tyson, D., Old, L. J., Larson, S. M., and Scheinberg, D. A., A phase 1B trial of humanized monoclonal antibody M195 (anti-CD33) in myeloid leukaemia: specific targeting without immunogenicity, *Blood*, 83, 1760, 1994.
37. Pietersz, G. A., Wenjun, L., Sutton, V. R., Burgess, J., McKenzie, I. F., Zola, H., and Trapani, J. A., *In vitro* and *in vivo* anti-tumor activity of a chimeric anti-CD19 antibody, *Cancer Immunol. Immunother.*, 41, 53, 1995.
38. Flavell, D. J., Bloehm, D. A., Emery, L., Noss, A., Ramsay, A., and Flavell, S. U., Therapy of human B-cell lymphoma bearing SCID mice is more effective with anti-CD19 and anti-CD38-saporin immunotoxins used in combination than either immunotoxin used alone, *Int. J. Cancer*, 62, 337, 1995.
39. Matthews, D. C., Appelbaum, F. R., Eary, J. F., Fisher, D. R., Durak, L. D., Bush, S. A., Hiu, T. E., Martin, P. J., Mitchell, D., Press, O. W., Badger, C. C., Storb, R., Nelp, W. B., and Bernstein, I. D., Development of a marrow transplant regimen for acute leukaemia using targeted haematopoietic irradiation delivered by 131-labeled anti-CD45 antibody, combined with cyclophosphamide and total body irradiation, *Blood*, 85, 1122, 1995.
40. Divgi, C. R., Welt, S., Kris, M., Real, F. X., Yeh, S. O. J., Gralla, R., Merchant, B., Schweighart, S., Unger, M., Larson, S. M., and Mendelsohn, J., Phase I and imaging trial of Indium-111-labeled anti-epidermal growth factor receptor monoclonal antibody 225 in patients with squamous cell lung carcinoma, *J. Natl. Cancer Inst.*, 83, 98, 1991.
41. De Santes, K., Slamon, D., Anderson, S. K., Shepard, M., Fendly, B., Maneval, D., and Press, O., Radiolabeled antibody targeting of the HER-2/neu oncoprotein, *Cancer Res.*, 52, 1916, 1992.
42. Hutzell, P., Kashmiri, S., Colcher, D., Primus, F. J., Horan Hand, P., Roselli, M., Finch, M., Yarranton, G. T., Bodmer, M., Whittle, N., King, D., Loullis, C. C., McCoy, D. W., Callahan, R., and Schlom, J., Generation and characterization of a recombinant/chimeric B72.3 (human γ1), *Cancer Res.*, 51, 181, 1991.
43. LoBuglio, A. F., Wheeler, R. H., Trang, J., Haynes, A., Rogers, K., Harvey, E. B., Syn, L., Ghrayeb, J., and Khazaeli, M. B., Mouse/human chimeric monoclonal antibody in man: kinetics and immune response, *Proc. Natl. Acad. Sci. U.S.A.*, 86, 4220, 1989.
44. Buchegger, F., Pelegrin, A., Delaloye, B., Bischoff-Delaloye, A., and Mach, J. P., Iodine-131-labeled MAb F(ab′)2 fragments are more effective and less toxic than intact anti-CEA antibodies in radioimmunotherapy of large colon carcinoma grafted in nude mice, *J. Nuclear Med.*, 31, 1035, 1990.
45. Yokota, T., Milenic, D. E., Whitlow, M., and Schlom, J., Rapid tumor penetration of a single-chain Fv and comparison with other immunoglobulin forms, *Cancer Res.*, 52, 3402, 1992.
46. Sharkey, R. M., Motta-Hennessy, C., Pawlyk, D., Siegal, J. A., and Goldenberg, D. M., Biodistribution and radiation dose estimates for yttrium and iodine labeled monoclonal antibody IgG and fragments in nude mice bearing human colonic tumor xenografts, *Cancer Res.*, 50, 2330, 1990.
47. King, D. J., Turner, A., Farnsworth, A. P. H., Adair, J. R., Owens, R. J., Pedley, R. B., Baldock, D., Proudfoot, K. A., Lawson, A. D. G., Beeley, N. R. A., Millar, K., Millican, T. A., Boyce, B., Antoniw, P., Mountain, A., Begent, R. H. J., Shochat, D., and Yarranton, G. T., Improved tumor targeting with chemically cross-linked recombinant antibody fragments, *Cancer Res.*, 54, 6176, 1994.
48. Welt, S., Durgi, C. R., Kemeny, N., Finn, R. D., Scott, A. M., Graham, M., Germain, J. S., Carswell-Richard, E., Larson, S. M., Oeltgen, H. F., and Old, L. J., Phase I/II study of iodine-131-labeled monoclonal antibody A33 in patients with advanced colon cancer, *J. Clin. Oncol.*, 12, 1561, 1994.

49. King, D. J., Antonio, P., Owens, R. J., Adair, J. R., Haines, A. M. R., Farnsworth, A. P. H., Finney, H., Lawson, A. D. G., Lyons, A., Baker, T. S., Baldock, D., Mackintosh, J., Gofton, C., Yarranton, G. T., McWilliams, W., Shochat, D., Leichner, P. K., Welt, S., Old, L. J., and Mountain, A., Preparation and pre-clinical evaluation of humanised A33 immunoconjugates for radioimmunotherapy, *Br. J. Cancer*, 72, 1364, 1995.
50. Behr, T. M., Sharkey, R. M., Juweid, M. E., Blumenthal, R. D., Dunn, R. M., Griffiths, G. L., Blair, H. J., Wolf, F. G., Becker, W. S., and Goldenberg, D. M., Reduction of the renal uptake of radiolabeled monoclonal antibody fragments by cationic amino acids and their derivatives, *Cancer Res.*, 55, 3825, 1995.
51. Delgardo, C., Francis, G. E., and Fisher, D., The uses and properties of PEG-linked proteins, *Crit. Rev. Ther. Drug Carrier Systems*, 9, 249, 1992.
52. Fragnani, R., Halpern, S., and Hagan, M., Altered pharmacokinetics and tumour localization properties of Fab' fragments of a murine monoclonal anti-CEA antibody by covalent modification with low molecular weight dextran, *Nuclear Med. Commun.*, 16, 362, 1995.
53. Mattes, M. J., Griffiths, G. L., Diril, H., Goldenberg, D. M., Ong, G. L., and Shih, L. B., Processing of antibody-radioisotope conjugates after binding to the surface of tumour cells, *Cancer*, 73, 787, 1994.
54. Ram, S. and Buchsbaum, D. J., Radioiodination of monoclonal antibodies D612 and 17-1A with 3-iodophenylisothiocyanate and their biodistribution in tumour-bearing nude mice, *Cancer*, 73, 808, 1994.
55. Stein, R., Goldenberg, D. M., Thorpe, S. R., Basin, A., and Mattes, M. J., Effects of radiolabeling monoclonal antibodies with a residualizing iodine radiolabel on the accretion of radioisotope in tumours, *Cancer Res.*, 55 3132, 1995.
56. Hird, V., Steward, J. S. W., Snook, D., Dhokia, B., Coulter, C., Lambert, H. E., Mason, W. P., Soulter, W. P., and Epenetos, A. A., Intraperitoneally administered ^{90}Y-labeled monoclonal antibodies as a third line of treatment in ovarian cancer. A phase 1-2 trial: problems encountered and possible solutions, *Br. J. Cancer*, 62, 48, 1990.
57. Harrison, A., Walker, C., Parker, D., Jankowski, K., Cox, J., Craig, A., Sanson, J., Beeley, N., Boyce, B., Chaplin, L., Eaton, M., Farnsworth, A., Millar, K., Millican, A., Randall, A., Secher, D., and Turner, A., The *in vivo* release of ^{90}Y from cyclic and acyclic ligand-antibody conjugates, *Nuclear Med. Biol.*, 18, 469, 1991.
58. Jain, K., Delivery of novel therapeutic agents in tumours: physiological barriers and strategies, *J. Natl. Cancer Inst.*, 81, 570, 1989.
59. Nakamura, K., and Kubo, A., Effect of interleukin-2 on the biodistribution of technetium-99m-labeled anti-CEA monoclonal antibody in mice bearing tumour xenografts, *Eur. J. Nuclear Med.*, 21, 924, 1994.
60. Rowlinson-Busza, G., Maraveyas, A., and Epenetos, A. A., Effect of tumour necrosis factor on the uptake of specific and control monoclonal antibodies in a human tumour xenograft model, *Br. J. Cancer*, 71, 660, 1995.
61. Dillman, R. O., Johnson, D. E., and Shawler, D. L., Comparisons of drugs and toxin immunoconjugates, *Antibod. Immunocon. Radiopharm.*, 1, 65, 1988.
62. Pietersz, G. A., Smyth, M. J., Kanellos, J., Cunningham, Z., Sacks, N. P. M., and McKenzie, I. F. C., Pre-clinical and clinical studies with a variety of immunoconjugates, *Antibod. Immunocon. Radiopharm.*, 1, 79, 1988.
63. Trail, P. A., Willner, D., Lasch, S. J., Henderson, A. J., Greenfield, R. S., King, D., Zoechler, M. E., and Braslawsky, G. R., Antigen-specific activity of carcinoma-reactive BR64-Doxorubicin conjugates evaluated *in vitro* and in human tumour xenograft models, *Cancer Res.*, 52, 5693, 1992.
64. Zein, N., Poncin, M., Nilakantan, R., and Ellestad, G. A., Calicheamicin γ_1 and DNA: molecular recognition process responsible for site-specificity, *Science*, 244, 697, 1989.

65. Nicolaou, K. C., Dai, W.-M., Tsay, S.-C., Estevez, V. A., and Wrasidlo, W., Designed enediynes: a new class of DNA-cleaving molecules with potent and selective anti-cancer activity, *Science*, 256, 1172, 1992.
66. Kitamura, K., Takahashi, T., Noguchi, A., Takashina, K.-I., Tsurumi, I. T., and Yamaguchi, T., Binding, internalisation and the cytotoxicity of monoclonal antibody A7-neocarzinostatin conjugates (A7 NCS) in target cells, *J. Exp. Med.*, 161, 199, 1990.
67. Yamaguchi, T., Tsurumi, H., Kotani, T., Yamaoka, N., Otsuji, E., Kitamura, K., and Takahashi, T., *In vivo* efficacy of neocarzinostatin coupled with Fab human/mouse chimeric monoclonal antibody A7 against human colorectal cancer, *Jpn. J. Cancer Res.*, 85, 167, 1994.
68. Kondo, S., Nakatsu, S., Sakahara, H., Kobayashi, H., Konishi, J., and Namba, Y., Anti-tumour activity of an immunoconjugate composed of anti-human astrocytoma monoclonal antibody and neocarzinostatin, *Eur. J. Cancer*, 29A, 420, 1993.
69. Chari, R. V., Jackel, K. A., Bourret, L. A., Derr, S. M., Tadayoni, B. M., Mattocks, K. M., Shah, S. A., Liu, C., Blattler, W. A., and Goldmacher, V. S., Enhancement of the selectivity and anti-tumour efficacy of a cc-1065 analogue through immunoconjugate formation, *Cancer Res.*, 55, 4079, 1995.
70. Chari, R. V., Martell, B. A., Gross, J. L., Cook, S. B., Shah, S. A., Blattler, W. A., McKenzie, S. J., and Goldmacher, V. S., Immunoconjugates containing novel maytansinoids: promising anti-cancer drugs, *Cancer*, 52, 127, 1992.

Chapter 4

Tumor Targeting by Antibody-Drug Conjugates

Itai Benhar and Ira H. Pastan

CONTENTS

0-8493-8547-4/97/$0.00+$.50

4.1 INTRODUCTION

The concept of selective targeted delivery of therapeutic agents to tumor sites has been extended by the introduction of the antibody-directed enzyme prodrug therapy (ADEPT) technique (Figure 1).[1-8] This technique consists of two or three stages. First, a monoclonal antibody (MAb) or an antibody fragment which is conjugated to an enzyme otherwise unique to the human extracellular environment is administered and allowed to localize to the tumor target and to clear from the circulation. Once localized the antibody-enzyme complex will activate a subsequently administered (relatively inactive) prodrug at the tumor site. The prodrug is converted to free active drug which is capable of penetrating into the adjacent tumor cells and eventually causing their death. Thus, a small highly toxic drug accumulates within the tumor at concentrations that are significantly higher than in other tissues. Such a small molecule will more readily diffuse into the inner mass of the tumor which is less accessible to larger antibody conjugates, overcoming problems of poor penetration and antigen heterogeneity which are common when the therapy of solid tumors is attempted. In addition, enzymes, being catalytic proteins with a high substrate turnover, are capable of generating many drug molecules for each antibody-enzyme conjugate bound at the tumor site, so their effect is amplified. The possible third step of ADEPT is the application of a clearing reagent aimed at disposing of circulating antibody-enzyme conjugates, and thereby minimizing prodrug activation away from the tumor site.[4]

ADEPT is intended to overcome some of the limitations inherent to other antibody-based therapeutics: limited distribution (which is inversely proportional to the size of the reagent);[9] limited specificity which is mainly due to the expression of antigen on normal cells;[10,11] and heterogeneity in the expression of the antigen by tumor cells.[12,13] In addition, ADEPT avoids some obstacles of non-targeted therapeutics: the high toxicity associated with conventional chemotherapy,[14] and the specificity limits to the use of prodrugs which are activated by enzymes naturally found in tumors, but are present in normal tissues as well.[15,16]

Most of the ADEPT systems described to date involve enzymes conjugated by chemical means to whole IgG molecules or to proteolytically produced Fab′ fragments. In a few cases, antibody fragments (Fv molecules) were employed as the targeting moiety, and the Fv-enzyme chimera was produced in *E. coli* as a wholly recombinant molecule. There are several recent reviews of the enzymes and the prodrugs used for ADEPT.[4-8] Antibodies and antibody fragments that were used as vehicles in ADEPT are the focus of this review.

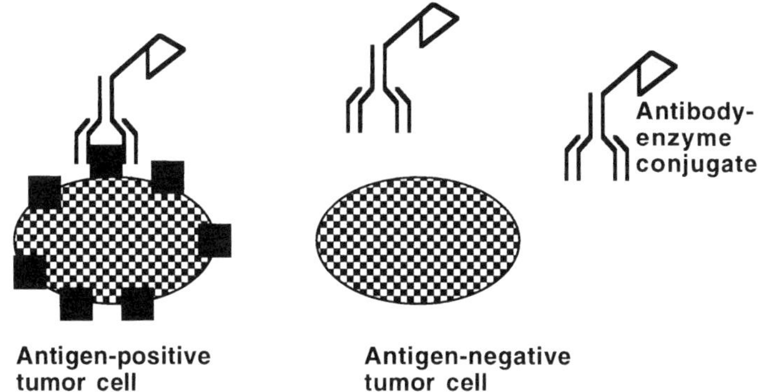

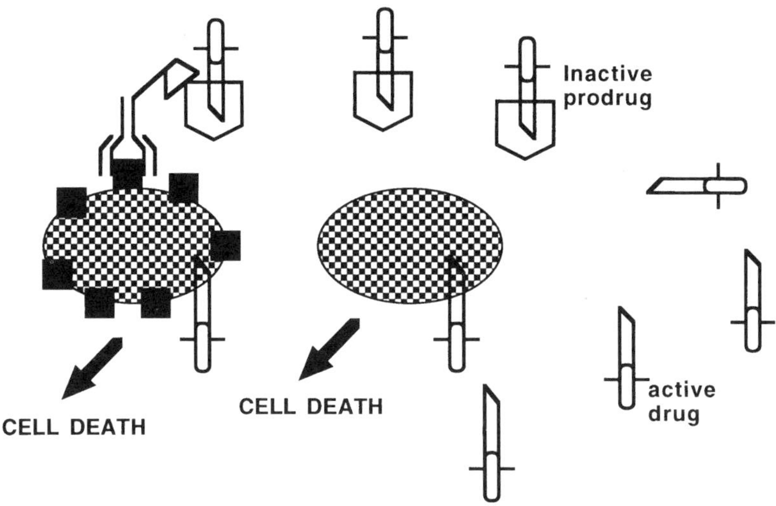

FIGURE 1
Antibody-directed enzyme prodrug therapy.

4.2 TARGET ANTIGENS AND ANTIBODIES

The repertoire of tumor-associated antigens that could be used as targets for ADEPT is larger and more diverse than the targets available for direct targeting of cytotoxic drugs or cytotoxins to cancer cells. The latter have to be internalized into the tumor cells upon binding of the targeting antibody, and should be expressed on the surface of each target cell to be killed at a high density. On the other hand, for ADEPT, a non-internalizing antibody is an advantage, and even an antigen that is secreted into the extracellular space of the tumor may be used as a target.[17] Moreover, the antigen used as an ADEPT target need not be expressed on all target cells, because of "the bystander effect," the prodrug which is being converted to active drug at the tumor site by enzyme-antibody molecules which are bound to antigen-positive cells accumulates at a relatively high local concentration. This in turn allows the drug to diffuse and affect the neighboring antigen-negative cells, as well as those cells which are distal from the vasculature of the tumor and are less accessible to the larger activating enzyme-antibody complex.

In fact, the antibodies that were utilized in ADEPT experiments were those already familiar to the targeted-therapy arena: antibodies against carcinoembryonic antigen (CEA), against cytokine receptors (epidermal growth factor; EGF, c-*erb*B2), and some antibodies that were raised against undefined extracellular antigens on melanoma and carcinoma cells were some of the tested candidates. Table 1 lists some of the antibodies that have been used to date as ADEPT vehicles, their targets, the conjugated enzyme, and the prodrug used.

Results from the cited studies and others suggested that an antibody of choice should have the following characteristics: (1) a high affinity, (bearing in mind the possibility of a very high-affinity reagent becoming "trapped" in the tumor periphery — the "binding site barrier"[33,34] and (2) contain a small targeting moiety — Fv or Fab' fragments localize better to tumors than IgG molecules. IgM molecules were never used, being relatively large, having lower affinities than IgG molecules, and being difficult to handle and chemically manipulate. The advantage of using a smaller antibody fragment can be nullified by the penalty paid in reduced affinity in comparison to the parental antibody, and in a more rapid clearance from the vascular system, which is desirable only after localization at the tumor has been achieved. Unfortunately, until now no attempt has been made to compare the efficacy of ADEPT systems employing an antibody and its (Fv or Fab') fragments in parallel.

Interestingly, the criteria applied for choosing antibodies as carriers of enzymes were similar to the criteria for choosing antibodies for immunotoxins and drug conjugates.[35,36] With a few exceptions, candidates were not tested *a priori* for internalization. Also, in most cases, murine antibodies were used, which were useful for the feasibility studies *in vitro* on cultured cancer cells and *in vivo* in xenograft mouse tumor models, but would be less useful in humans, mainly due to the

TABLE 1

Antibodies Used for ADEPT

	Antibody	Antigen	Enzyme	Prodrug	Ref.
1.	W14 (Fab)	bhCG (human chorionic gonadotropin)	Carboxypeptidase G2	para-*N*-bis(2-chloroethyl) aminobenzoyl-glutamate	18
2.	L6 (IgG2a)	Antigen on human carcinomas	Alkaline phosphatase (calf intestinal)	*p*-[*N,N*-bis(2-chloroethyl)amino] phenyl phosphate	19
3.	CEM-231 Fab′	CEA (carcinoembrionic antigen)	β-Lactamase (*E. cloacae*)	DAVLBHYD prodrug	20
4.	L6 (F(ab′)$_2$)	Antigen on human carcinomas	β-Lactamase (*B. cereus* and *E. coli*)	Cephalosporin mustard (CM)	21
5.	12.8 (F(ab′)$_2$)	Antigen on human colon cancer (Colo205) cells	β-Glucoronidase	Glucoronid prodrug of *p*-hydroxyaniline mustard (BHAMG)	22
6.	RH1	Antigen on AS-30D rat hepatoma cells	β-Glucoronidase	BHAMG glucoronide prodrug	23
7.	FRP5 (scFv)	c-*erb*B2	Alkaline phosphatase	Not tested	24
8.	L6 (IgG2a)	Antigen on human carcinomas	Penicillin G Amidase	Doxorubicin and melphalan *N*-phenylacetamido derivatives	24
9.	L6 (scFv)	Antigen on human carcinomas	β-Lactamase	Cephalosporin mustard (CM) (*B. cereus*)	25
10.	007B (Fab′) CEM-231 (Fab′) CC-49 (Fab′)	KS1/4 CEA TAG-72	β-Lactamase (*E. cloacae*)	DAVLBHYD prodrug	26
11.	A5B7 (F(ab′)$_2$)	CEA	Carboxypeptidase G2 A1T mutant	Not tested	27
12.	ICR12 (IgG2a)	c-*erb*B2	Carboxypeptidase G2	4-[(2-chloroethyl)(2-mesyloxy-ethyl)amino]benzoyl-glutamate	29
13.	ZCE025 (Fab′)	CEA	β-Lactamase	Not tested	30
14.	hum4D5 (dsFv)	c-*erb*B2	β-Lactamase	Cephalothin doxorubicin prodrug	31
15.	L6 (Fab′) P1.17 (Fab′) 96.5 (Fab′)	All three are nonspecified carcinoma antigens	β-Lactamase (*B. cereus*)	Cephalosporin derivative of doxorubicin	32

immunogenicity problem.[2,5,7] Only in a couple of cases were Fab'[37] or disulfide-stabilized Fv (dsFv)[31] fragments of humanized antibodies used.[31,37]

4.3 ANTIBODY PREPARATION AND CONJUGATION TECHNIQUES

Most of the antibody-enzyme conjugates were prepared using MAbs which were produced by standard hybridoma technology.[7,38] No particular IgG subclass was preferred, and IgG1 or IgG2 were equally employed. A few conjugates were made by conjugation of the enzyme to the whole antibody, while others were prepared by coupling the enzyme to antibody fragments. These were produced by limited proteolysis by pepsin,[20,21] yielding the bivalent $F(ab')_2$, which was in some cases reduced to the monovalent Fab' form with a free cysteinyl residue available for conjugation. In a handful of cases, genetically engineered antibody fragments were used as the enzyme carriers; these will be discussed in the next section. With one exception,[22] in which the antibody and enzyme were held together by a disulfide bond, the chemical conjugation techniques that were used utilized heterobifunctional reagents and resulted in stable non-reducible linkages (thioether bonds).[6,19-21,23,25-27,29,32,39,40]

In a few cases, the antibody or the enzyme was tailored for efficient site-specific conjugation using recombinant DNA techniques; Werlen et al., modified both the $F(ab')_2$ and the carboxypeptidase G2 (CPG2) for site-specific conjugation between the C terminus of the former and the (substituted) N terminus of the latter.[28] Mikolajczyk et al., modified the N terminus of a recombinant β-lactamase so it could be site specifically conjugated to an Fab' fragment.[30]

4.4 ANTIBODY ENGINEERING AND ADEPT

A few of the enzyme carriers tested in ADEPT systems were antibody fragments that were constructed using recombinant DNA techniques. Bosslet et al.[37] constructed a fully humanized recombinant fusion protein consisting of the Fab' of high-affinity anti-CEA MAb BW431 fused to a human β-glucoronidase gene. Their aim was to overcome the inability to readminister an antibody-enzyme conjugate to humans due to the development of HAMA (human anti-mouse) and human anti-enzyme antibodies in patients following treatment with a murine anti-CEA antibody coupled to *Pseudomonas* CPG2[41] (which was the only ADEPT clinical trial attempted to date). Their approach was to use the V_H and CH1 regions of humanized BW431 as building blocks,[42] and fuse them through a synthetic linker to human β-glucoronidase cDNA[43]. A plasmid carrying this construct was co-transfected into BHK cells together with a second plasmid carrying the humanized BW431 kappa chain. Protein recovered from transfectoma supernatants had antigen-binding affinity which was similar to that of the parental murine antibody and the ability to catalyze the cleavage of 4-methylumberilliferyl-glucuronide prodrug to 4-methylumberilliferone.

Wels et al.[24] constructed genes expressing a single-chain Fv (scFv)-alkaline phosphatase fusion. This group isolated MAbs which specifically bind to the extracellular domain of c-*erb*bB2,[44] and developed one of them, FRP5, as the targeting moiety of a wholly recombinant Fv-enzyme fusion protein, which was presented as a tool for immunohistochemical detection of c-*erb*B2 positive cells. The V_H and V_L domains of FRP5 were isolated from hybridoma RNA by reverse transcription followed by polymerase chain reaction (PCR) amplification, and subcloned into an *E. coli* expression vector in which V_H was linked to V_L via a flexible $(Gly_4Ser)_3$ linker.[45] The *E. coli* alkaline-phosphatase (*pho*A) gene was fused at the 3′ end of V_L, completing the single-chain expression cassette. The protein product was isolated from bacterial lysates by affinity chromatography, utilizing a flag epitope that was incorporated into the construct. The purified FRP5 (Fv)-phoA protein showed specific binding to c-*erb*B2 positive cells, and was capable of facilitating their immunohistochemical detection using Fast Red as a substrate. The possibility of employing FRP5 (Fv)-phoA as an ADEPT reagent was not addressed.

Goshorn et al.[26] followed up on encouraging results from phase I trials which were performed using MAb L6 or its $F(ab')_2$ fragments, showing its ability to localize and to deliver radionuclides to human tumors.[46-48] The same antibody was already tested in an ADEPT system, where its $F(ab')_2$ fragment was conjugated to β-lactamase, and was able to eliminate tumor cells bearing L6 antigen by converting the prodrug cephalosporin mustard (CM) to the cytotoxic drug phenyldiamine mustard (CDPM).[21] The goal of these investigators was to prepare a homogeneous reagent (in contrast to the heterogeneous chemical conjugates) which could be produced in *E. coli*. The L6 V_H and V_L clones were obtained by PCR amplification of L6 genomic clones.[49] The Fv was assembled by connecting V_H and V_L via a synthetic flexible linker,[45] and inserted 3′ to a *pel*B leader sequence for secretion, and 5′ of a *Bacillus cereus* β-lactamase gene. The fusion protein was recovered in active form from culture supernatant and cell paste by chromatography on an anti-idiotype 13B immunoaffinity column. It was found to render L6 antigen-positive cancer cells sensitive to the effects of the prodrug CM in a dose-dependent fashion.

Rodrigues et al.[31] used a similar approach in which they constructed a disulfide-stabilized anti-p185^{HER2} Fv-β-lactamase fusion protein. Their work was based on results from studies of the anti c-*erb*B2 (HER2/*neu*) humanized antibody HumAb4D5 which is now in phase II/III clinical trials for the treatment of metastatic breast cancer. In addition to testing HumAb4D5 F(ab')$_2$ for retargeting cytotoxic T lymphocytes[50,51] and stealth liposomes for drug delivery,[52] these investigators aimed to incorporate it into a potent ADEPT system.

The expression cassette was constructed by standard subcloning and mutagenesis techniques as a bicistronic operon encoding the humAb4D5 V_L followed by the humAb4D5 V_H-β-lactamase gene fusion. *Pho*A signal sequences were inserted 5' of each cistron to facilitate secretion of the protein product. Cysteine codons replaced codons of residues in the framework region of V_H and V_L, at positions that facilitated the formation of an intermolecular disulfide bond that would stabilize the Fv, according to principles developed by Glockshuber et al.,[53] Brinkmann et al.,[54] and Reiter et al.[55] The recombinant protein was secreted and assembled as a double-chain protein in the periplasm of *E. coli* and was purified by several chromatographic steps. The product was capable of converting a cephalosporin-doxorubicin prodrug into doxorubicin, and to target it to tumor cells overexpressing p185^{HER2}. The serum pharmacokinetics of hum4D5 dsFv in mice were also investigated, and the reagent was found to clear rapidly from the circulation. This demonstrates the advantage of the relatively small molecule over larger antibody-enzyme or Fab'-enzyme conjugates which persist for longer time periods, making it necessary to wait longer prior to prodrug administration, or to apply a clearing reagent[56] to avoid undesirable activation of the drug away from the tumor site.

4.5 CLINICAL STUDIES

The feasibility of the ADEPT approach has been demonstrated in preclinical studies using tumor xenograft rodent models.[1,7,8,19,25,27,29,32,54,56a-58,60] To date, a single clinical trial has been reported. In this trial, the toxicity of galactosylated anti-CPG2 antibody SB43 (SB43-gal) and the prodrug 4-[(2-chloroethyl) (2-mesyloxyethyl)amino] benzoyl-L-glutamic acid (CMDA) in combination with an anti-CEA Fab'-CPG2 conjugate was evaluated in patients with drug-resistant colorectal carcinoma.[3,41] Administration of approximately 350 mg of enzyme-drug conjugate was well tolerated and gave plasma concentrations which were similar to those found optimal in the mouse studies. Toxicities were prodrug related and were mostly transient myelosuppression. All patients developed antibodies against both the mouse antibody and the bacterial enzyme CPG2.[59] Cyclosporin delayed the development of host antibodies allowing up to three weekly cycles of therapy.[3] Of the 17 patients treated, 8 received a dose of CMDA prodrug which was considered potentially therapeutic. Of these, four patients had partial remission and one had a partial response. This demonstrates the feasibility of the ADEPT approach for human anti-cancer treatment.

4.6 CONCLUSION

Antibody-directed enzyme prodrug therapy seems to be a valuable addition to other immunotherapeutic methods which are currently being evaluated. When tested *in vitro* on cultured cancer cells, most of the antibody-enzyme conjugates demonstrated an ability to selectively target and activate the corresponding prodrug. *In vivo* efficacy studies using mouse tumor xenograft models provide valuable data confirming the validity of the concept.[4,6]

Only one phase I clinical trial has been performed thus far and it used $F(ab')_2$ of the anti-CEA monoclonal antibody A5B7 linked to CPG2.[3] It was used to treat colorectal carcinoma patients with the prodrug CMDA. Partial responses were observed in some of the patients, and side effects including an immune response against the antibody-enzyme conjugate were also recorded.

Taken together, the *in vivo* studies demonstrate the feasibility of ADEPT systems and also highlight some of the obstacles which still lie ahead. Among these are the need to accelerate the clearance of the reagent from the circulation and its possible immunogenicity. Both problems have already been addressed by applying antibody engineering so that smaller and humanized antibody fragments rather than the larger murine antibodies are used for enzyme targeting. More studies are required to further advance the ADEPT concept, and undoubtedly antibody technology and antibody engineering will be key players in this process.

REFERENCES

1. Bagshawe, K. D., Antibody directed enzymes revive anticancer prodrugs concept, *Br. J. Cancer*, 56, 531, 1987.
2. Bagshawe, K. D., Towards generating cytotoxic agents at cancer sites, *Br. J. Cancer*, 60, 275, 1989.
3. Bagshawe, K. D., Antibody-directed enzyme prodrug therapy (ADEPT), *Clin. Rep. Dis. Markers*, 9, 233, 1991.
4. Bagshawe, K. D., Antibody-directed enzyme prodrug therapy, *Clin. Pharmacol.*, 27, 368, 1994.

5. Huennekens, F. M., Tumor-targeting: activation of prodrugs by enzyme-monoclonal antibody conjugates, *Trends Biotechnol.*, 12, 234, 1994.
6. Deonarain, M. P. and Epenetos, A. A., Targeting enzymes for cancer therapy: old enzymes in new roles, *Br. J. Cancer*, 70, 786, 1994.
7. Bagshawe, K. D., Sharma, S. K., Springer, C. J., and Rogers, G. T., Antibody-directed enzyme prodrug therapy (ADEPT): a review of some theoretical, experimental and clinical aspects, *Ann. Oncol.*, 5, 879, 1994.
8. Bagshawe, K. D., Antibody-directed enzyme prodrug therapy: a Review, *Drug Dev. Res.*, 34, 220, 1995.
9. Jain, R. K. and Baxter, L. T., Mechanism of heterogeneous distribution of monoclonal antibodies and other macromolecules in tumours. Significance of increased interstitial pressure, *Cancer Res.*, 48, 7022, 1988.
10. Begent, R. H. J., Ledermann, J. A., Green, A. J., Bagshawe, K. D., Riggs, S. J., Searle, F., Keep, P. A., Adam, T., Dale, R. G., and Glaser, M. D., Antibody distribution and dosimetry in patients receiving radiolabelled antibody therapy for colorectal cancer, *Br. J. Cancer*, 60, 406, 1989.
11. Del-Viccio, S., Reynolds, J. C., Carrasquillo, J. A., Blasberg, R. G., Neumann, R. D., Lotze, M. T., Bryant, G. J., Franks, R. J., and Larson, S. M., Local distribution and concentration of intravenously injected ^{131}I-9.2.27 monoclonal antibody in human malignant melanoma, *Cancer Res.*, 49, 2783, 1989.
12. Primus, F. J., Kuhns, W. J., and Goldenberg, D. M., Immunological heterogeneity of carcinoembrionic antigen: immuno-histochemical detection of carcinoembrionic antigen determinants in colonic tumors with monoclonal antibodies, *Cancer Res.*, 43, 693, 1983.
13. Edwards, P. A. W., Heterogeneous expression of cell surface antigens in normal epithelia and their tumors revealed by monoclonal antibodies, *Br. J. Cancer*, 51, 149, 1985.
14. Valeriote, F. and Putten, L., Proliferation-dependent cytotoxic action of anti-cancer agents: a review, *Cancer Res.*, 35, 2619, 1975.
15. Paul, B. D., Serrano, J. A., Friedman, A. E., Sarlos, I. J., Sternberger, N. J., Wasserkrug, H. L., and Seligman, A. M., New agents for prostatic cancer activated specifically by prostatic acid phosphatase, *Cancer Treatment Rep.*, 61, 259, 1977.
16. Connors, T. A., Antitumor drugs with latent activities, *Biochimie*, 60, 979, 1978.
17. Mason, D. W. and Williams, A. F., The kinetics of antibody binding to membrane antigens in solution and at the cell surface, *Biochem. J.*, 187, 1, 1980.
18. Bagshawe, K. D., Springer, C. J., Searle, F., Antoniw, P., Sharma, S. K., Melton, R. G., and Sherwood, R. F., A cytotoxic agent can be generated selectively at cancer sites, *Br. J. Cancer*, 58, 700, 1988.
19. Wallace, P. M. and Senter, P. D., *In vitro* and *in vivo* activities of monoclonal antibody-alkaline phosphatase conjugates in combination with phenol mustard phosphate, *Bioconj. Chem.*, 2, 349, 1991.
20. Meyer, D. L., Jungheim, L. N., Mikolajczyk, S. D., Shepherd, T. A., Starling, J. J., and Ahlem, C. N., Preparation and characterization of a β-Lactamase-Fab′ conjugate for the site-specific activation of oncolytic agents, *Bioconj. Chem.*, 3, 42, 1992.
21. Svensson, H. P., Kadow, J. F., Vrudhula, V. M., Wallace, P. M., and Senter, P. D., Monoclonal antibody-β-lactamase conjugates for the activation of a cephalosporin mustard prodrug, *Bioconj. Chem.*, 3, 176, 1992.
22. Roffler, S. R., Wang, S.-M., Chern, J.-W., Yeh, M.-Y., and Tung, E., Anti-neoplastic glucorinide prodrug treatment of human tumor cells targeted with a monoclonal antibody-enzyme conjugate, *Biochem. Pharmacol.*, 42, 2062, 1991.
23. Wang, S.-M., Chern, J.-W., Yeh, M.-Y., Ng, J. C., Tung, E., and Roffler, S. R., Specific activation of glucoronide prodrugs by antibody-targeted enzyme conjugates for cancer therapy, *Cancer Res.*, 52, 4484, 1992.

24. Wels, W., Harwerth, I.-M., Zwickl, M., Hardman, N., Groner, B., and Hynes, N. E., Construction, bacterial expression and characterization of a bifunctional single-chain antibody-phosphatase fusion protein targeted to the human *erb*B-2 receptor, *Bio/Technology*, 10, 1128, 1992.
25. Vrudhula, V. M., Senter, P. D., Fischer, K. J., and Wallace, P. M., Prodrugs of doxorubicin and melphalan and their activation by a monoclonal antibody-penicillin-G amidase conjugate, *J. Med. Chem.*, 36, 919, 1993.
26. Goshorn, S. C., Svensson, H. P., Kerr, D. E., Somerville, J. E., Senter, P. D., and Perry Fell, H., Genetic construction, expression, and characterization of a single-chain anti-carcinoma antibody fused to β-lactamase, *Cancer Res.*, 53, 2123, 1993.
27. Meyer, D. L., Jungheim, L. N., Law, K. L., Mikolajczyk, S. D., Shepherd, T. A., Mackensen, D. G., Briggs, S. L., and Starling, J. J., Site-specific prodrug activation by antibody β-lactamase conjugates: regression and long-term growth inhibition of human colon carcinoma xenograft models, *Cancer Res.*, 53, 3956, 1993.
28. Werlen, R. C., Lankinen, M., Rose, K., Blakey, D., Shuttleworth, H., Melton, R., and Offord, R. E., Site-specific conjugation of an enzyme and antibody fragment, *Bioconj. Chem.*, 5, 411, 1994.
29. Eccles, S. A., Court, W. J., Box, G. A., Dean, C. J., Melton, R. G., and Springer, C. J., Regression of established breast carcinoma xenografts with antibody-directed enzyme prodrug therapy against c-*erb*B2 p185, *Cancer Res.*, 54, 5171, 1994.
30. Mikolajczyk, S. D., Meyer, D. L., Starling, J. J., Law, K. L., Rose, K., Dufour, B., and Offord, R. E., High yield, site-specific coupling on N-terminally modified β-lactamase to a proteolytically derived single-sulfhydryl murine Fab', *Bioconj. Chem.*, 5, 636, 1994.
31. Rodrigues, M. L., Presta, L. G., Kotts, C. E., Wirth, C., Mordenti, J., Osaka, G., Wong, W. L. T., Nuijens, A., Blackburn, B., and Carter, P., Development of a humanized disulfide-stabilized anti-p185^{HER2} Fv-β-lactamase fusion protein for activation of a cephalosporin doxorubicin prodrug, *Cancer Res.*, 55, 63, 1995.
32. Svensson, H. P., Vrudhula, V. M., Emswiler, J. E., MacMaster, J. F., Cosand, W. L., Senter, P. D., and Wallace, P. M., *In vitro* and *in vivo* activities of a doxorubicin prodrug in combination with monoclonal antibody β-lactamase conjugates, *Cancer Res.*, 55, 2357, 1995.
33. Weinstein, J. N., Eger, R. R., Covell, D. G., Black, C. D., Mulshine, J., Carrasquillo, J. A., Larson, S. M., and Keenan, A. M., The pharmacology of monoclonal antibodies, *Ann. N. Y. Acad. Sci.*, 507, 199, 1987.
34. Juweid, M., Newmann, R., Paik, C., Perez-Bacete, M. J., Sato, J., Van Osdol, W., and Weinstein, J. N., Micropharmacology of monoclonal antibodies in solid tumors: direct experimental evidence for a binding site barrier, *Cancer Res.*, 52, 5144, 1992.
35. Brinkmann, U. and Pastan, I., Immunotoxins against cancer, *Biochim. Biophys. Acta*, 1198, 27, 1994.
36. Pastan, I., Pai, L. H., Brinkmann, U., and FitzGerald, D. J., Recombinant toxins: new therapeutic agents for cancer, *Ann. N. Y. Acad. Sci.*, in press.
37. Bosslet, K., Czech, J., Lorenz, P., Sedlacek, H. H., Schermann, M., and Seeman, G., Molecular and functional characterization of a fusion protein suited for tumour specific prodrug activation, *Br. J. Cancer*, 65, 234, 1992.
38. Kohler, G. and Milstein, C., Continuous culture of fused cells secreting antibody of predefined specificity, *Nature* (*London*) 256, 495, 1975.
39. Searle, F., Bier, C., and Buckley, R. G., The potential of carboxypeptidase G2 antibody conjugate as anti-tumour agents. Preparation of anti-human chorionic gonadotropin carboxypeptidase G2 and cytotoxicity of the conjugates against JAR choriocarcinoma cells *in vitro*, *Br. J. Cancer*, 53, 377, 1986.

40. Melton, R. G., Boyle, J. M. B., Rogers, G. T., Burke, P., Bagshawe, K. D., and Sherwood, R. F., Optimization of small scale coupling of A5B7 monoclonal antibody to carboxypeptidase G2, *J. Immunol. Methods*, 158, 49, 1993.
41. Bagshawe, K. D., Sharma, S. K., Springer, C. J., Antoniw, P., Boden, J. A., Rogers, G. T., Burke, P. J., Melton, P. G., and Sherwood, R. F., Antibody-directed enzyme prodrug therapy (ADEPT). Clinical report, *Antibod. Immunoconj. Radiopharm.*, 4, 204, Abstract 0-11, [year].
42. Güssow, D. and Seeman, G., Humanization of monoclonal antibodies, *Methods Enzymol.*, 203, 99, 1991.
43. Oshima, A., Kyle, J. W., Miller, R. D., Hoffman, J. W., Powell, P. P., Grobb, J. H., Sly, W. S., Tropak, M., Guise, K. S., and Gravel, R. A., Cloning, sequencing and expression of cDNA for human β-glucuronidase, *Proc. Natl. Acad. Sci. U.S.A.*, 84, 685, 1987.
44. Harwerth, I.-M., Wels, W., Marte, B., and Hynes, N. E., Monoclonal antibodies against the extracellular domain of the *erb*B-2 receptor function as partial ligand agonists, *J. Biol. Chem.*, 267, 15160, 1992.
45. Huston, J. S., Levinson, D., Mudgett-Hunter, M., Tai, M.-S., Novotny, J., Margolies, M. N., Ridge, R. J., Bruccoleri, R. E., Haber, E., Crea, R., and Oppermann, H., Protein engineering of antibody binding sites: recovery of specific activity in an anti-digoxin single-chain Fv analogue produced in *E. coli*, *Proc. Natl. Acad. Sci. U.S.A.*, 85, 5879, 1988.
46. Goodman, G. E., Hellström, I., Nicaise, C., Brodzinsky, L., Hummel, D., and Hellström, K. E., Phase I clinical trial of murine monoclonal antibody L6 in breast, colon, ovarian, and lung cancer, *J. Clin. Oncol.*, 8, 1083, 1990.
47. Denardo, S. J., O'Grady, L. F., Macey, D. J., Kroger, L. A., Denardo, G. L., Lambon, K. R., Levy, N. B., Mills, S. L., Hellström, I., and Hellström, K. E., Quantitative imaging of mouse L6 monoclonal antibody in breast cancer patients to develop a therapeutic strategy, *Nuclear Med. Biol.*, 18, 621, 1991.
48. Denardo, S. J., Warhoe, K. A., O'Grady, L. F., Hellström, I., Hellström, K. E., Mills, S. L., Macey, D. J., Goodnight, J. E., and Denardo, G. L., Radioimmunotherapy for breast cancer: treatment of a patient with I-131 L6 chimeric monoclonal antibody, *Int. J. Biol. Markers*, 6, 221, 1991.
49. Skerra, A. and Plückthun, A., Assembly of a functional immunoglobulin Fv fragment in *Escherichia* coli, *Science*, 240, 1038, 1988.
50. Shalabi, M. R., Shepard, H. M., Presta, L., Rodrigues, M. L., Beverley, P. C. L., Feldmann, M., and Carter, P., Development of humanized bispecific antibodies reactive with cytotoxic lymphocytes and tumor cells overexpressing the *HER*2 protooncogene, *J. Exp. Med.*, 175, 217, 1992.
51. Rodrigues, M. L., Shalabi, M. R., Werther, W., Presta, L., and Carter, P., Engineering of a humanized bispecific $F(ab')_2$ fragment for improved binding to T cells, *Int. J. Cancer*, 7, 45, 1992.
52. Park, J. W., Hong, K., Carter, P., Asgari, H., Guo, L. Y., Shalabi, M. R., Wirth, C., Kotts, C., Keller, G. A., Wood, W. I., Papahajopoulos, D., and Benz, C. C., Development of anti-$p185^{HER2}$ immunoliposomes for cancer therapy, *Proc. Natl. Acad. Sci. U.S.A.*, 92, 1327, 1995.
53. Glockshuber, F., Malia, M., Pfityzinger, I., and Plückthun, A., A comparison of strategies to stabilize immunoglobulin Fv-fragments, *Biochemistry*, 29, 1362, 1990.
54. Brinkmann, U., Reiter, Y., Jung, S.-H., Lee, B. K., and Pastan, I., A recombinant immunotoxin containing a disulfide-stabilized Fv fragment, *Proc. Natl. Acad. Sci. U.S.A.*, 90, 7538, 1993.
55. Reiter, Y., Brinkmann, U., Webber, K. O., Jung, S.-H., and Pastan, I., Engineering interchain disulfide bonds into conserved framework regions of Fv fragments: improved biochemical characteristics of recombinant immunotoxins containing disulfide-linked Fv, *Prot. Eng.*, 33, 5451, 1994.

56. Marshall, D., Pedley, R. B., Melton, R. G., Boden, J. A., Boden, R., and Begent, R. H. J., Galactosylated streptavidin for improved clearance of biotinylated intact and $F(ab')_2$ fragments of an anti-tumour antibody, *Br. J. Cancer*, 71, 18, 1995.

56a. Kerr, D. E., Schreiber, G. J., Vrudhula, V. M., Svensson, H. P., Hellström, I., Hellström, K. E., and Senter, P. D., Regressions and cures of melanoma xenografts following treatment with monoclonal antibody β-lactamase conjugates in combination with anticancer prodrugs, *Cancer Res.*, 55, 3558, 1995.

57. Meyer, D. L., Jungheim, L. N., Law, K. L., Mikolajczyk, S. D., Shepherd, T. A., Mackensen, D. G., Briggs, S. L., and Starling, J. J., Site-specific prodrug activation by antibody β-lactamase conjugates: regression and long-term growth inhibition of human colon carcinoma xenograft models, *Cancer Res.*, 53, 3956, 1993.

58. Meyer, D. L., Law, K. L., Payne, J. K., Mikolajczyk, S. D., Zarrinmayeh, H., Jungheim, L. N., King, J. K., Shepherd, T. A., and Starling, J. J., Site-specific prodrug activation by antibody β-lactamase conjugates: preclinical investigation of the efficacy and toxicity of doxorubicin delivery by antibody directed catalysis, *Bioconj. Chem.*, 5, 440, 1995.

59. Sherma, S. K., Bagshawe, K. D., Melton, R. G., and Sherwood, R. F., Human immune response to monoclonal antibody-enzyme conjugates in ADEPT pilot clinical trial, *Cell Biophys.*, 21/22, 109, 1993.

60. Svensson, H. P., Wallace, P. M., and Senter, P. D., Synthesis and characterization of monoclonal antibody β-lactamase conjugates, *Bioconj. Chem.*, 5, 262, 1994.

61. Vrudhula, V. M., Svensson, H. P., Kennedy, K. A., Senter, P. D., and Wallace, P. M., Antitumor activity of a cephalosporin prodrug in combination with monoclonal antibody-β-lactamase conjugates, *Bioconj. Chem.*, 4, 334, 1993.

Part II

Application of Antibody Therapeutics

Chapter 5

THERAPEUTIC ANTIBODIES IN INFECTIOUS DISEASE

William J. Harris

CONTENTS

0-8493-8547-4/97/$0.00+$.50

5.1 INTRODUCTION

Treatment of infectious disease was the very first target of antibody-based therapies when Behring and Kitasato[1] in 1890 described the presence of anti-toxins in animals immunized with sublethal doses of diphtheria and tetanus toxoid and demonstrated that these anti-toxins could be transferred from one animal to another through serum. Treatment of children with anti-diphtheria sheep sera began in 1893. Before the advent of serum therapy over half of all children died of diphtheria, but this figure had dropped to 24% after 6 months of use of this antisera. The clinical value of serotherapy has therefore been established for over 100 years.[2] However, difficulties were encountered with these pioneering studies in standardizing antisera and it was found that repeated injection of foreign serum sometimes caused serum sickness and anaphylactic reactions. The latter was reduced by active immunization with a mixture of diphtheria toxin and antisera and then the discovery that formalin-treated diphtheria toxin could effect immunization without causing disease provided the universal immunization procedures used today. Anti-tetanus serotherapy was introduced more gradually but was a major lifesaving treatment in the Great War.

The risk of serum sickness was finally overcome with the introduction of human immunoglobulin preparations in 1944 (standard immunoglobulin) and then hyperimmunoglobulins possessing particularly high antibody levels against bacteria or viral components were introduced in the

1970s.[3] Intravenous administration of immunoglobulin can have severe side effects due to Fc-mediated activation of complement though this can be eliminated by a variety of enzymic or chemical treatments.[2] However, the level of any specific anti-infective antibody in polyclonal preparations is low and the efficacy of treatment is limited by the amount of immune globulin that can be delivered. Monoclonal antibodies (MAbs) therefore represent a major advance in the levels of active antibody that can be delivered, and the ability to select MAbs of high neutralizing ability has provided a new era in serotherapy against infectious disease.

5.2 IMMUNE RESPONSES TO INFECTION

5.2.1 Bacteria

Defenses against bacterial infection are related to the structure of the invading microorganism and its pathogenic profile which also determines the relative importance of antibody-mediated protection and cure. Most bacteria cause general toxic effects through the release of toxins and specific tissue damage through invasiveness. In cases where toxin damage predominates, exemplified by *Vibrio cholerae*, *Corynebacterium diphtheriae*, *Streptococcus pyogenes*, and *Bordetella pertussis*, antibody-mediated neutralization of toxins is often sufficient for therapy as underlined by the early success of serotherapy and vaccination against these diseases.

There are a number of general defense mechanisms against invasion by bacteria which are often responsible for reducing the rate of early multiplication in the host. A main defense is with defensins, cationic oligopeptides concentrated within phagocytic vacuoles and secreted into body fluids and epithelial surfaces. They act by increasing membrane permeability to bacteria and enveloped viruses. Other defenses recognize bacterial components and affect their removal independent of the B- and T-cell immune system and thus provide the first line of defense against invasiveness. These act by activation of the alternate complement lysis pathway, activation of macrophages, triggering of cytokine release, and mast cell degranulation.[4]

5.2.1.1 Mode of Action of Antibodies

Antibody plays a major role in the next line of defense through interference with a number of events during bacterial infection.[5] Antibody therapy could be targeted to block any of these events though the different bacterial infection processes usually define the most susceptible event for any particular bacteria. The major sites of action can be summarized as follows:

1. Antibodies which bind to fimbriae or bacterial surface components can block their attachment to host cells or tissues, and by binding directly to bacterial surfaces, they effectively target complement-mediated killing and enhance phagocytosis via Fc and C3 receptors.
2. Many organisms evade complement-mediated destruction by adsorbing serum complement factors such as C3b with lipopolysaccharides present either as capsules distal from the susceptible bacterial membrane or secreted into the serum. Antibodies can be generated to block C3b binding to these factors.
3. Tissue invasion by bacteria is frequently mediated by their secretion of destructive enzymes such as proteases and hyaluronidase. Neutralization by antibody can delay tissue penetration allowing more time for phagocytic killing of bacteria.

While such humoral responses represent major defense mechanisms for the majority of bacteria, a minority rely more upon T-cell-mediated responses and are less obviously susceptible to antibody-based therapy approaches. These include *Legionella pneumophila*, *Chlamydia*, and *Mycobacteria*.

5.2.2 Viruses

The first line of defense against viral infection is production of interferon-α and -β (IFN-α, IFN-β) which act to reduce the permissiveness of non-infected cells and inhibit viral replication in cells which are already infected.

The immune response is a complex of interactions of B and T lymphocytes resulting in the generation of antiviral antibody by B cells and virus-specific delayed type hypersensitivity (DTH) and cytotoxic responses by T lymphocytes.[6] Specific B-cell-mediated antibody production in response to viral infection was the first effector function mechanism of antiviral immunity to be recognized, and for many years it was considered that antibody-mediated defense mechanisms (humoral immunity) were the major and only source of viral immunity after natural infection or vaccination. Antiviral antibodies can reduce virus spread by (1) preventing viral attachment to the cell surface by blocking cellular receptors, (2) aggregate viral particles, (3) inhibiting viral internalization, (4) inhibiting virus uncoating, (5) enhancing viral removal by increasing uptake into phagocytes through Fc receptors on phagocytes, and (6) enhancing virolysis or cytolysis of infected cells by complement or antibody-dependent cellular cytotoxicity (ADCC).

Cell-mediated immunity through T-cell activation is also critical for defense against many viral infections and in some cases is the major defense mechanism. The relative roles of humoral and cell-mediated immunity then depend on viral pathology and life cycle. For some virus families such as picorna- and myxoviruses antibody production is a critical factor while cell-mediated responses predominate with some herpesvirus or retrovirus infections. It is therefore important to define the potential and limitations of humoral defense mechanisms for any particular virus family in selecting those which offer opportunities for antibody therapy. Further, specific antibodies can be of little relevance in recovery from a primary infection but can be very important in preventing re-infections or reactivation.

There are a number of factors which can be considered strong evidence for antibody-mediated therapy. These include data showing that passive transfer of specific antibody from mother to newborn provides protection to small infants, as has been demonstrated for influenza A[7] and respiratory syncytial virus (RSV).[8] Patients with constitutional hypogammaglobulinemia show increased susceptibility to picornavirus, including polio[9] and echoviruses, but are not exceptionally sensitive to herpes simplex, measles, or vaccinia infections.[6] In some case the combination of IFN-α and antibody to clear virus released from cells may be sufficient to control infection.

5.2.2.1 T-Cell-Mediated Immunity

T lymphocytes play a major role in defense against many viruses both as helper cells in permitting the optimal production of antibody by B lymphocytes and/or directly as effector cells permitting clearance of intracellular viruses. Two classes of T cells can be distinguished: the CD8+ cytotoxic T lymphocyte (Tc) and CD4+ T lymphocyte (helper Th2 or inflammatory Th1). Tc cells kill virally infected cells by programming them for apoptosis through the release of cytotoxins such as perforin and proteases.[10] CD4+ Th2 provides IL-4 and IL-5 accessory factors in the activation of B cells and CD4+ Th1 secrete IL-2, TNF-β and IFN-γ to mediate the recruitment of inflammatory macrophages into the lesion.[11] In many cases viral epitopes which are recognized by T cells to stimulate specific B-cell populations differ from those recognized by protective antibodies and this accounts for the often low titer of neutralizing antibodies to total antiviral response in immune polyclonal sera. This may also contribute to the failure of vaccines of recombinant viral proteins or peptides selected on the bases that they are epitopes to neutralizing antibodies.

CD8+ cytotoxic T lymphocytes (CTLs) recognize virally derived peptides displayed on the surface of infected cells in association with major histocompatibility complex (MHC) class I molecules and cause direct cell lysis. A striking feature of CTLs is that as with T helper cells, they recognize predominantly viral epitopes from internal often nonstructural viral proteins. It is common for CTLs to recognize proteins synthesized early in infection, thus permitting T-cell-mediated inhibition of virus growth at an early stage. In this way then CTL responses complement antibody mediated responses which are principally aimed at structural proteins to clean up virus particles released into the extracellular milieu.

5.2.2.2 Mode of Action of Antibodies

There is usually a good correlation between the ability of monoclonal or polyclonal antibodies to neutralize a virus *in vitro* and *in vivo* efficacy and rodent MAb technology has allowed the delineation of critical neutralizing epitopes on many viruses. Immunization of rodents with viruses can elicit neutralizing antibodies against epitopes which are not immunodominant or prevalent during natural human infection and such antibodies can offer good prospects for therapy even with some viral families where humoral immunity is not normally a major defense. However, *in vivo* additional epitopes may provide more effective targets for therapy. Transfer of MAbs to nonstructural proteins of yellow fever virus are protective *in vivo*, apparently through a mechanism of recognition of the infected cell and not virus particles.[12] Such antibodies are likely to destroy infected cells in collaboration with killer cells in an ADCC manner.

5.3 IMMUNE GLOBULINS

Table 1 lists the major human immune globulin preparations currently available.[13]

5.3.1 Intravenous Immune Globulin

Intravenous immune globulin (IVIG) is a preparation of human immune globulins pooled from at least 1000 donors and contains antibodies to several diseases including hepatitis A, hepatitis B, and measles. It aims to provide a broad spectrum of opsonic and neutralizing IgG antibodies for the prevention or attenuation of a wide variety of infections.[14] A primary use of IVIG is in the treatment of primary humoral immunodeficiency states such as congenital agammaglobulinemias, common variable immunodeficiency, Wiskott-Aldrich syndrome,

TABLE 1

Anti-Infective Human Immunoglobulins

Anti-Infective Human Immunoglobulins
Standard Immune Globulin (SSG)
Intravenous Immune Globulin (IVIG)
Hyperimmune IVIG:
Aids
Clostridium perfringens toxin
Cytomegalovirus
Diphtheria
Hepatitis A
Hepatitis B
Measles
Mumps
Polio
Pertussis
Rabies
Respiratory syncytial virus
Rubella
Tetanus
Vaccinia

X-linked immunodeficiency, and severe combined immunodeficiency. The effectiveness for this indication is implied since children receiving regular and adequate injections can enjoy relative freedom from a variety of common viral infections. Intramuscular formulations are effective in preventing hepatitis A when administered within 14 days of exposure and larger doses will provide protection to travelers for up to 8 weeks. IVIG also prevents or modifies measles if administered within 6 days of exposure and is particularly suitable for passive immunization of immunosuppressed cancer patients who come into contact with measles.

5.3.2 Hepatitis Immune Globulin

Hepatitis immune globulin (HBIG) is prepared from plasma prescreened for high titers of hepatitis B surface antigen (HbsAg), generally at titers greater than 1:100,000. It is recommended for use in post-exposure for individuals who have been exposed by infected sexual partners or to blood containing HbsAg, and for infants born to HbsAg-positive women.[15] In one study, it prevented disease in 75% of people with needle stick exposure[16] and prevented maternofetal transfer in 85–95% of mothers.[17] The combined use of HBIG and vaccine has been reported to be useful for post-exposure prophylaxis by avoiding the lag of several months that occurs in 10–45% of vaccine recipients before antibody can be detected.[18]

5.3.3 Tetanus Immune Globulin

This hyperimmune globulin is indicated for management of tetanus-prone wounds in individuals with no history of tetanus immunization. It is usually given simultaneously with combined tetanus-diphtheria toxoid vaccine.[19]

5.3.4 Rabies Immune Globulin

Rabies immune globulin (RIG) is a hyperimmune sera prepared from volunteers who have been immunized against rabies with standard vaccine and is designed for management of individuals who have been exposed to rabid animals. RIG is given in conjunction with the vaccine and data suggests the combination to be 100% successful.[20]

5.3.5 Varicella-Zoster Immune Globulin

Varicella-zoster immune globulin (ZIG) is prepared by selecting high titer sera from volunteers and is used for susceptible immunocompromised individuals and others recently exposed to varicella zoster. It is given to babies who have no maternal antibody, to newborns whose mothers develop chickenpox within 5 days of birth, and all premature babies of less than 28 weeks gestation. If administered within 96 h of exposure, ZIG modifies the severity of chickenpox but does not prevent infection. Due to very limited supplies and expense its use has been limited to life-threatening situations. ZIG is recommended for seronegative recipients of transplants.[21]

5.3.6 Cytomegalovirus Immune Globulin

IVIG has been widely used over the last 10 years for the prevention and treatment of cytomegalovirus (CMV) infection in solid organ and bone marrow transplants[21] with varying reports of efficacy. More recently, the combination of ganciclovir and IVIG has been used to treat diagnosed CMV interstitial pneumonia and data showed significantly improved short-term survival when compared to historical controls; however, long-term survival may be compromised.[22] It is likely that the level of effective anti-CMV titer in IVIG preparations varies considerably in different preparations[23-24] and this is likely a factor in some of the poorer clinical results.

More convincing data of efficacy has been obtained using hyperimmune anti-CMV antisera in liver transplant patients,[25] bone marrow,[26-27] and such hyperimmune IVIG (CytoGam:Cytotect), which must contain at least fivefold higher levels of reactive antibody, and has been formally approved in many countries for management of CMV infections in renal transplant patients.

5.3.7 RSV Immune Globulin

Several studies using IVIG to treat infants and young children hospitalized with RSV disease have been carried out.[28-30] Reductions in nasal virus titer and improved oxygenation were noted with those trials using IVIG with a significant anti-RSV neutralizing titer, but mean duration of hospitalization was not reduced.

Due to the unreliability and difficulty of obtaining IVIG with acceptable anti-RSV neutralizing titers, a hyperimmune anti-RSV IVIG has recently been specifically developed and a reduction in rates of RSV infections and hospitalization has been described in a 3-year trial of high risk infants and children.[31] An application for an Investigational New Drug License was recently approved by the U.S. Food and Drug Administration (FDA).

5.3.8 Human Immunodeficiency Virus (HIV) Immune Globulin

Hyperimmune sera derived from donors who are HIV positive but clinically healthy have been evaluated in phase I/II studies with inconclusive results.[32-34] In one study[35] of 21 patients who received a high dose of antisera only one died during the treatment period (5%) compared to 6 out of 30 deaths (20%) in controls. In a more extensive phase II study, 86 patients showed a significant reduction in CD4 counts and AIDS-defining clinical events. While the control group had a mean of 1.25 AIDS-defining events per patient, the treatment group had 0.43 events per patient.[36] However, HIV-infected individuals can possess antibodies which enhance viral infection either via complement or Fc receptors (reviewed in Reference 37) and this concern may limit future treatments using polyclonal antisera.

5.3.9 Gram-Negative Bacteria Immune Globulin

Nearly 3000 cases of sepsis occur annually in the U.S. with approximately 40% of patients developing shock. The lethal component of Gram-negative bacteria is the lipopolysaccharide (LPS) of the bacterial cell surface. Since the lipid A portion (core) of LPS is highly conserved across bacterial species, much effort has been expended in identifying common conserved immunogenic epitopes (for review see Reference 38). Several clinical studies have been carried out with immune sera derived from volunteers vaccinated with *E. coli* J5 with equivocal results.[38-41]

TABLE 2

Human and Humanized MAbs Against Viral Targets

Cytomegalovirus
Rabies
Rubella
Hepatitis A
Hepatitis B
Influenza
Herpes simplex
Measles (SSPE)
Varicella zoster
Epstein-Barr virus
Human T-cell leukemia virus
HIV
Respiratory syncytial virus
Junin virus
Vaccinia

Adapted from Harris, W. J. and Cunningham, C. C., *Antibody Therapeutics,* Springer/R. G. Landes Co., Austin, 1995; Larrick, J.W., *Immunotherapy and Vaccines,* Cryz, S. J., Ed., VCH Weinheim, 1991, 129; and Emery, S. C. and Adair, J. R., *Exp. Opin. Invest. Drugs,* 3, 241, 1994.

5.4 MAb-BASED THERAPIES

5.4.1 Antiviral Antibodies

A list of human and humanized MAbs with potential therapeutic applications is described in Table 2.[13,42] A number of these have only limited commercial interest at present and are therefore not discussed further.

5.4.1.1 Hepatitis B

Hepatitis due to hepatitis B (HBV) is one of the world's major illnesses with an estimated 300 million carriers of whom 25–30% will die from HBV-induced cirrhosis or hepatocellular carcinoma. The high frequency of carriers is due to the propensity of the virus to cause persistent infection of the liver and shed high concentrations of viral antigen consisting of complete and incomplete viral particles into the blood continuously for many years. HBV is not itself cytopathic and the resulting liver damage is due to viral antigens on the surface of the infected hepatocyte being targeted by cytotoxic T cells.

The chronic carrier state can arise through several routes. Of babies born to HBV "e" antigen-positive mothers 90% become infected and over 90% of these will develop a carrier state.[43] This very high frequency of development of the chronic state probably arises through the children receiving a large inoculum of virus from maternal blood before or during birth at a time when their immune system is still underdeveloped. In contrast only 10% of adults develop the chronic state following primary infection. Acute self-limiting infections extend over 10–20 weeks and are accompanied by continual release of HBV antigens, s, e, or c, into the blood. This is usually accompanied by the appearance of antibodies to s, e, and c which decline on recovery. The presence of anti-HBs in the serum of convalescents, particularly of anti-a specificity, usually confers almost complete resistance to re-infection.[44] Patients who remain HBsAg positive for 20 weeks or more are likely to become chronic carriers who still retain levels of anti-HBc and anti-HBe titers.

There are no antivirals that are effective against hepatitis B infection making the disease a prime candidate for antibody-based therapy. Further, the success achieved in preventing disease with hepatitis immune globulin[16-17] provides great encouragement that a MAb-based product will be therapeutically effective.

Antibodies directed against the "a" determinant of HB surface antigen are potentially suitable for therapy, and with the ready availability of sources of primed peripheral blood lymphocytes from vaccinees, several groups have successfully isolated human-mouse heterohybridomas and human-human hybridomas.[45-46] Ostberg[46] isolated a trioma (OST 577) by fusing peripheral blood lymphocytes from a volunteer vaccinated with HBV vaccine. This has been evaluated in two clinical settings:[47]

1. Chronic active hepatitis B. Twelve patients received 7–8 doses over 35 to 37 day periods and reductions of the order of 50% were noted for serum levels of liver enzymes, HBsAg, and viral DNA. Minimal side effects were noted.
2. Liver transplant in hepatitis B patients. Five patients received a total of 70–90 mg of OST 577 just before, during, and after liver transplantation and maintenance doses of 10 mg were given for up to 23 months. While one patient died of causes unrelated to hepatitis, 2 of 4 of the remaining were free of any evidence of HB infection 3 years later. The remaining 2 patients seroconverted 250 days after transplantation but had no clinical signs of infection after 3 years.

These data are very encouraging since one would expect 100% of control patients to be re-infected under these conditions.

5.4.1.2 Cytomegalovirus

Cytomegalovirus is a member of the herpes group of viruses whose name is derived from its cytopathic effect expressed as formation of giant cells with typical intranuclear and cytoplasmic inclusions resembling owls eyes. Primary CMV infection occurs in 60–70% of the population throughout the world with in most cases, little clinical effect. The virus then remains latent in tissues and can be reactivated later in life. In the immunocompromised or immunosuppressed individual, however, both primary infection and reactivation can cause serious diseases including CMV pneumonia, enteritis, retinitis, viremia, hepatitis, and leukopenia. CMV infection is therefore a significant problem in newborns, elderly, transplant patients, cancer patients receiving chemotherapy, and individuals infected with the HIV virus.[48] Approximately 70% of transplant patients will endure a period of active infection with about 40% experiencing serious and life-threatening illness. At least 25% of AIDS patients will suffer from CMV-induced retinitis.

Prior to 1983, there were no antivirals effective against CMV infections. Currently, the antivirals acyclovir, ganciclovir, and foscarnet which are broadly active against herpesviruses are available, but none of these are particularly potent against CMV and all have undesirable or toxic side effects which make them especially unattractive therapeutic candidates for the immunosuppressed. Also, there is increasing concern at the spread of drug-resistant mutants. On the other hand, the promising results reported with IVIG or CMV immune globulin offers support for the provision of a MAb-based therapy.[22-24] Data that supports the likely efficacy of an antibody-based product arises from extensive studies of the risks of virus transmission from mother to fetus, which show that congenital CMV infection is more likely to be symptomatic if the mother has a primary infection during pregnancy rather than a recurrent infection when the mother carries pre-existing antibodies to CMV which can be transferred transplacentally.[49]

The envelope proteins of CMV, gB(gCI), gCII, and gH/gL(gCIII) are the main targets for human humoral immune responses. While most CMV seropositive individuals have detectable antibody to gB, only 5–10% carry anti-gH antibodies. Neutralizing antibody response against gB is particularly high in some individuals[50] with multiple epitopes upon gB being involved in virus neutralization and inhibition of cell-to-cell spread.[51] By contrast, only a single epitope upon gH seems to be associated with neutralization. The latter epitope on gH is highly conserved among CMV strains while the epitopes of gB show a significant level of heterogeneity between strains.[52-55] Also, there is evidence that gH plays an important role in acute infection and the absence of antibodies to gH relates to symptomatic infection.[56] Neutralizing antibodies against gH therefore offers the most promising basis for a therapeutic reactive against all clinical strains of CMV.

5.4.1.2.1 *Anti-gH MAbs*

A neutralizing MAb, MuHCMV16, was produced by immunization of mice with purified hCMV strain AD169 and shown to bind to gH.[57] This antibody has been humanized (HuHCMV 16) and shown to bind to 13 different clinical strains confirming the gH epitope to be well conserved. The humanized antibody also retains the ability to effectively neutralize laboratory and clinical isolates of CMV *in vitro*.[58] This antibody has been expressed in a high-yielding mammalian cell line and is expected to enter clinical trials shortly. An additional humanized antibody, CMV-5, has been described.[59]

MSL 109 (formerly SDZ89-109) is a human anti-gH IgG1/κ MAb derived from a mouse-human heterotrioma with an ED_{50} of the order of 0.5 μg/ml for clinical isolates of CMV.[47] Preclinical studies with nonhuman primates showed the antibody to be essentially free of toxicity up to 16 mg/kg and doses of 0.5 mg/kg for up to 1 year did not induce any immune responses.[60] Clinical studies have been carried out for two applications:

1. Two phase I clinical trials in bone marrow transplant patients have shown the antibody to be free of toxicity and devoid of HAMA responses. The highest dosing regimes were 0.5 mg/kg every 3 weeks for up to 6 months, and 2 mg/kg every 2 weeks for 12 weeks.[61-62] Serum half-lives up to 17 days were recorded.
2. Two phase I/II trials have been carried out in AIDS patients. Safety and tolerance was established in a study of up to 10 mg/kg every 2 weeks for up to 24 weeks in CMV seropositive patients with viruria.[47] In the second trial MSL 109 was given concurrently with ganciclovir or foscarnet to AIDS patients with documented CMV retinitis. The median time of progression to retinitis was 202 days in patients given MSL 109 and antiviral compared with an estimate of 100 days with patients receiving antiviral alone. The latter was calculated from historical data.[59]

5.4.1.2.2 *Anti-gB MAbs*

A human MAb (C23) derived from a mouse-human heterohybridoma has been evaluated in a phase I clinical trial in healthy volunteers at doses up to 80 mg/head. Half-life was of the order of 22–26 days and no immune responses were observed.[63] Neutralizing anti-gB MAb SDZ89-104, derived from a mouse-human heterotrioma, was tested in 5 patients undergoing bone marrow transplantation with no deleterious effects.[61] Murine MAb HCMV 37 which recognizes a range of clinical isolates[57,64] has been humanized.[65]

5.4.1.3 *Varicella-Zoster Virus*

Varicella-zoster virus (VZV) is the herpesvirus responsible for chickenpox and shingles. After the primary infection (chickenpox) VZV lies dormant in a dorsal root ganglion and when reactivated migrates along the sensory nerves to the skin, giving rise to the rash of zoster (shingles). Chickenpox is a common disease predominantly of children with the rate of serious complications after infection being low in the normal individual. However, primary infection in the adult or immunocompromised can be a rapidly fatal infection with pneumonia, pancreatitis, hepatitis, and encephalitis.[66] Reactivation giving rise to zoster is equally serious in the immunocompromised and, with the decline in their immune system, in the elderly.

Three approaches are used to treat VZV infections. Oral and intravenous acyclovir are effective in reducing the severity of VZV infections and reduces the risk of visceral dissemination and duration of shedding in the immunocompromised.[67] A vaccine consisting of an attenuated (OKA) strain of VZV has been available in Japan and Europe for many years and has been approved recently in the U.S. Widespread use of the vaccine for normal children has not generally been practiced due to the low incidence of serious complications in this patient group and the length of protection provided by the vaccine (7–10 years) is less than that acquired from natural infection. Finally, passive immunotherapy with ZIG within 4 days of acute exposure has been shown to prevent or reduce the severity of disease in immunocompromised patients.[68]

In view of the inappropriateness of vaccination and the undesirable side effects of high doses of antivirals[69] in a number of clinical settings and the observed efficacious effects of ZIG, anti-VZV MAbs may have a role in preventing and/or treating VZV infection, either alone or in combination with antiviral agents.

The human immune response to VZV infection predominates against virally encoded glycoproteins which localize on the surface of infected cells. The three major glycoproteins are designated gpI, gpII, and gpIII. Murine and human MAbs which neutralize VZV *in vitro* have been identified against all of these antigens.[70-73] It has been found that anti-gpIII, in contrast to anti-gpI and anti-gpII MAbs, not only neutralize virus without complement but also inhibit the spread of virus from cell to cell. Anti-gpIII MAbs are therefore the antibodies of choice as therapeutics. gpIII is the homologue of herpes simplex virus and cytomegalovirus glycoproteins gH emphasizing the similarities in biology of these viruses. Anti-gpIII murine MAb 206 has very potent activity with respect to complement-independent neutralization of VZV infection *in vitro*,[74] blocks the entry and egress of virus, and prevents syncytial formation *in vitro*.[75] This antibody has been humanized[76] in preparation for clinical trials.

Human MAb V3 is derived from a mouse-human heterohybridoma cell line prepared after *in vitro* immunization of human lymphocytes. It is reactive against gpIII and has a neutralization titer *in vitro* 15,000-fold greater than normal human serum gammaglobulin (NHSG).[77]

5.4.1.4 Herpes Simplex Virus

Acute infections by herpes simplex virus (HSV) principally involves skin, mucous membranes, and corneal epithelium in the case of HSV-1 and the skin of the genital area and vaginal mucous membranes in the case of HSV-2. After the initial infectious cycle, the virus migrates along nerve axons to associated somas in the sensory ganglia where it either continues to replicate with neuronal destruction or establishes latent infection with neuronal survival. In the latter case, the viral genome can be repeatedly reactivated later in life with transfer of viral genomes from axon to epithelium where lesions develop.[78] A number of neutralizing murine MAbs have been described, one of which has been humanized.[79-80]

5.4.1.5 Human Immunodeficiency Virus

The biology and pathology of HIV has been one of the most studied topics in research in recent years (reviewed in Reference 81). Targets for neutralizing MAbs have been identified in the V3 loop, V2, CD4-binding domain, and C terminal regions of the envelope gp120, and the C terminal region of gp41.[81] AIDS patients do not generally carry high levels of neutralizing antibodies against their homologous strain though some do show high levels of antiviral activity against laboratory strains of HIV. Also, neutralizing antibodies appear to be replaced by enhancing antibodies as the disease progresses. These observations emphasize that care needs to be taken in the use of hyperimmune human polyclonal sera and candidate therapeutic MAbs need to be screened against clinical isolates of the virus. Neutralizing murine MAbs against gp120 were evaluated in eleven late-stage AIDS patients who received 125 mg twice monthly for 3 months.[82] The MAbs had a short serum half-life of 30 h. Five out of eleven patients showed a decrease in serum p24 antigen and 3 out of 11 developed a HAMA response. Fourteen murine MAbs with promising *in vitro* neutralization activity have been compared in the WHO-NIAID sponsored Antibody Serological Project whereby samples of all MAbs were sent to a variety of laboratories for confirmatory *in vitro* neutralization studies and ranking with respect to potency.[83] The most potent are prime therapeutic candidates though whether they should be taken to clinical trial as murine antibodies is debatable. AIDS-439 is an IgG1 mouse human chimeric antibody with specificity for the V3 region of gp120 which neutralizes both 111B and NM laboratory strains of HIV.[84] A phase I/IIa study was carried out in 12 advanced AIDS patients who received 20 mg of antibody every 3 weeks for up to 6 months. Three out of eight patients showed a clear decrease in viral load as measured by p24 antigen levels and polymerase chain reaction (PCR) detection of viral RNA. A broadly neutralizing antibody murine NM-01 which recognizes a relatively well-conserved peptide in the V3 loop has been described.[85] This antibody has been humanized and showed fourfold increased *in vitro* neutralization potency.[86] This is expected to enter clinical trial shortly. Heterohybridomas expressing human antibodies against the V3 loop and CD4 binding domains of gp120 with *in vitro* viral neutralizing activity have been described.[87]

5.4.1.6 Rabies

Rabies is a significant disease throughout the world. About 500,000 receive anti-rabies treatment and 40,000–50,000 people are reported to die of rabies each year in India.[88-89] Standard treatment is vaccination along with anti-rabies hyperimmune sera and there is evidence that anti-rabies antibodies are an important aspect to therapy. Hyperimmune anti-rabies sera is in limited supply and expensive. A number of groups have isolated murine MAbs against rabies antigens and shown them to neutralize rabies virus both *in vitro* and *in vivo*.[90-91] In particular, MAbs recognizing neutralizing epitopes upon the rabies virus G protein have successfully protected and treated mice against lethal doses of virus.[91]

5.4.1.7 RSV

RSV is the major cause of acute respiratory illness in young children admitted to hospitals, and general practice will treat at least five times the number admitted to hospitals. The virus causes annual epidemics of bronchiolitis and pneumonia in children throughout the world. Efforts to produce an effective vaccine have been unsuccessful and the only antiviral drug, ribavirin (Virazole, ICN) is restricted to use in high-risk or severely ill infants. A humanized antibody RSHZ19 has been developed and shown efficacy in mice, rats, and cynomolgous monkeys and in phase I human clinical trial was well tolerated with no human anti-mouse response and had an extended half-life equivalent to human immunoglobulin. This humanized MAb is well advanced in clinical trials and is discussed in detail later in Chapter 13.

TABLE 3
Human and Humanized MAbs Against Bacterial Targets

Tetanus toxoid
Diphtheria toxoid
Clostridium perfringens toxin
Gram-negative endotoxins
Pseudomonas aeruginosa
Lipolysaccharides
Exotoxin A
Outer membrane protein
Haemophilus influenzae
Mycobacterium leprae
Neisseria meningitidis
Pneumococcus

Adapted from Harris, W. J. and Cunningham, C. C., *Antibody Therapeutics*, Springer/R. G. Landes Co., Austin, 1995; Larrick, J.W., *Immunotherapy and Vaccines*, Cryz, S. J., Ed., VCH Weinheim, 1991, 129; and Emery, S. C. and Adair, J. R., *Exp. Opin. Invest. Drugs*, 3, 241, 1994.

5.4.2 Antibacterial Therapeutic Antibodies

Human MAbs against a number of bacterial antigens are summarized in Table 3. Anti-tetanus and anti-diphtheria toxoid neutralizing antibodies are unlikely to be of commercial value due to universal vaccination procedures and antibiotics are likely to remain the therapeutics of choice for many bacterial infections. However, antibody-based treatments may be important with the increasing spread of multiple drug resistance and the undesirability of widespread prophylactic use of antibiotics.

5.4.2.1 Gram-Negative Bacterial Infections

The majority of nosocomial Gram-negative bacillary infections are caused by *Escherichia coli*, *Klebsiella* species, and *Pseudomonas aeruginosa* against which broad-spectrum antibiotics are the major treatment. However, their effectiveness is compromised by innate and acquired antibiotic resistance. Immunological therapy has therefore been evaluated in combination with antibiotics using antibodies directed against either the LPS of *E. coli* and *Ps. aeruginosa* or the capsular polysaccharide (CPS) of *Klebsiella*. A number of human and murine MAbs against these components have been described (reviewed in Reference 38). Several clinical trials have provided evidence for a protective effect of sero-specific anti-*Ps. aeruginosa* LPS[92] sera and anti-*E. coli* core glycolipid (anti-J5) antibodies have successfully inhibited shock in septic patients.[93-94]

MAb therapy would seem on first consideration to present a formidable task since there are innumerable serotypes of *E. coli, Klebsiella, and Ps. aeruginosa*. Even bacteremic isolates include 24 capsular types of *Klebsiella*, 9 serotypes of *Ps. aeruginosa*, and 12 serotypes of *E. coli*.[95] A number of murine and human MAbs that recognize conserved groups in the core-lipid A region of *E. coli* have been described and tested *in vivo* in animals, but protection was either absent or detectable only after very large dosing.[95-99] In contrast serotype-specific antibodies are protective at low doses[95,100-102] against their parent. Therapy based upon cocktails would therefore seem an effective strategy; however, any such trials are likely to be extended and expensive to meet regulatory authorities demands for such cocktail products.

Exotoxin-A of *Ps. aeruginosa* is largely responsible for the virulence and pathogenicity of this bacterium and passive immunization with anti-Exotoxin A antibodies may have therapeutic potential. A human IgM anti-Exotoxin A with neutralizing activity *in vitro* and which exerts a therapeutic effect in mouse models has been described.[103]

5.4.2.2 Septic Shock

LPS's, particularly the lipid A moiety, are the endotoxin moieties released from Gram-negative bacteria during septicemic periods and cause activation of monocytes and macrophages and massive release of cytokines such as TNF, IL-1, platelet-activating factor, and thromboxane-A2 which in turn trigger disseminated intravascular coagulation, respiratory distress syndrome, acute renal failure, and shock. Specific therapies based upon inhibition of these factors are being examined (reviewed in References 104 and 105). Since LPS is the most powerful and broadest spectrum activator of the sepsis cascade,[106] MAbs against lipid A components have been evaluated for treatment of septic shock.[107]

Murine IgM MAb E5 (XOMA) raised against the J5 rough mutant of *E. coli* has undergone considerable clinical development.[108-110] Initial trial studies suggested that E5 improved the survival of patients two- to three-fold providing the antibody was administered before the patients entered shock. Larger scale trials, however, did not provide sufficient evidence of efficacy and the product did not receive an FDA license in 1991. About 50% of the patients also mounted a HAMA response and the antibody was rapidly cleared with a serum half-life of only 20 h.

HA-1A is a human monoclonal IgM antibody derived from a mouse-human heterohybridoma cell line established from Epstein-Barr virus (EBV) transformed lymphocytes from a volunteer immunized with *E. coli* J-5 vaccine.[111] HA-1A also recognizes lipid A and displays broad reactivity against a range of naturally occurring rough mutants of Gram-negative bacteria. Despite being an IgM, it shows binding affinities of the order of 10^{-8} M for bacteria previously treated with antibiotics to expose antigen. Five phase I safety trials have been carried with HA-1A (Centoxin) and initial phase II trials were interpreted to demonstrate a reduction in mortality from 47 to 30% in 200 cases.[112] 4000 patients were enrolled on a compassionate-use basis in the U.S.[113] but the data did not provide sufficient evidence of efficacy to receive FDA approval in 1992. A further clinical trial was halted in 1993 because the death rate among those receiving Centoxin was higher than in the placebo group, and the product was taken off the market in countries where it had been approved. A more focused trial in meningococcemia is ongoing. The problems arising from clinical studies with these two antibodies have been reviewed.[107]

Human TNF is an inflammatory cytokine which plays a central role in defense against pathogens, but overproduction leads to inflammatory responses which can accentuate pathogenesis of many disease states. Animal studies have confirmed that anti-TNF MAbs can be effective both prophylactically and therapeutically and prevent shock during lethal bacteremia.[114] A humanized anti-TNF monoclonal (CDP571) has completed phase I trials in healthy volunteers at doses between 0.1 to 10 mg/kg and was well tolerated with a mean serum half-life of 13 days. This product is described in detail in Chapter 14.

5.4.2.3 Bacterial Toxoids

Human MAbs G2 and G6 recognize the C and B domains of tetanus toxoid, respectively. A mixture of these two MAbs had a 150-fold higher toxin neutralizing activity than the commercial polyclonal preparation Tetanobulin (Green Cross Co., Japan).[115] *Clostridium perfringens* causes severe infection of muscle and gas gangrene (myonecrosis). The alpha toxin, a zinc-metallo phospholipase C, is a crucial determinant of pathogenesis and makes a significant contribution to the development of gas gangrene.[116] A murine MAb which specifically binds at or near the active site has been described and humanized.[117] Alpha toxin from *Staphylococcus aureus* has multiple biological activities including causing lethality, dermonecrosis, and hemolysis. It is one of the major virulence factors in staphylococcal infections. A murine MAb 12E has been described that protects rabbits against dermonecrotic effects and mice against the lethal effects of alpha toxin.[118] This antibody has recently been humanized.[119]

5.5 FUTURE PROSPECTS

5.5.1 Antibacterial MAbs

The natural antibody response to microbial antigens is frequently influenced by T cells. In particular, T suppressor cells (Ts) limit the extent to which specific populations of B cells expand in response to antigens such as the polysaccharides of *Streptococcus pneumoniaie, Neisseria meningitidis, Ps. aeruginosa, Streptococcus mutans, Serratia marcesans,* and *E. coli.*[120] In contrast, T-helper cells (Th) stimulate an antibody response to protein antigens and there is the possible existence of amplifier T cells (Ta) which promote clonal expansion of antigen-stimulated B cells.[121] These regulatory influences then may place severe limitations on the normal ability of antibody repertoires to exert their maximal therapeutic effect. Antibody therapy, however, is independent of such regulatory influences and offers the opportunity to treat patients with doses of antibodies manyfold greater than achieved in the endogenous response and to maintain very high levels for extended time periods. There is therefore considerable scope for antibacterial monoclonal treatments particularly for prophylaxis of opportunistic infection.

The incidence of *Candida albicans* disseminated infection is rising exponentially due mainly to the rise in the AIDS and other immunocompromised populations. *C. albicans* is now the fourth most frequent cause of nosocomial infections. Only a few drugs are available, the most potent being amphotericin B but this must be administered by continual intravenous infusion and has toxic effects upon the kidney. Alternative formulations are being designed to reduce toxicity, however, a more serious problem is the increase in drug resistance. One study reported resistance in about 13% of patients.[122] T-cell-mediated immunity and non-specific cellular immunity are often described as the main natural defenses against fungal infection, however, there is increasing evidence that protective antibodies also play an important role. Several studies have demonstrated that administration of antibodies can protect mice against the lethal effects of *C. albicans* and *Cryptococcus neoformans* (for a review see Reference 123). In human studies, antibodies against heat shock protein 90 (hsp90) have been found to be associated with recovery from *C. albicans* infection and protection against disseminated disease in patients with AIDS [124-125] and IVIG may reduce *C. albicans* infections in patients receiving liver transplants.[126]

Pneumocystis carinii is recognized as an important cause of pneumonia in immunocompromised patients but rarely causes primary infection in immunocompetent hosts.[127] Prior to the use of antipneumocystic prophylaxis, up to 80% of AIDS patients would develop pneumonia mostly through reactivation of latent infections. Clearly then, impaired immune function is the most important susceptibility factor. The likelihood of *P. carinii* infection is increased during cyclosporin or corticosteroid therapy. Current therapy uses pentamidine, trimethoprim-sulfamethoxazole or trimethoprim-dapsone.[128] All have some undesirable side effects such as nephrotoxicity which limits the desirability of their use prophylactically. The selection of resistant strains, not only of *P. carinii* but also of other bacteria, is equally worrying.

5.5.2 Antiviral MAbs

Major viral targets to date are members of the herpes group of viruses and it is likely that antibody therapy could be extended to additional members of this family and other families who display latent infection and cause disease by reactivation. Epstein-Barr virus (EBV), because of its clinical and oncogenic importance, is the most studied member of the herpes group. Primary infection results in infectious mononucleosis and it is implicated in Burkitt's lymphoma, nasopharyngeal carcinoma, and polyclonal lymphomas in immunocompromised patients (for review see Reference 129). Transplant patients who develop primary EBV infection within 3 months of transplantation run a high risk of developing EBV-related lymphoproliferative syndrome. EBV is carried for life in the circulating lymphocytes of the immune host. The natural *in vivo* humoral response to EBV infection is against the gp85 component of the virus while experimentally raised neutralizing antibodies are directed against the gp350/220 glycoprotein complex, and vaccination with gp350 has been shown in animals to block tumor outgrowth.[130] There is no antiviral therapy for either infectious mononucleosis or lymphoproliferative syndromes. While antibody-mediated protection is not therefore a major natural protection mechanism, there may be potential clinical application for anti-gp350 neutralizing MAbs.

Human herpesvirus 6 (HHV-6) is a T-lymphotropic human herpesvirus present in patients with lymphoproliferative disorders and AIDS.[131] At least 90% of individuals are infected by HHV-6 by the age of 2 years and it can reactivate in immunocompromised hosts and cause pneumonia.[132] The possible significance of the virus as a cause of serious disease is a topic of current discussion.[133]

The possibility that viruses in the latent state or endogenous retroviruses may play a role in the etiology of many autoimmune, neurological, or mental diseases has been the topic of much discussion for many years. In many cases, these viruses may exert their pathogenic effect in the absence of active viral nucleic acid replication or spread of viral particles. Under these circumstances the vast majority of current and future antivirals, which are targeted to prevent virus growth, will be ineffective.

The immune secondary response which ideally prevents infection or leads to faster elimination of infected cells, includes both B cells that bind viral proteins and T cells that recognize viral peptides presented in association with the MHC. Stimulation or mimicking of either process may be routes to therapy for these disease states. However, neurons, especially sensory neurons appear to be permanently class I MHC negative leaving antibody-based elimination of viruses as potentially vital for central nervous system therapy.

5.6 CONCLUSIONS

Antibody-based therapy to treat infectious disease has been successful for over 100 years. The historical limitations on this therapy are: (1) inability to isolate those antibodies which most effectively neutralize infectivity and virulence, (2) inability to achieve high serum levels of antibody which neutralize infection, (3) side effects through use of nonhuman antibodies, and (4) very short serum half-life of nonhuman antibodies. The ready availability of human and humanized MAbs has provided the solution to all of these problems. Antibodies which target antigens unique to bacteria or viruses will not cross-react with normal body constituents and can in practice be given in unlimited quantities without any toxic or deleterious side effects. Antiviral neutralizing MAb preparations are 5000 to 15,000 more potent than hyperimmune sera. Therapy and prophylaxis can then target logarithmically higher infectious loads. Further, with expected serum half-lives of 15–25 days, single-dose regimes can provide extended protection. By contrast, traditional drug therapy requires multiple daily dosing regimes with potential toxicity. A major concern in the (particularly prophylactic) use of chemical drugs is the rapid development of drug resistance. Antibody-based therapies, if directed at conformational epitopes will not easily give rise to resistant mutants.

Pathogen-host interactions are complex and regulated. It is not in the invading organisms interest to kill its host too quickly, nor does the host "overreact" and focus its entire defense capabilities upon a pathogen. The immune response is a complex interaction of B and T cells, cytokines, and cytokine receptors. In many cases the antibody-mediated response is muted. MAb therapy offers the opportunity to override natural host regulation and to effectively treat infectious diseases which do not make use of antibodies during normal defense.

The major drawbacks to antibody therapy are the cost of materials and mode of delivery. Cost of manufacture of antibodies in mammalian cells limits their application to life-threatening disease states as does intravenous administration. However, intramuscular formulations can be designed and the future use of antibody fragments manufactured in microorganisms or plants offers an opportunity for antibody-based therapy to be provided at costs approaching those of traditional chemical drugs.

REFERENCES

1. Behring, E. A. and Kitasato, S., Uber das Zustandekommen der Diphtherie-Immunitat und der Tetanus-Immunitat bei Thieren, *Dtsch. Med. Wochenschr.*, 49, 1113, 1990.
2. Gronski, P., Seiler, F. R., and Schwick, H. G., Discovery of antitoxins and development of antibody preparations for clinical uses from 1890 to 1990, *Mol. Immunol.*, 28, 1321, 1991.
3. Finlayson, J. A., in *Medical Microbiology*, Vol. 1., Easmon, C. S. D. F. and Jeljaszewicz, J., Eds., [publishers name, address] 1982, 129.
4. Janeway, C. A. and Travers, P., *Immunobiology: The Immune System in Health and Disease*, Blackwell Scientific Publications, Oxford, 1994.
5. Joiner, K. A., Brown, E. F., and Frank, M. M., Complement and bacteria: chemistry and biology in host defence, *Annu. Rev. Immunol.*, 2, 461, 1984.
6. Dimmock, N. J. and Minor, P. D., Eds. *Immune Responses, Virus Infections and Disease*, IRL Press, Oxford, 1989.
7. Puck, J. M., Glezen, W. P., and Franck, A. L., Protection of infants from infection with influenza A virus by transplacentally acquired antibody, *J. Infect. Dis.*, 142, 844, 1980.
8. Ogilvie, M. M., Vathenen, A. S., Radford, M., Codd, J., and Key, S., Maternal antibody and respiratory syncytial virus infection in infancy, *J. Med. Virol.*, 7, 263, 1981.
9. Wyatt, H., Poliomyelitis in hypogammaglobulinemics, *J. Infect. Dis.*, 128, 802, 1973.
10. Apasov, S., Redegeld, F., and Sitkovsky, M., Cell-mediated cytotoxicity: contact and secreted factors, *Curr. Opin. Immunol.*, 5, 404, 1993.
11. Moller, G., Ed., T helper cell subpopulation, *Immunol. Rev.*, 123, 1, 1991.
12. Schlessinger, J. J., Brandriss, M. W., and Walsh, E. E., Protection against 17D yellow fever encephalitis in mice by passive transfer of monoclonal antibodies to the nonstructural glycoprotein gp48 and by active immunization with gp48, *J. Immunol.*, 135, 2805, 1985.
13. Harris, W. J. and Cunningham, C. C., *Antibody Therapeutics*, Springer/R. G. Landes Co., Austin, 1995.
14. Cross, A. S., Immunotherapy, in *Immunotherapy and Vaccines*, Cryz, S. J., Ed., VCH, Weinheim, 1991, 97.
15. Centers for Disease Control, Recommendation of the Immunization Practices Advisory Committee (ACIP): recommendation for prevention against viral hepatitis, *MMWR*, 34, 313, 1985.
16. Seeff, L. B., Wright, E. C., Zimmerman, H. J., Alter, H. J., Dietz, A. A., Felsher, B. F., Finkelstein, J. D., Garcia-Pont, P., Gerin, J. L., Greenlee, H. B., Hamilton, J., Holland, P. V., Kaplan, P. M., Kiernan, T., Koff, R. S., Leevy, C. M., McAuliffe, V. J., Nath, N., Purcell, R. H., Schiff, E. R., Schwartz, C. C., Tamburro, C. H., Vlahcevic, Z., Zemel, R., and Zimmon, D. S., Type B hepatitis after needlestick exposure: prevention with hepatitis B immune globulin, final report of the Veterans Administration cooperative study, *Ann. Intern. Med.*, 88, 285, 1978.
17. Centers for Disease Control, Protection against viral hepatitis, *MMWR*, 39, 1, 1990.
18. Szmuness, W., Stevens, C. E., Oleszko, W. R., and Goodman, A., Passive-active immunization against hepatitis B: immunogenicity studies in adult Americans, *Lancet*, 1, 575, 1981.
19. Centers for Disease Control, Recommendations of the Immunization Practices Advisory Committee (ACIP): diphtheria, tetanus and pertussis: guidelines for vaccine prophylaxis and other preventative measures, *MMWR*, 6, 281, 1985.
20. Centers for Disease Control, Recommendations of the Immunization Practices Advisory Committee (ACIP): rabies prevention in the United States, *MMWR*, 33, 393, 1984.

21. Bean, B., Antiviral therapy: current concepts and practices, *Clin. Microbiol. Rev.*, 5, 146, 1992.
22. Emmanuel, D., The use of passive immune therapy with intravenous immunoglobulin for the prevention and treatment of cytomegalovirus infections following solid organ and marrow transplantation, in *Multidisciplinary Approach to Understanding Cytomegalovirus Disease,* Michelson, S. and Plotkin, S. A., Eds., Excerpta Medica, Amsterdam, 1993, 295.
23. Foung, S. K., Bradshaw, P. A., and Emanuel, D., Uses of human monoclonal antibodies to human cytomegalovirus and varicella-zoster virus, in *Therapeutic Monoclonal Antibodies,* Borrabaeck, C. A. and Larrick, J. W., Eds., Stockton Press, New York, 1990, 173.
24. Roy, D. M. and Grundy, J. E., Evaluation of neutralizing antibody titers against human cytomegalovirus in intravenous gammaglobulin preparations, *Transplantation*, 54, 1109, 1992.
25. Snydman, D. R., Werner, B. G., Dougherty, N. N., Griffith, J., Rubin, R. H., Dienstag, J. L., Rohrer, R. H., Freeman, R., Jenkins, R., Lewis, W. D., Hammer, S., O'Rourke, E. O., Grady, G. F., Fawaz, K., Kaplan, M. M., Hoffman, M. A., Katz, A. T., Doran, M., and the Boston Center for Liver Transplantation CMVIG study group, Cytomegalovirus immune globulin prophylaxis in liver transplantation: a randomized double-blind placebo-controlled trial, *Ann. Intern. Med.*, 119, 984, 1993.
26. O'Reilly, R. J., Reich, L., Gold, J., Kirkpatrick, D., et al., A randomised trial of intravenous hyperimmune globulin for the prevention of cytomegalovirus (CMV) infections following marrow transplantation: preliminary results, *Transplant. Proc.*, XV, 1405, 1983.
27. Blacklock, H. A., Griffiths, P., Stirk, P., and Prentice, H. G., Specific hyperimmune globulin for cytomegalovirus pneumonitis, *Lancet,* ii, 152, 1985.
28. Hemming, V. G., Rodriguez, W., Kim, H. W., Brandt, C. D., Parrott, R. H., Burch, B., Prince, G. A., Baron, P. A., Fink, R., and Reaman, G., Intravenous immunoglobulin treatment of respiratory syncytial virus infection in infants and young children, *Antimicrob. Agents Chemother.*, 31, 1882, 1987.
29. Groothuis, J. R., Levin, M. J., Rodriguez, W., Hall, C. B., Long, C. E., Kim, H. W., Lauer, B. A., and Hemming, V. G., Use of intravenous gamma globulin to passively immunize high-risk children against respiratory syncytial virus: safety and pharmacokinetics. The RSVIG Study Group, *Antimicrob. Agents Chemother,* 35, 1469, 1991.
30. Meissner, H. C., Fulton, D. R., Groothuis, J. R., Geggel, R. L., Marx, G. R., Hemming, V. G., Hougen, T., and Snydman, D. R., Controlled trial to evaluate protection of high-risk infants against respiratory syncytial virus disease by using standard intravenous immune globulin, *Antimicrob. Agents Chemother.*, 37, 1655, 1993.
31. Hemming, V. G., Prince, G. A., Groothuis, J. R., and Siber, G. R., Hyperimmune globulins in prevention and treatment of respiratory syncytial virus infections, *Clin. Microbiol. Rev.*, 8, 22, 1995.
32. Jackson, G. G., Perkins, J. T., Rubenis, M., Paul, D. A., Knigge, M., Despotes, J. C., and Spencer, P., Passive immunoneutralization of human immunodeficiency virus in patients with advanced AIDS, *Lancet,* ii, 647, 1988.
33. Karpas, A., Hewlett, I. K., Hill, F., Gray, J., Byron, N., Gilgen, D., Bally, V., Oates, J. K., Gazzard, B., and Epstein, J. E., Polymerase chain reaction evidence of human immunodeficiency virus 1 neutralization by passive immunization in patients with AIDS and AIDS-related complex, *Proc. Natl. Acad. Sci. U.S.A.*, 87, 7613, 1990.

34. Vittecoq, D., Mattlinger, B., Barre-Sinoussi, F., Courouce, A. M., Rouzioux, C., Doinel, C., Bary, M., Viard, J. P., Bach, J. F., Rouger, P., and Lefrere, J. J., Passive immunotherapy in AIDS: a randomised trial of serial human immunodeficiency virus-positive transfusions of plasma rich in p24 antibodies versus transfusions of seronegative plasma, *J. Infect. Dis.*, 165, 364, 1992.
35. Levy, J. L., Anti-HIV hyperimmune plasma: a new weapon in the anti-AIDS armoury is under trial, in *The Biotechnology Report 1994/95*, Price, E., Ed., Campden Publishing Ltd., Hong Kong, 1994, 98.
36. Jacobson, J. M., Colman, N., Ostrow, N. A., Simson, R. W., Tomesch, D., Marlin, L., Rao, M., Mills, J. L., Clemens, J., and Prince, A. M., Passive immunotherapy in treatment of advanced HIV infection, *J. Infect. Dis.*, 168, 298, 1993.
37. Levy, J. A., Pathogenesis of human immunodeficiency virus infection, *Microbiol. Rev.*, 57, 183, 1993.
38. Larrick, J. W., Treatment of Infectious Disease with monoclonal antibodies, in *Immunotherapy and Vaccines*, Cryz, S. J., Ed., VCH Weinheim, 1991, 129.
39. Ziegler, E. J., Protective antibody to endotoxin core: the emperor's new clothes, *J. Infect. Dis.*, 158, 286, 1988.
40. Baumgartner, J. D., Immunotherapy with antibodies to core lipopolysaccharides: a critical appraisal, *Infect. Dis. Clin. N. Am.*, 5, 915, 1991.
41. Cross, A. S. and Opal, S., Therapeutic intervention in sepsis with antibody to endotoxin: is there a future?, *J. Endotoxin Res.*, 1, 57, 1994.
42. Emery, S. C. and Adair, J. R., Humanized monoclonal antibodies for therapeutic applications, *Exp. Opin. Invest. Drugs*, 3, 241, 1994.
43. Thomas, H. C., The immune response to hepatitis B virus, in *Immune Responses, Virus Infections and Disease*, Dimmock. N. J. and Minor, P. D., Eds., Oxford University Press, Oxford, 1989, 105.
44. Szmuness, W., Alter, H. J., and Maynard, J. E., Eds., *Viral Hepatitis*, The Franklin Institute, Philadelphia, 1981.
45. Harada, K., Ichimori, Y., Sasano, K., Sasai, S., Kiatano, K., Iwasa, S., Tsukamoto, K., and Sugino, Y., Human-Human hybridomas secreting hepatitis B virus-neutralizing antibodies, *Bio/Technology*, 7, 374, 1989.
46. Ehrlich, P. H., Moustafa, Z. A., Justice, J. C., Harfeldt, K. E., Kelley, R. L., and Ostberg L., Characterization of human monoclonal antibodies directed against the hepatitis B surface antigen, *Hum. Antibod. Hybridomas*, 3, 27, 1992.
47. Cornett, J. B., Clinical results with humanized and human monoclonal antibodies, in *Animal Cell Technology. Basic and Applied Aspects*, Kobayashi, T., Kitagawa, Y., and Okumura, K., Eds., Kluwer Academic Publishers, The Netherlands, 6, 63, 1994.
48. Forbes, B. A., Acquisition of cytomegalovirus infection: an update, *Clin. Microbiol. Rev.*, 2, 204, 1989.
49. Fowler, K. B., Stagno, S., Pass, R. F., Britt, W. J., Boll, T. J., and Alford, C. A., The outcome of congenital cytomegalovirus infection in relation to maternal antibody status, *N. Engl. J. Med.*, 326, 663, 1992.
50. Marshall, G. S., Rabalais, G. P., Stout, G. G., and Waldeyer, S. L., Antibodies to recombinant derived glycoprotein B after natural human cytomegalovirus infection correlate with neutralizing activity, *J. Infect. Dis.*, 165, 381, 1992.
51. Rasmussen, L., Progress in the development of a human cytomegalovirus glycoprotein subunit vaccine, in *Multidisciplinary Approach to Understanding Cytomegalovirus Disease*, Michelson, S. and Plotkin, S. A., Eds., Excerpta Medica, Amsterdam, 1993, 311.
52. Urban, M., Britt, W., and Mach, M., The dominant linear neutralizing antibody binding site of glycoprotein gp86 of human cytomegalovirus is strain specific, *J. Virol.*, 66, 1303, 1992.

53. Simpson, J. A., Chow, J. C., Baker, J., Avdalovic, N., Yuan, S., Au, D., Co, M. S., Vasquez, M., Britt, W. J., and Coelingh, K. L., Neutralizing monoclonal antibodies that distinguish three antigenic sites on human cytomegalovirus glycoprotein H have conformationally distinct binding sites, *J. Virol.*, 67, 489, 1993.
54. Chou, S. and Dennison, K. M., Analysis of interstrain variation in cytomegalovirus glycoprotein B sequences encoding neutralization related epitopes, *J. Infect. Dis.*, 163, 1229, 1991.
55. Darlington, J., Super, M., Patel, K., Grundy, J. E., Griffiths, P. D., and Emery, V. C., Use of polymerase chain reaction to analyse sequence variation within a major neutralizing epitope of glycoprotein B in clinical isolates of human cytomegalovirus, *J. Gen. Virol.*, 72, 1985, 1991.
56. Rasmussen, L., Morris, M., Wolitz, R., Dowling, A., Fessell, J., Holodniy, M., and Merigan, T. C., Deficiency in antibody response to human cytomegalovirus glycoprotein gH in human immunodeficiency virus-infected patients at risk from cytomegalovirus retinitis, *J. Infect. Dis.*, 170, 673, 1994.
57. Cranage, M. P., Kouzarides, T., Bankier, A. T., Strachwell, S., Weston, K., Tomlinson, P., Barrell, B., Hart, H., Bell, S. E., Minson, A. C., and Smith, G. L., Identification of the human cytomegalovirus glycoprotein B gene and induction of neutralizing antibodies via its expression in recombinant vaccinia virus, *EMBO J.*, 5, 3057, 1986.
58. Grundy, J. E., Hamilton, A., Roy, D., King, S., Turner, A., and Harris, W. J., A humanized cytomegalovirus specific monoclonal antibody for prophylaxis and therapy, Abstr. 8th International Symposium on Infections in the Immunocompromised Host, Davos, Switzerland, 1994.
59. Nadler, P., Wood, D. L., Ostberg, L., and Co, M. S., The use of human and genetically engineered humanized antibodies for the prophylaxis and treatment of cytomegalovirus infection, *Transplant Immunol. Lett.*, IX: 13, 1994.
60. Ehrlich, P. H. and Ostberg, L., Characterisation of human anti-cytomegalovirus monoclonal antibodies, in *Therapeutic Monoclonal Antibodies*, Borrebaeck, C. A. and Larrick, J. W., Eds., Stockton Press, New York, 1990, 209.
61. Autlitsky, W. E., Schulz, T. F., Tilg, H., Niederweiser, D., Larcher, K., Ostberg, L., Scriba, M., Martindale, J., Stern, A. C., Grass, P., Mach, M., Dierich, M. P., and Huber, C., Human monoclonal antibodies neutralizing cytomegalovirus (CMV) for prophylaxis of CMV disease: report of a phase I trial in bone marrow transplant patients, *J. Infect. Dis.*, 163, 1344, 1991.
62. Drobyski, W. R., Gottlieb, M., Carrigan, D., Ostberg, L., Greenbau, M., Schran, H., Magid, P., Ehrlich, P., Nadler, P. I., and Ash, R. C., Phase I study of safety and pharmacokinetics of a human anti-cytomegalovirus monoclonal antibody in allogeneic bone marrow transplant recipients, *Transplantation*, 51, 1190, 1991.
63. Masuho, Y., Matsumoto, J., Sugano, T., Tomiyama, T., Sasaki, S., and Koyama, T., Development of a human monoclonal antibody against cytomegalovirus with the aim of a passive immunotherapy, in *Therapeutic Monoclonal Antibodies*, Borrebaeck, C. A. and Larrick, J. W., Eds., Stockton Press, New York, 1990, 187.
64. Cranage, M. P., Smith, G. L., Bell, S. E., Hart, H., Brown, C., Bankier, A. T., Tomlinson, P., Barrell, B. G., and Minson, T. C., Identification and expression of a human cytomegalovirus glycoprotein with homology to the Epstein-Barr virus BXLF2 product, varicella zoster gpIII, and Herpes simplex virus type 1 glycoprotein H, *J. Virol.*, 62, 1416, 1988.
65. Tempest, P. R., White, P., Buttle, M., Carr, F. J., and Harris, W. J., Identification of framework residues required to restore antigen binding during reshaping of a monoclonal antibody against the glycoprotein gB of human cytomegalovirus, *Int. J. Biol. Macromol.*, 17, 37, 1995.

66. Whitley, R. J. and Schlitt, M., Encephalitis caused by herpesviruses, including B virus, in *Infections of the Central Nervous System*, Scheld, W. M., Whitley, R. J., and Durack, D. T., Eds., Raven Press. New York, 1991, 41.
67. Whitley, R. J. and Gnann, J. W., Acyclovir: a decade later, *N. Engl. J. Med.*, 11, 782, 1992.
68. Zaia, J. A., Levin, M. J., Preblud, S. R., Leszczynski, J., Wright, G. G., Ellis, R. J., Curtis, A. C., Valerio, M. A., and LeGore, J., Evaluation of varicella zoster immune globulin: protection of immunosuppressed children after household exposure to varicella, *J. Infect. Dis.*, 147, 737, 1983.
69. Bean, B., Antiviral therapy: Current concepts and practices, *Clin. Microbiol. Rev.*, 5, 146, 1992.
70. Forghani, B., Dupuis, K. W., and Schmidt, N. J., Varicella zoster viral glycoproteins analysed with monoclonal antibodies, *J. Virol.*, 52, 5, 1984.
71. Foung, S. K. H., Perkins, S., Koropchak, C., Fishwild, D. M., Wittek, A. E., Engleman, E. G., Grumet, F. C., and Arvin, A. M., Human monoclonal antibodies neutralizing varicella zoster virus, *J. Infect. Dis.*, 152, 280, 1985.
72. Keller, P. M., Neff, B. J., and Ellis, B. W., Three major glycoprotein genes of varicella zoster whose products have neutralizing epitopes, *J. Virol.*, 52, 293, 1984.
73. Sugano, T., Matsumoto, Y., Miyamoto, C., and Masuho, Y., Hybridomas producing human monoclonal antibodies against varicella zoster virus, *Eur. J. Immunol.*, 17, 359, 1987.
74. Montalvo, E. A. and Grose, C., Neutralization epitope of varicella zoster virus on native viral glycoprotein gp118 (VZV glycoprotein gpIII), *Virology*, 149, 230, 1986.
75. Rodriguez, J. E., Mininger, T., and Grose, C., Entry and egress of varicella virus blocked by the same anti-gH monoclonal antibody, *Virology*, 196, 840, 1993.
76. Moss, M., Grose, C., Carr, F., Fitzek, M., and Harris, W. J., Reshaping of an anti-varicella zoster virus antibody. Abstr. 2nd International Conference on the Varicella Zoster Virus, 1994.
77. Sugano, T., Tomiyama, T., Matsumoto, Y., Sasaki, S., Kimura, T., Forghani, B., and Masuho, Y., A human monoclonal antibody against varicella zoster virus glycoprotein III, *J. Gen. Virol.*, 72, 2065, 1991.
78. Stevens, J. G., Human Herpesviruses: a consideration of the latent state, *Microbiol. Rev.*, 53, 318, 1989.
79. Balachandran, N., Bacchetti, S., and Rawls, W. E., Protection against lethal challenge of Balb/c mice by passive transfer of monoclonal antibodies to five glycoproteins of herpes simplex virus type 2, *Infect. Immun.*, 37, 1132, 1982.
80. Co, M. S., Deschamps, M., Whitley, R. J., and Queen, C., Humanized antibodies for antiviral therapy, *Proc. Natl. Acad. Sci. U.S.A.*, 88, 2869, 1991.
81. Levy, J. A., Pathogenesis of human immunodeficiency virus infection, *Microbiol. Rev.*, 57, 183, 1993.
82. Hinkula, J., Bratt, G., Gilljam, G., Nordlund, S., Broliden, P. A., Holmberg, V., Olausson-Hansson, E., Albert, J., Sandstrom, E., and Wahren, B., Immunological and virological interactions in patients receiving passive immunotherapy with HIV-1 neutralizing monoclonal antibodies, *J. Acquired Immune Deficiency Syndrome*, 7, 940, 1994.
83. D'Souza, M. P., Geyer, S. J., Hanson, C. V., Hendry, R. M., and Milman, G., Evaluation of monoclonal antibodies to HIV-1 envelope by neutralization and binding assays: an international collaboration, *AIDS*, 8, 169, 1994.
84. Loveless, M. D., Early clinical trial of anti-HIV antibodies in AIDS. What lessons can we learn, in *Antibody Based Therapeutics: The Latest Clinical Trial and Applications Strategies*, IBC conference, Washington, June 1994.
85. Nakamura, M., Sasaki, H., Terada, M., and Ohno, T., Complement-dependent virolysis of HIV-1 with monoclonal antibody NM-01, *Aids Res. Hum. Retroviruses*, 9, 619, 1993.

86. Armour, K., Terada, M., Nakamura, M., Sasaki, H., Carr, F. J., Ohno, T., and Harris, W. J., Virolysis and *in vitro* neutralization of HIV by humanized monoclonal antibody hNM-01, Abstr. Tenth International Congress Aids, 1994.
87. Gorny, M., Conley, A. J., Karwowski, S. B., Buchbinder, A., Xu, J. Y., Emini, E. A., Koenig, S., and Zolla-Pazner, S., Neutralization of diverse human immunodeficiency virus type 1 variants by an anti-V3 human monoclonal antibody, *J. Virol.*, 66, 7538, 1992.
88. Steele, H. H., Rabies in the Americas and remarks on global aspects, *Rev. Infect. Dis.*, 10, (Suppl. 4), 585, 1988.
89. Baer, G. M., Research towards rabies prevention: overview, *Rev. Infect. Dis.*, 10 (Suppl. 4), 576, 1988
90. Dietschold, B., Tollis, M., Lafon, M., Wunner, W. H., and Koporowski, H., Mechanisms of rabies virus neutralization by glycoprotein-specific monoclonal antibodies, *Virology*, 161, 29, 1987.
91. Schumacher, C. L., Dietzschold, B., Ertl, H. C., Niu, H. S., Rupprecht, C. E., and Koprowski, H., Use of mouse anti-rabies monoclonal antibodies in post exposure treatment of rabies, *J. Clin. Invest.*, 84, 971, 1989.
92. Bodey, G. P., Bolivar, R., Fainstein, V., and Jadeja, L., Infections caused by *Pseudomonas aeruginosa, Rev. Infect. Dis.*, 5, 279, 1983.
93. Ziegler, E., McCutchan, J. A., Fierer, J., Glauser, M. P., Sadoff, J. C., Douglas, H., and Braude, A. I., Treatment of gram-negative bacteraemia and shock with a human antiserum to a mutant *Escherichia coli, N. Engl. J. Med.*, 307, 1225, 1982.
94. Baumgartner, J. D., Glauser, M. P., McCutchan, J. A., Ziegler, E. J., van Melle, G., Klauber, M. R., Vogt, M., Muehlen, E., Luethy, R., Chiolero, R., and Geroulanos, S., Prevention of Gram-negative shock and death in surgical patients by antibody to endotoxin core glycolipid. *Lancet*, 2, 59, 1985.
95. Lang, A. B., Bruderer, U., Fuerer, E. Larrick, J. W., and Cryz, S. J., Immunoprotective capacities of human and murine monoclonal antibodies recognizing serotype-specific and common determinants of Gram-negative bacteria, in *Therapeutic Monoclonal Antibodies*, Borrabaeck, C. A. and Larrick, J. W., Eds., Stockton Press, New York, 1990, 223.
96. Dunn, D. L., Bogard, W. C., and Cerra, F. B., Efficacy of type-specific and cross-reactive murine monoclonal antibodies directed against endotoxin during experimental sepsis, *Surgery*, 98, 283, 1985.
97. Young, L. S., Monoclonal antibodies: technology and application to Gram negative infections. *Infection*, 13, Suppl. 2, S224, 1985.
98. Miner, K. M., Manyak, C. L., Williams, E., Jackson, J., Jewell, M., Gammon, M. T., Ehrenfreund, C., Hayes, E., Callahan, L. T. III, Zweerink, H., and Sigal, N. H., Characterization of murine monoclonal antibodies to *Escherichia coli* J5, *Infect. Immun.*, 52, 56, 1986.
99. Salles, M. F., Mandine, E., Zalisz, R., Guenounou, M., and Smets, P., Protective effects of murine monoclonal antibodies in experimental septicemia: *E. coli* antibodies protect against different serotypes of *E. coli, J. Infect. Dis.*, 159, 641, 1989.
100. Stoll, B. J., Pollack, M., Young, L. S., Koles, N., Gascon, R., and Pier, G. B., Functionally active monoclonal antibody that recognizes an epitope on the O-side chain of *Pseudomonas aeruginosa* immunotype-1 lipopolysaccharide, *Infect. Immun.*, 53, 656, 1986.
101. Sawada, S., Kawamura, T., and Masuho, Y., Immunoprotective human monoclonal antibodies against five major serotypes of *Pseudomonas aeruginosa, J. Gen. Microbiol.*, 133, 3581, 1987.
102. Zweerink, H. J.,Gammon, M. C., Hutchison, C. F., Jackson, J. J., Lombardo, D., Miner, K. M., Puckett, J. M., Sewell, T. J., and Sigal, N. H., Human monoclonal antibodies that protect mice against challenge with Pseudomonas aeruginosa, *Infect. Immun.*, 56, 1873, 1988.

103. Nakatani, T., Nomura, N., Horigome, K., Ohtsuka, H., and Noguchi, H., Functional expression of human monoclonal antibody genes directed against pseudomonal exotoxin A in mouse myeloma cells, *Bio/Technology*, 7, 805, 1989.
104. Cohen, J. and Glauser, M. P., Septic shock: treatment, *Lancet*, 338, 736, 1991.
105. Giroir, B. P., Mediators of septic shock: new approaches for interrupting the endogenous inflammatory cascade, *Crit. Care. Med.*, 21, 780, 1993.
106. Corriveau, C. C. and Danner, R. L., Endotoxin as a therapeutic target in septic shock, *Infect. Agents Dis.*, 2, 35, 1993.
107. Warren, H. S., Danner, R. L., and Munford, R. S., Anti-endotoxin monoclonal antibodies, *N. Engl. J. Med.*, 326, 1153, 1992.
108. Wood, D. M., Parent, J. B., Gazzano-Santoro, H., Lim, E., Pruyne, P. T., Watkins, J. M., Spoor, E. S., Reardan, D. T., Trown, P. W., and Conlon, P. J., Reactivity of monoclonal E5 with endotoxin: 1. Binding to lipid A and rough polysaccharides, *Circ. Shock*, 38, 55, 1992.
109. Parent, J. B., Gazzano-Santoro, H., Wood, D. M., Lim, E., Pruyne, P. T., Trown, P. W., and Conlon, P. J., Reactivity of monoclonal antibody E5-11 binding to short and long chain smooth lipopolysaccharides, *Circ. Shock*, 38, 63, 1992.
110. Greenman, R. L., Schein, R. M., Martin, M. A., Wenzel, R. P., MacIntyre, N. R., Emmanuel, G., Chmel, H., Kohler, R. B., McCarthy, M., Plouffe, J., Russell, J. A., and the XOMA Sepsis Study Group, A controlled clinical trial of E5 murine monoclonal IgM antibody to endotoxin in the treatment of gram negative sepsis, *JAMA*, 266, 1097, 1991.
111. Baumgartner, J. D., Monoclonal anti-endotoxin antibodies for the treatment of gram negative bacteremia and septic shock, *Eur. J. Clin. Microbiol. Inf. Dis.*, 9, 711, 1990.
112. Smith, C., Wortler, C., Dixon, W., and Ziegler E., Monoclonal antibody HA-1A for gram negative shock, *Lancet*, 338, 695, 1991.
113. McCloskey, R. V., Straube, R. C., Sanders, C., Smith, S. M., and Smith, C. R., Treatment of septic shock with human monoclonal antibody Ha-1A. A randomised, double-blind placebo-controlled trial, *Ann. Intern. Med.*, 121, 1, 1994.
114. Tracey, K. J. Y., Fong, D. G., Hesse, K. R. Manogue, A. T., Lee, A. T., Kuo, G. C., Lowry, S. F., and Cerami, A., Anti-cachectin/TNF monoclonal antibodies prevent septic shock during lethal bacteremia, *Nature*, 330, 662,1987.
115. Hashizume, S., Sato, S., Kato, M., Mamei, M. et al., Clinical applications of human monoclonal antibodies, in *Animal and Cell Technology: Basic and Applied Aspects*, Kobayashi, T., Kitagawa, Y., and Okumura, K., Eds., Kluwer Academic Publishers, The Netherlands, 6, 75, 1994.
116. Williamson, E. D. and Titball, R. W., A genetically engineered vaccine against the alpha-toxin of Clostridium perfringens protects mice against experimental gas gangrene, *Vaccine*, 11, 1253, 1993.
117. Tempest, P. R., White, P., Williamson, E. D., Titball, R. W., Kelly, D. C., Kemp, G. J. L., Gray, P. M. D., Forster, S. J., Carr, F. J., and Harris, W. H., Efficient generation of a reshaped human antibody specific for the α-toxin of *Clostridium perfringens*, *Prot. Engng.*, 7, 2501, 1994.
118. Blomqvist, L. and Sjorgen, A. M., Production and characterisation of monoclonal antibodies against *Staphylococcus aureus* α-toxin, *Toxicon*, 26, 265, 1988.
119. Puentes, E. and Harris, W. J., unpublished, 1996.
120. Baker, P. J., Regulation of magnitude of antibody response to bacterial polysaccharide antigens by thymus-derived lymphocytes, *Infect. Immun.*, 58, 3465, 1990.
121. Baker, P. J., Suppressor T cells, *ASM News*, 59, 123, 1993.
122. Anon., Rising fungal disease provoke new treatment strategies, *ASM News*, 61, 281, 1995.
123. Casadevall, A., Antibody immunity and invasive fungal infections, *Infect. Immun.*, 63, 4211, 1995.

124. Matthews, R. and Burnie, J., The role of hsp90 in fungal infection, *Immunol. Today,* 13, 345, 1992.
125. Matthews, R., Burnie, J., Smith, D., Clark, I., Midgley, J., Conolly, M., and Gazzard, B., Candida and AIDS: evidence for protective antibody, *Lancet, ii,* 263, 1988.
126. Stratta, R. J., Shaefer, M. S., Cushing, K. A., Markin, R. S., Reed, E. C., Langnas, A. N., Pillen, T. J., and Shaw, B. W., Jr., A randomised prospective trial of acyclovir and immune-globulin prophylaxis in liver transplant recipients receiving OKT3 therapy, *Arch. Surg.,* 127, 55, 1992.
127. Bartlett, M. S. and Smith, J. W., *Pneumocystis carinii,* an opportunist in immunocompromised patients, *Clin. Microbiol. Rev.,* 4, 137, 1991.
128. Varthalitis, I. and Meunier, F., *Pneumocystis carinii* pneumonia: the pathogen, the diagnosis and recent advances in management, *Int. J. Antimicrob. Agents,* 1, 97, 1991.
129. Khanna, R., Burrows, S. R., and Moss, D. J., Immune regulation in Epstein-Barr virus associated diseases, *Microbiol. Rev.,* 59, 387, 1995.
130. Morgan, A. J., Mackett, M., Finerty, S., Arrand, J. R., Scullion, F. T., and Epstein, M. A., Recombinant vaccinia expressing Epstein-Barr virus glycoprotein gp340 protects cottontop tamarins against EBV-induced malignant lymphomas, *J. Med. Virol.,* 25, 189, 1988.
131. Salahuddin, S. Z., Ablashi, D. V., Markham, P. D., Josephs, S. F., Sturzenegger, S., Kaplan, M., Halligan, G., Biberfeld, P., Wong-Staal, F., Kramarsky, B., and Gallo, R. C., Isolation of a new virus, HBLV, in patients with lymphoproliferative disorders, *Science,* 234, 596, 1986.
132. Carrigan, D. R., Crodyski, W. R., Russler, S. K., Tapper, M. A., Knox, K. K., and Ash, R. C., Interstitial pneumonitis associated with human herpesvirus-6 infection in marrow transplantation, *Lancet,* 338, 147, 199l.
133. Pellet, P. E., Black, J. B., and Yamamoto, M., Human herpesvirus-6: the virus and search for its role as a human pathogen, *Adv. Virus Res.,* 41, 1, 1992.

Chapter 6

ANTIBODY THERAPEUTICS: APPLICATION TO AUTOIMMUNITY

Lucienne Chatenoud

CONTENTS

0-8493-8547-4/97/$0.00+$.50

6.1 INTRODUCTION

Under physiological conditions the immune system does not develop destructive autoimmune reactions against self-tissues.[1] Nevertheless, it is now very extensively documented that, in normal individuals, although deletion mechanisms ensure the elimination of most autoreactive T and B lymphocytes, this purging is far from complete.[2,3] It is presently accepted that lymphocytes may escape deletion if their T-cell receptor is specific for self-peptides which are not processed and presented within the thymus (i.e., cryptic peptides). Another possibility is that of peripheral antigens that can only promote central deletion if brought and processed in sufficient amounts within the thymus. Even though it has been established that under particular conditions cell deletion may also occur outside the thymus,[4] substantial progress has been made in our understanding of non-deletion dynamic mechanisms that operate in the periphery to refrain from potentially destructive autoreactivity. Concepts like anergy,[5] cytokine-mediated immune deviation,[6] suppression,[7] vetoing,[8] and anti-idiotypic network regulation,[1] have thus emerged for which the precise cellular and molecular basis remains controversial.

One must also emphasize that a fundamental but unfortunately still unresolved issue is our inability to distinguish in a reliable way a pathogenic from a nonpathogenic autoreactive B or T lymphocyte. In particular, especially in the case of organ-specific autoimmune diseases, it has not yet been fully established if so-called "natural" autoreactive B and T lymphocytes, present in normal individuals, express immunoglobulin or T-cell receptors with adequate epitope specificity, affinity, and/or avidity to give rise to pathological autoimmune reactions. The situation is somewhat different in the case of non-organ-specific autoimmune diseases in which there is evidence for a "natural" hyperautoreactivity.[9]

Effective and durable treatment of ongoing autoimmune diseases still represents a major challenge. Conventional treatments mostly rely on chemical immunosuppressants, i.e., corticosteroids, azathioprine, methotrexate, cyclophosphamide, and cyclosporin. Two major drawbacks of such therapies are their relative long-term ineffectiveness with consequent recurrence of the destructive immunopathologic processes, and the well-documented infectious and tumorigenic risks linked to chronic administration.

Fifteen years of experience in using immunosuppressive monoclonal antibodies (MAbs) for studies mainly in clinical transplantation has clearly demonstrated their potency in both preventing and reversing ongoing lesional immune reactions, i.e., graft rejection.[10-11] In addition, data from a variety of experimental models have well established that some MAbs may also express therapeutic activities not shared by conventional chemical immunosuppressants. Thus, antibodies or genetically engineered molecules to distinct functionally relevant T-cell receptors (CD3, CD4, CD28/CTLA4Ig, adhesion receptors, or adhesins) can promote immune tolerance not only to foreign tissue alloantigens but also to autoantigens.[12-30]

The aim of this review is to present data from clinical studies that have used MAbs in the treatment of autoimmunity trying to concentrate on the situations for which the results are more promising. In addition, on the basis of available experimental data the author shall discuss the possibility of applying MAb therapy as a means to restore self-tolerance.

6.2 POTENTIAL TARGETS OF THERAPEUTIC MAbs

Immune responses are the result of an effective cooperation between functionally distinct cell types that are antigen presenting cells (APC), B and T lymphocytes. Cell cooperation is mediated through the interaction of cell membrane receptors and soluble mediators namely, cytokines, that are all potentially attractive targets for therapeutic MAbs.

Among T lymphocytes CD4+ cells play a major role in several autoimmune diseases and have thus constituted a privileged target for antibody-mediated intervention. In particular, antibodies to CD4, CD3, the constant portion of the T-cell receptor (TCR) and major histocompatibility complex (MHC) class II products were applied to selectively act on the molecular entities selectively engaged in antigen recognition.[16-20,30-32] Antibodies to adhesion molecules that enhance the affinity of cell-to-cell interactions have also been investigated such as ICAM-1.[33] The possibility of acting on activated T cells drove the interest in antibodies to the interleukin (IL-2) receptor (CD25), a strategy that when applied to autoimmune diseases only had moderate success.[34] More recently, very interesting data have been obtained by interfering with cell receptors involved in the delivery of costimulatory signals such as CD28 and CTLA4 for T cells and CD40 for B cells.[35-36] Various studies have in fact demonstrated that T cells require two signals for activation: signal 1 is provided by stimulation through TCR, and signal 2 (the costimulatory signal) is provided by ligation of one or more T-cell-surface receptors. Engagement of TCR alone, i.e., delivery of signal 1 without signal 2, promotes T-cell-specific unresponsiveness (anergy).[5] The first costimulatory pathway to be characterized is transduced through the CD28 molecule, whose specific ligands B7.1 and

B7.2 are present at the surface of APCs.[35] CTLA-4 is the product of a gene closely related to CD28, that also acts as a B7 ligand. A recently described soluble recombinant fusion protein, CTLA-4Ig, competes for CD28 engagement and blocks T-cell-dependent responses *in vitro*.[24] *In vivo*, CTLA4Ig blocks T-cell-dependent antibody production effectively prevents xenogeneic pancreatic islet and allogeneic cardiac allograft rejection and can also reverse established murine lupus.[25-26,37]

Cytokines are essential mediators of immunity and inflammation, two mechanisms that operate to a variable extent during the course of autoimmune diseases. To neutralize the biological effect of cytokines, one must inhibit their binding to specific receptors. In theory, this can be achieved in various ways, including treatment with anti-cytokine antibodies, soluble cytokine receptors, antagonists of cytokine receptors (as in the case of IL-1), and genetically engineered immunoadhesins, including two soluble receptor fragments linked to an immunoglobulin constant frame.[38-40]

Proinflammatory cytokines may represent privileged targets in the treatment of some autoimmune diseases and this is very well illustrated by the impressive clinical results recently reported in patients presenting with rheumatoid arthritis treated with a MAb to tumor necrosis factor (TNF).[41-43]

Cytokine-producing T cells are heterogeneous. Thus two distinct T helper CD4+ subsets have been characterized first in mice and then in humans termed TH1 and TH2.[44] TH1 clones that are interferon-γ (IFN-γ) producers preferentially support macrophage activation and cell-mediated delayed type hypersensitivity responses. TH2 clones synthesizing IL-4, IL-6, IL-10, and IL-13 provide efficient help for B-cell proliferation and differentiation as well as for antibody production.[44-45] *In vivo* the key regulatory role of TH1- and TH2-type cells was deduced from the study of experimental and clinical situations involving strong or persistent antigen stimulation as seen in certain infectious diseases (i.e., murine leishmaniasis or human leprosy). TH1- and TH2-type cells have profound cytokine-mediated counter-regulatory effects on each other, which explains why humoral and cellular responses to a given antigen often alternate in reciprocal dominance.[44-45] Thus IFN-γ is produced by TH1 cells and inhibits TH2 cell proliferation whereas IL-10, which is produced by TH2 cells, inhibits TH1 cell function. IL-12, produced by monocyte/macrophages, was recently shown to be important for driving the response toward TH1. Moreover, the presence of IL-4 at the time of antigen triggering may be essential to shift the balance toward TH2. The enormous efforts being made to delineate the pathophysiological role in autoimmune diseases of a polarization of specific responses toward a preferential TH1 or TH2 phenotype may lead to new therapeutic strategies in the very near future.[6,44-45]

6.3 CLINICAL STUDIES

The application of MAbs for the treatment of autoimmune diseases is less widespread compared with their extensive use in clinical transplantation. With some exceptions the vast majority of the conducted trials are pilot phase I/II studies to assess the safety of the product and to define therapeutic dose ranges on the basis of pharmacokinetics and biological studies.

Antibodies to CD4, to CD52, and more recently antibodies to TNF have been the subject of interesting studies in rheumatoid arthritis, multiple sclerosis, psoriasis, and systemic vasculitis and the data obtained deserve some detailed discussion.

6.3.1 CD4 Antibodies

An enormous body of data has accumulated over the last 10 years on the remarkable capacity of MAbs to CD4 to suppress immune responses to soluble and tissue antigens, i.e., alloantigens and autoantigens.[14-22,46-47] Such an effect was further proof of the key role played by CD4+ lymphocytes in T-cell-mediated autoimmunity. The therapeutic effectiveness of MAbs was evident in experimental models of both spontaneous or induced autoimmune diseases.[16-20,47-48] CD4 also represented the first antibody specificity for which a tolerance-promoting effect was described. [27-28,47]

In humans, CD4 is expressed not only at the surface of a subset of lymphocytes but also on monocytes, macrophages, Langerhans' cells, eosinophils, endothelial cells of hepatic sinusoids, sperm and brain cells.[47] Only in lymphocytes is the intracytoplasmic carboxy terminal domain of CD4 non-covalently linked to the protein-tyrosine kinase $p56^{lck}$, a T-cell-specific member of the *src* family involved in signal transduction.[49] In addition to its role as an adhesion molecule specifically binding MHC class II-bearing targets, CD4 acts as a coreceptor for the TCR/CD3 complex and contributes to its signaling function.[49-51] Studies using bispecific antibodies in comodulation and coclustering experiments have provided evidence of a physical interaction between CD4 and TCR/CD3.[50-51] In contrast, the independent ligation of the two receptors, using soluble CD4 antibodies, inhibits the capacity of resting T cells to respond to physiological stimuli.[52] Thus, a decreased proliferation and lymphokine production was observed upon stimulation with soluble antigens, alloantigens, lectins, and antibodies to TCR/CD3, which was not explained by simple blockade of adhesion to MHC class II.[47,53] One hypothesis is that anti-CD4 binding interferes with the physical proximity between CD4 and TCR/CD3 needed for optimal signal transduction. Alternatively, some authors claim that a "negative signal," whose molecular basis remains elusive, could be transduced upon anti-CD4 binding, independently of TCR/CD3 ligation.[47,50-51,54]

The first pilot trials used mouse antibodies to human CD4 applied to patients presenting with long-standing rheumatoid arthritis, psoriasis, inflammatory bowel disease, or uveitis.[47,55-60] The treatment was well tolerated, only rare cases of mild side effects after the first injection (linked to minor cytokine release) have been reported.[47] The antibodies used essentially induced partial and transient disappearance of circulating CD4+ cells; coating of CD4+ cells was also observed with dose-dependent saturation of CD4 binding sites.[47,55-60] When present, antigenic modulation only affected a minor proportion of CD4 receptors. The results were encouraging in terms of therapeutic effectiveness, but in most cases the effects were short-lasting.[47,55-60]

The drawback in all these trials was the sensitizing effect of the murine monoclonals, which justified trials of humanized CD4 antibodies. Several of the published studies focused on the use of the chimeric cM-T412 antibody (human IgG1). In rheumatoid arthritis results from open studies seemed encouraging especially when cumulative doses of 350–700 mg were used.[61] There were no major signs of acute toxicity reported; some authors describe self-limited adverse events such as fever associated with myalgia, malaise and asymptomatic hypotension that appear to correlate with transient elevations of serum IL-6.[62,63] Mild sensitization was reported in a majority of the patients.[61-63] However, the major problem was that the therapeutic effect could not be confirmed in the context of a large randomized, double-blind placebo controlled study including patients with early rheumatoid arthritis.[64] Also of concern was the very profound and long-lasting CD4+ cell depletion (up to 60% from baseline for over 18-30 months)[65] noted with cM-T412 contrary to what was initially reported with the parental mouse M-T151 anti-CD4 antibody.[60] It has been proposed that apoptosis could mediate, at least in part, this massive depletion.[66]

Results from open pilot studies suggest that CD4 antibody therapy either alone or in combination (i.e., with antibodies to CD52) could be effective in treating severe forms of psoriasis, inflammatory bowel disease, uveitis, and severe vasculitis.[58-59,67-70] One may hope that controlled studies will be actively promoted in these sorts of indications to determine the validity of at least some of these indications.

6.3.2 Antibodies to TNF

The results of a randomized double-blind study have recently been reported showing the effectiveness of a neutralizing antibody to human

TNF in the treatment of rheumatoid arthritis. TNF is one of the various cytokines that are produced in abundance by cells infiltrating synovial membranes from rheumatoid arthritis patients. It was also demonstrated that the production of many of the detected cytokines and mainly IL-1, IL-6, IL-8, and GM-CSF was dependent on the presence of TNF since their levels were significantly decreased when neutralizing antibodies to TNF were added to the *in vitro* cultures.[71] Based on these studies the key role of TNF in rheumatoid arthritis was proposed; the main source of TNF in affected joints was macrophages. The *in vivo* relevance of this hypothesis was validated in two experimental settings. Mice expressing a human TNF transgene develop a chronic arthritis that may be fully prevented by treament with antibodies to TNF.[71] In addition, in a model of collagen type II-induced arthritis in which the animals develop an erosive form of chronic arthritis, CD4 antibodies can prevent disease but are ineffective once the inflammatory and destructive process is established.[71] At variance, neutralizing antibodies to murine TNF applied once the disease has started are able to decrease the severity of objective and histopathological symptoms (e.g., swollen joints, bone erosions).[71] Another unexpected but potentially relevant observation was that in established arthritis combining a suboptimal dose of antibody to TNF, which per se had no significant effect, with CD4 antibody therapy greatly improved paw swelling, limb involvement, and joint erosion. Furthermore, optimal anti-TNF combined with CD4 antibody significantly improved the results obtained with anti-TNF alone.[72] Thus, in this model anti-TNF and anti-CD4 are synergistic in ameliorating established disease. One interpretation of these results is that in order to "sensitize" the system to the effect of T-cell-directed immunointervention it is mandatory to neutralize the inflammation that is the hallmark of self-perpetuating ongoing autoimmunity. In terms of strategy this could be relevant for most autoimmune diseases and not only for established arthritis.

All these data provided the rationale for evaluating the effect of the blocking chimeric (IgG1) antibody to TNF cA2 in patients with long-standing rheumatoid arthritis. Results from the initial phase I/II open trial on 20 patients showed that treatment with cA2 showed no acute toxicity and significant improvement of the clinical and laboratory parameters.[41] Subsequently, results of a multicenter controlled trial including 73 patients provided direct evidence for a significant therapeutic benefit lasting for several weeks after the end of treatment.[42] Some of the patients having disease relapse underwent 2 to 4 cycles of retreatment.[43] Disease flares were sensitive to retreatment but the mean duration of the induced remissions progressively diminished probably due to the appearance of an anti-allotypic sensitization.[43] (See also Chapter 14.)

6.3.3 Antibodies to CD52

CD52 is a low molecular weight (12 amino acids) glycosylphosphatidylinositol (GPI)-anchored protein expressed at the surface of human B cells and T cells as well as monocyte/macrophages.[73] The first rat MAb to CD52, CAMPATH-1, was characterized in 1983[74] and was initially used to deplete mature T cells from bone marrow transplants. A fully reshaped humanized version, CAMPATH-1H (human IgG1), was derived by genetic engineering.[75] (See Chapter 1.) This antibody is highly depleting *in vivo*; CD4+ cells do not return to normal for several consecutive months. Upon the first injection CAMPATH-1H triggers an acute self-limited cytokine release that is the cause for a transient flu-like syndrome. This antibody has been applied in patients with rheumatoid arthritis. At 3 and 6 months of treatment an improvement in the Paulus score was observed in about half of the patients.[77]

Another indication in which CAMPATH-1H seems to be very effective is severe systemic vasculitis.[69-70] The antibody was initially applied to rare forms of vasculitis in which pathogenesis is thought to involve mainly T-cell-mediated mechanisms. Subsequently, patients with Wegener's granulomatosis have also been treated with success. Particularly impressive in this clinical context were the long-term remissions that could be obtained when combining antibodies to CD52 and to CD4.[69-70]

Very promising results have also been obtained in multiple sclerosis.[78] In the vast majority of patients a stabilization of the clinical symptoms has been observed. Over a 6–12 months followup the long-lasting lymphocyte depletion seemed to correlate with a marked decrease in the appearance of new lesions in the central nervous system as assessed by NMR scanning.

As a whole CAMPATH-1H seems quite unique in its capacity to promote long-lasting remission of life-threatening autoimmune diseases that are unresponsive to conventional treatments. Results from ongoing trials will help to draw more definite conclusions.

6.4 LESSONS FROM EXPERIMENTAL MODELS: IS IT POSSIBLE TO RESTORE SELF-TOLERANCE IN OVERT AUTOIMMUNITY?

Autoimmune diseases may be induced by immunizing animals with more or less purified antigenic preparations from various organs in the presence of complete Freunds adjuvant. Thus, experimental allergic encephalomyelitis, thyroiditis, or myasthenia are induced upon the immunization with myelin basic protein, thyroglobulin, or acethylcholine receptor. Much effort has been devoted to device strategies to specifically prevent these disorders, namely to restore self-tolerance.

Several of the strategies proposed use the administration of the antigen itself under particular conditions. Thus, injecting thyroglobulin to normal mice precludes further development of experimental thyroiditis by injecting the antigen in complete Freunds adjuvant. Similarly, one may prevent experimental allergic encephalomyelitis by pretreating the animals with myelin basic protein in incomplete Freunds adjuvant. In addition, it was recently shown that some routes of administration including intrathymic and oral delivery are particularly favorable for inducing tolerance.[79] This was initially shown in the case of induced autoimmune diseases and was subsequently extended to spontaneous autoimmune diseases. Thus, in non-obese diabetic (NOD) mice that spontaneously develop a T-cell-mediated autoimmune insulin-dependent diabetes (IDDM), disease development is prevented by the oral, intravenous, or intrathymic delivery of some of the putative autoantigens, i.e., glutamic acid decarboxylase (GAD), insulin, hsp60.[80]

These models have been an extremely rich source of fundamental information but one may still question their direct clinical application. There are two main reasons for that. First, in most human autoimmune diseases the triggering autoantigen(s) are ill defined. Second, the strategies we alluded to are mostly effective in preventing but not in reversing established autoimmunity which is the situation one must face in the clinic.

At this point I would like to discuss in some detail recent and somewhat unexpected data obtained in NOD mice which suggest that MAbs to T cells, and in particular to CD3, are very promising tools to restore self-tolerance in established autoimmunity.

NOD mice, originally described by Makino et al.[81] are an accurate experimental model of human IDDM. Overt metabolic disturbances (glycosuria and hyperglycemia) spontaneously appear by 15 weeks of age and are preceeded by a progressive infiltration of the islets of Langerhans' with mononuclear cells termed "insulitis."[81] Insulitis appears by 5 weeks of age and is observed both in NOD males and females. Depending on the colony, the cumulative incidence of overt IDDM reaches 60–80% in females and 10–80% in males. There is compelling evidence to confirm the essential role of T-cell-mediated immunity in the pathogenesis of IDDM: (1) neonatal thymectomy prevents the onset of disease[82] and athymic NOD nude mice are free of insulitis and IDDM,[83] (2) IDDM can be adoptively transferred to NOD neonates, irradiated adult NOD mice and, more recently, to athymic NOD nude mice, by injection of splenic T cells from diabetic animals; both CD4+ and CD8+ lymphocytes are needed to achieve effective transfer of disease,[80,84] and (3) different immunointervention strategies specific for T cells are effective in preventing IDDM.[80]

A number of immunosuppressive agents have been shown to prevent IDDM in NOD mice when administered before the onset of the insulitis and/or the clinical manifestations.[80] These include cyclosporin A[85] and different MAbs such as, anti-CD3,[86] anti-CD4,[87] and anti-T-cell receptor (TcR) αβ.[88] In contrast, the treatment of mice with established metabolic disease, which is the situation encountered in clinical practice, still represents a major challenge. A recent report by Maki et al.[89] showed that stable remission of overt IDDM could be achieved by complete *in vivo* T-cell debulking, induced by treatment with a rabbit anti-lymphocyte polyclonal antiserum or a mixture of depleting antibodies to CD4 and CD8 at high doses (approximately 5 mg cumulated MoAb dose/mouse), applied within 14 days of disease onset.[89] In this study, the profound and prolonged T-cell depletion that was required to achieve the long-term remission totally precludes applying this protocol to the clinical situation.

CD3 antibodies are potent immunosuppressants that essentially act by reversibly clearing CD3/TCR complexes due to the antigenic modulation they promote.[90-92] Low-dose anti-CD3 treatment is thus particularly adapted to short-term immunosuppression as it avoids the long-term T-cell depletion. We first determined the dose of anti-CD3 (145 2C11, hamster IgG1) that was well tolerated by adult male and female NOD mice of various ages. The poor tolerance, in adult mice of most strains, of the first anti-CD3 injections is in fact related to a massive cell activation and cytokine release which it promotes.[93] A dose of 5–20 μg was defined.[30] We then assessed the immunosuppressive efficacy of this dose by testing its capacity to influence the course of established spontaneous insulitis in NOD mice. Spontaneous diabetes in our breeding colony appears at 15–28 weeks of age, and is preceded by insulitis which develops by 5–8 weeks. Although more than 80% of males and females show signs of insulitis by 10 weeks of age, only 10–15% of males normally become diabetic, compared with 50–60% of females at 25 weeks. A 5-day course of anti-CD3 (5 μg/day) in 10-week-old NOD females induced a major reduction of the insulitis. By the time of the last injection, only 27.5% of the islets examined showed insulitis, as compared to 59% in the control group. This effect was transient, disappearing within two weeks of the last injection.[30]

The same protocol was used to determine whether anti-CD3 could stop the progression of spontaneous ongoing autoimmune IDDM.[30] Overtly diabetic mice (glycemia >4 g/l) were randomized to receive either anti-CD3 or irrelevant hamster immunoglobulins. Diabetes regressed in 64–80% of the mice treated with anti-CD3, as reflected by the disappearance of glycosuria and a return to normal glycemia. The event was significantly more frequent than spontaneous remission in control NOD mice treated with the irrelevant hamster immunoglobulins. The anti-CD3-induced remissions presented a number of unexpected features: (1) 2–4 weeks were required for the effect to occur, while the reversal of spontaneous insulitis is far more rapid; (2) the effect was durable (until sacrifice at > 4 months); (3) the effect was specific for β-cell-associated antigens, since mice showing anti-CD3-induced remission rejected histoincompatible skin grafts normally while they did not destroy syngeneic islet grafts, unlike control untreated overtly diabetic NOD females; (4) remission was associated with only partial and transient T-cell depletion; CD3+ cell counts returned to normal 5–10 days after the end of treatment, i.e., 1–3 weeks before remissions started to occur; and (5) clinical remission was maintained despite the persistence of CD3+ αβ+ CD4+ and CD8+ insulitis.[30] Our results provide the first indication that a short course of anti-CD3 given alone can induce long-term and possibly permanent remission from spontaneous autoimmune diabetes in adult mice with active disease. The effect was obtained at a very advanced stage of the pathologic process, when more than 70% of β cells had been destroyed.

As a whole these data provide the first evidence that tolerance may be restored in the context of overt autoimmunity by means of T-cell-specific MAbs and in the absence of exogenous antigen administration.

6.5 CONCLUSIONS

The future for MAbs is exciting as enormous progress has been made in the last 15 years and it is likely that before a similar time period has elapsed they will have become standard tools, no longer shrouded in mystique, in various clinical settings. Despite the different problems surrounding their production and preclinical/clinical development (i.e., high cost, side effects namely, acute cytokine-related syndrome, xenosensitization), continued effort in pursuing the study of therapeutic MAbs appears worthwhile. With the development of humanized antibodies their potential therapeutic uses are set to expand. Already they have spread from the field of transplantation to the fields of autoimmunity, infectious diseases, and cancer.

Moreover, from a more fundamental point of view, an understanding of the molecular basis of the unique tolerogenic properties of some MAbs would clear the way for development of more easily accessible therapeutic strategies, i.e., simple chemicals or recombinant receptor agonist and/or antagonist ligands that would mimic the desired therapeutic effect. The real challenge for the future for both immunologists and pharmacologists, will be to dissect the intimate molecular and cellular mechanisms through which antibodies express these subtle modulatory effects.

REFERENCES

1. Schwartz, R. H., Immunological tolerance, in *Fundamental Immunology*, Paul, W. E., Ed., Raven Press Ltd., New York, 1993, 677.
2. Schluesner, H. J. and Wekerle, H., Autoaggressive T lymphocyte lines recognizing the encephalitogenic region of myelin basic protein: *in vitro* selection from unprimed rat T lymphocyte populations, *J. Immunol.*, 135, 3128, 1985.
3. Burns, J., Rosenzweig, A., Zweiman, B., and Lisak, R. P., Isolation of myelin basic protein-reactive T-cell lines from normal human blood, *Cell. Immunol.*, 81, 435, 1983.
4. Jones, L. A., Chin, L. T., Longo, D. L., and Kruisbeek, A. M., Peripheral clonal elimination of functional T cells, *Science*, 250, 4988, 1990.
5. Schwartz, R. H., A cell culture model for T lymphocyte clonal anergy, *Science*, 248, 1349, 1990.
6. Mason, D. and Fowell, D., T-cell subsets in autoimmunity, *Curr. Opin. Immunol.*, 4, 728, 1992.
7. Jensen, P. E. and Kapp, J. A., Genetics of insulin-specific helper and suppressor T cells in non-responder mice, *J. Immunol.*, 135, 2990, 1985.
8. Miller, R. G., The veto phenomenon and T cell regulation, *Immunol. Today*, 7, 112, 1986.
9. Schwartz, R., Autoimmunity in *Fundamental Immunology*, Paul, W. E., Ed., Raven Press Ltd., New York, 1993, 1033.
10. Cosimi, A. B., Colvin, R. B., Burton, R. C., Rubin, R. H., Goldstein, G., Kung, P. C., Hansen, W. P., Delmonico, F. L., and Russell, P. S., Use of monoclonal antibodies to T-cell subsets for immunologic monitoring and treatment in recipients of renal allografts, *N. Engl. J. Med.*, 305, 308, 1981.
11. Cosimi, A. B., Burton, R. C., Colvin, R. B., Goldstein, G., Delmonico, F. L., Laquaglia, M. P., Tolkoff-Rubin, N., Rubin, R. H., Herrin, J. T., and Russell, P. S., Treatment of acute renal allograft rejection with OKT3 monoclonal antibody, *Transplantation*, 32, 535, 1981.
12. Nicolls, M. R., Aversa, G. G., Pearce, N. W., Spinelli, A., Berger, M. F., Gurley, K. E., and Hall, B. M., Induction of long-term specific tolerance to allografts in rats by therapy with an anti-CD3-like monoclonal antibody, *Transplantation*, 55, 459, 1993.
13. Wofsy, D., Mayes, D. C., Woodcock, J., and Seaman, W. E., Inhibition of humoral immunity *in vivo* by monoclonal antibody to L3T4: studies with soluble antigens in intact mice, *J. Immunol.*, 135, 1698, 1985.
14. Qin, S. X., Wise, M., Cobbold, S. P., Leong, L., Kong, Y. C., Parnes, J. R., and Waldmann, H., Induction of tolerance in peripheral T cells with monoclonal antibodies, *Eur. J. Immunol.*, 20, 2737, 1990.
15. Weyand, C. M., Goronzy, J., Swarztrauber, K., and Fathman, C. G., Immunosuppression by anti-CD4 treatment *in vivo*. Cellular and humoral responses to alloantigens, *Transplantation*, 47, 1039, 1989.
16. Brostoff, S.W. and Mason, D.W., Experimental allergic encephalomyelitis: successful treatment *in vivo* with a monoclonal antibody that recognizes T helper cells, *J. Immunol.*, 133, 1938, 1984.
17. Christadoss, P. and Dauphinee, M. J., Immunotherapy for myasthenia gravis: a murine model, *J. Immunol.*, 136, 2437, 1986.
18. Wofsy, D. and Seaman, W. E., Reversal of advanced murine lupus in NZB/NZW F1 mice by treatment with monoclonal antibody to L3T4, *J. Immunol.*, 138, 3247, 1987.
19. Waldor, M. K., Sriram, S., Hardy, R., Herzenberg, L. A., Lanier, L., Lim, M., and Steinman, L., Reversal of experimental allergic encephalomyelitis with monoclonal antibody to a T-cell subset marker, *Science*, 227, 415, 1985.

20. Shizuru, J. A., Taylor-Edwards, C., Banks, B. A., Gregory, A. K., and Fathman, C. G., Immunotherapy of the nonobese diabetic mouse: treatment with an antibody to T-helper lymphocytes, *Science*, 240, 659, 1988.
21. Pearson, T. C., Madsen, J. C., Larsen, C. P., Morris, P. J., and Wood, K. J., Induction of transplantation tolerance in adults using donor antigen and anti-CD4 monoclonal antibody, *Transplantation*, 54, 475, 1992.
22. Qin, S., Cobbold, S. P., Pope, H., Elliott, J., Kioussis, D., Davies, J., and Waldmann, H., "Infectious" transplantation tolerance, *Science*, 259, 974, 1993.
23. Isobe, M., Yagita, H., Okumura, K., and Ihara, A., Specific acceptance of cardiac allograft after treatment with antibodies to ICAM-1 and LFA-1, *Science*, 255, 1125, 1992.
24. Linsley, P. S., Wallace, P. M., Johnson, J., Gibson, M. G., Greene, J. L., Ledbetter, J. A., Singh, C., and Tepper, M. A., Immunosuppression *in vivo* by a soluble form of the CTLA-4 T cell activation molecule, *Science*, 257, 792, 1992.
25. Lenschow, D. J., Zeng, Y., Thistlethwaite, J. R., Montag, A., Brady, W., Gibson, M. G., Linsley, P. S., and Bluestone, J. A., Long-term survival of xenogeneic pancreatic islet grafts induced by CTLA4Ig, *Science*, 257, 789, 1992.
26. Lin, H., Bolling, S. F., Linsley, P. S., Wei, R. Q., Gordon, D., Thompson, C. B., and Turka, L. A., Long-term acceptance of major histocompatibility complex mismatched cardiac allografts induced by CTLA4Ig plus donor-specific transfusion, *J. Exp. Med.*, 178, 1801, 1993.
27. Benjamin, R. J., Cobbold, S. P., Clark, M. R., and Waldmann, H., Tolerance to rat monoclonal antibodies. Implications for serotherapy, *J. Exp. Med.*, 163, 1539, 1986.
28. Benjamin, R. J. and Waldmann, H., Induction of tolerance by monoclonal antibody therapy, *Nature*, 320, 449, 1986.
29. Gutstein, N. L., Seaman, W. E., Scott, J. H., and Wofsy, D., Induction of immune tolerance by administration of monoclonal antibody to L3T4, *J. Immunol.*, 137, 1127, 1986.
30. Chatenoud, L., Thervet, E., Primo, J., and Bach, J. F., Anti-CD3 induces long-term remission of overt autoimmunity in non-obese diabetic mice, *Proc. Natl. Acad. Sci. U.S.A.*, 91, 123, 1994.
31. Boitard, C., Bendelac, A., Richard, M. F., Carnaud, C., and Bach, J. F., Prevention of diabetes in non-obese diabetic mice by anti-I-A antibodies: Transfer of protection by splenic T cells, *Proc. Natl. Acad. Sci. U.S.A.*, 85, 9719, 1988.
32. Sempe, P., Bedossa, P., Richard, M. F., Bach, J. F., and Boitard, C., Anti-alpha/beta T cell receptor monoclonal antibody provides an efficient therapy for autoimmune diabetes in nonobese diabetic (NOD) mice, *Eur. J. Immunol.*, 21, 1163, 1991.
33. Springer, T. A., Dustin, M. L., Kishimoto, T. K., and Marlin, S. D., The lymphocyte function-associated LFA-1, CD2, and LFA-3 molecules: cell adhesion receptors of the immune system, *Annu. Rev. Immunol.*, 5, 223,1987.
34. Anlot, P., The clinical and experimental use of monoclonal antibodies to the IL-2 receptor, in *Monoclonal Antibodies in Transplantation*, Chatenoud, L., Ed., Landes Company, Austin, 1995, 53.
35. Linsley, P. S., Brady, W., Urnes, M., Grosmaire, L. S., Damle, N. K., and Ledbetter, J. A., CTLA-4 is a second receptor for the B cell activation antigen B7, *J. Exp. Med.*, 174, 561, 1991.
36. van den Eertwegh, A. J., Noelle, R. J., Roy, M., Shepherd, D. M., Aruffo, A., Ledbetter, J. A., Boersma, W. J., and Claassen, E., *In vivo* CD40-gp39 interactions are essential for thymus-dependent humoral immunity. I. *In vivo* expression of CD40 ligand, cytokines, and antibody production delineates sites of cognate T-B cell interactions, *J. Exp. Med.*, 178, 1555, 1993.
37. Finck, B. K., Linsley, P. S., and Wofsy, D., Treatment of murine lupus with CTLA4Ig, *Science*, 265, 1225, 1994.

38. Ozmen, L., Gribaudo, G., Fountoulakis, M., Gentz, R., Landolfo, S., and Garotta, G., Mouse soluble IFN gamma receptor as IFN gamma inhibitor. Distribution, antigenicity, and activity after injection in mice, *J. Immunol.*, 150, 2698, 1993.
39. Dinarello, C. A. and Thompson, R. C., Blocking IL-1: interleukin 1 receptor antagonist *in vivo* and *in vitro*, *Immunol. Today*, 12, 404, 1991.
40. Peppel, K., Crawford, D., and Beutler, B., A tumor necrosis factor (TNF) receptor-IgG heavy chain chimeric protein as a bivalent antagonist of TNF activity, *J. Exp. Med.*, 174, 1483, 1991.
41. Elliott, M. J., Maini, R. N., Feldmann, M., Long-Fox, A., Charles, P., Katsikis, P., Brennan, F. M., Walker, J., Bijl, H., Grayeb, J., and Woody, J., Treatment of rheumatoid arthritis with chimeric monoclonal antibodies to tumor necrosis factor alpha, *Arthritis Rheum.*, 36, 1681, 1993.
42. Elliott, M. J., Maini, R. N., Feldmann, M., Kalden, J. R., Antony, C., Smolen, J. S., Leeb, B., Breedveld, F. C., Macfarlane, J. D., Bijl, H., and Woody, J., Randomised double-blind comparison of chimeric monoclonal antibody to tumor necrosis factor alpha (cA2) versus placebo in rheumatoid arthritis, *Lancet*, 344, 1105, 1994.
43. Elliott, M. J., Maini, R. N., Feldmann, M., Long-Fox, A., Charles, P., Bijl, H., Grayeb, J., and Woody, J., Repeated therapy with monoclonal antibody to tumor necrosis factor alpha (cA2) in patients with rheumatoid arthritis, *Lancet*, 344, 1125, 1994.
44. Mosmann, T. R. and Coffman, R. L., TH1 and TH2 cells: different patterns of lymphokine secretion lead to different functional properties, *Annu. Rev. Immunol.*, 7, 145, 1989.
45. Reiner, S. L. and Seder, R. A., T helper cell differentiation in immune response, *Curr. Opin. Immunol.*, 7, 360, 1995.
46. Cobbold, S., Adatis, E., Marshall, S., Waldman, H., Mechanisms of peripheral tolerance and suppression induced by monoclonal antibodies to CD4 and CD8, *Immunol. Rev.*, in press.
47. Emmrich, F. and Bach, J. F., Therapeutic anti-CD4 antibodies, in *T-Cell-Directed Immunointervention*, Bach, J. F., Ed., Blackwell, Oxford, 1993, 176.
48. Gilkeson, G. S., Spurney, R., Coffman, T. M., Kurlander, R., Ruiz, P., and Pisetsky, D. S., Effect of anti-CD4 antibody treatment on inflammatory arthritis in MRL-lpr/lpr mice, *Clin. Immunom. Immunopathol.*, 64, 166, 1992.
49. Julius, M., Maroun, C. R., and Haughn, L., Distinct roles for CD4 and CD8 as coreceptors in antigen receptor signalling, *Immunol. Today*, 14, 177, 1993.
50. Anderson, P., Blue, M. L., and Schlossman, S. F., Comodulation of CD3 and CD4. Evidence for a specific association between CD4 and approximately 5% of the CD3:T cell receptor complexes on helper T lymphocytes, *J. Immunol.*, 140, 1732, 1988.
51. Emmrich, F., Rieber, P., Kurrle, R., and Eichmann, K., Selective stimulation of human T lymphocyte subsets by heteroconjugates of antibodies to the T cell receptor and to subset-specific differentiation antigens, *Eur. J. Immunol.*, 18, 645, 1988.
52. Biddison, W. E., Rao, P. E., Talle, M. A., Goldstein, G., and Shaw, S., Possible involvement of the OKT4 molecule in T cell recognition of class II HLA antigens. Evidence from studies of cytotoxic T lymphocytes specific for SB antigens, *J. Exp. Med.*, 156, 1065, 1982.
53. Wilde, D. B., Marrack, P., Kappler, J., Dialynas, D. P., and Fitch, F. W., Evidence implicating L3T4 in class II MHC antigen reactivity; monoclonal antibody GK1.5 (anti-L3T4a) blocks class II MHC antigen-specific proliferation, release of lymphokines, and binding by cloned murine helper T lymphocyte lines, *J. Immunol.*, 131, 2178, 1983.
54. Bank, I. and Chess, L., Perturbation of the T4 molecule transmits a negative signal to T cells, *J. Exp. Med.*, 162, 1294, 1985.

55. Herzog, C., Walker, C., Muller, W., Rieber, P., Reiter, C., Riethmuller, G., Wassmer, P., Stockinger, H., Madic, O., and Pichler, W. J., Anti-CD4 antibody treatment of patients with rheumatoid arthritis: I. Effect on clinical course and circulating T cells, *J. Autoimmun.*, 2, 627, 1989.
56. Horneff, G., Burmester, G. R., Emmrich, F., and Kalden, J. R., Treatment of rheumatoid arthritis with an anti-CD4 monoclonal antibody, *Arthritis Rheum.*, 34, 129, 1991.
57. Wendling, D., Widjenes, J., Racadot, E., and Morel-Fourrier, B., Therapeutic use of monoclonal anti-CD4 antibody in rheumatoid arthritis, *J. Rheumatol.*, 18, 325, 1991.
58. Nicolas, J. F., Chamchick, N., Thivolet, J., Widjenes, J., Morel, P., and Revillard, J. P., CD4 antibody treatment of severe psoriasis, *Lancet*, 338, 321, 1991.
59. Emmrich, J., Seyfarth, M., Fleig, W. E., and Emmrich, F., Treatment of inflammatory bowel disease with anti-CD4 monoclonal antibody, *Lancet*, 338, 570, 1991.
60. Reiter, C., Kakavand, B., Rieber, P., Schattenkirchner, M., Riethmuller, G., and Kruger, K., Treatment of rheumatoid arthritis with monoclonal CD4 antibody M-T151. Clinical results and immunopharmacologic effects in an open study, including repeated administration, *Arthritis Rheum.*, 34, 525, 1991.
61. van-der-Lubbe, P. A., Reiter, C., Breedveld, F. C., Kruger, K., Schattenkirchner, M., Sanders, M. E., and Riethmuller, G., Chimeric CD4 monoclonal antibody cM-T412 as a therapeutic approach to rheumatoid arthritis, *Arthritis Rheum.*, 36, 1375, 1993.
62. Moreland, L. W., Pratt, P. W., Sanders, M. E., and Koopman W. J., Experience with a chimeric monoclonal anti-CD4 antibody in the treatment of refractory rheumatoid arthritis, *Clin. Exp. Rheumatol.*, 11, S153, 1993.
63. van-der-Lubbe, P. A., Reiter, C., Miltenburg, A. M., Kruger, K., de-Ruyter, A. N., Rieber, E. P., Bijl, H., Riethmuller, G., and Breedveld, F. C., Treatment of rheumatoid arthritis with a chimeric CD4 monoclonal antibody (cM-T412): immunopharmacological aspects and mechanisms of action, *Scand. J. Immunol.*, 39, 286, 1994.
64. van-der-Lubbe, P. A., Dijkmans, B. A., Markusse, H. M., Nassander, U., and Breedveld, F. C., A randomized, double-blind, placebo controlled study of CD4 monoclonal antibody therapy in early rheumatoid arthritis, *Arthritis Rheum.*, 38, 1097, 1995
65. Moreland, L. W., Pratt, P. W., Bucy, R. P., Jackson, B. S., Feldman, J. W., and Koopman, W. J., Treatment of refractory rheumatoid arthritis with a chimeric anti-CD4 monoclonal antibody. Long-term followup of CD4+ T cell counts, *Arthritis Rheum.*, 37, 834, 1994.
66. Choy, E. H., Adjaye, J., Forrest, L., Kingsley, G. H., and Panayi, G. S., Chimaeric anti-CD4 monoclonal antibody cross-linked by monocyte Fc gamma receptor mediates apoptosis of human CD4 lymphocytes, *Eur. J. Immunol.*, 23, 2676, 1993.
67. Prinz, J., Braun-Falco, O., Meurer, M., Daddona, P., Reiter, C., Rieber, P., and Riethmuller, G., Chimaeric CD4 monoclonal antibody in treatment of generalised pustular psoriasis, *Lancet*, 338, 320, 1991.
68. Morel, P., Revillard, J. P., Nicolas, J. F., Widjenes, J., and Thivolet, J., Anti-CD4 monoclonal antibody therapy in severe psoriasis, *J. Autoimmun.*, 5, 465, 1992.
69. Mathieson, P. W., Cobbold, S. P., Hale, G., Clark, M. R., Oliveira, D. B., Lockwood, C. M., and Waldmann, H., Monoclonal-antibody therapy in systemic vasculitis, *N. Engl. J. Med.*, 323, 250, 1990.
70. Lockwood, C. M., Thyru S., Isaacs, J. D., Hale, G., and Waldmann, H., Long-term remission of intractable systemic vasculitis with monoclonal antibody therapy, *Lancet*, 341, 1620, 1993.
71. Brennan, F. M., Cope, A. P., Katsikis, P., Gibbons, D. L., Maini, R. N., and Feldmann, M., Selective immunosuppression of tumour necrosis factor-alpha in rheumatoid arthritis, in *Selective Immunosuppression: Basic Concepts and Clinical Applications*, Adorini, L., Ed., Karger A.G., Basel, 1995, 48.

72. Williams, R. O., Mason, L. J., Feldmann, M., and Maini, R. N., Synergy between anti-CD4 and anti-tumor necrosis factor in the amelioration of established collagen-induced arthritis, *Proc. Natl. Acad. Sci. U.S.A.*, 91, 2762, 1994.
73. Xia, M. Q., Tone, M., Packman, L., Hale, G., and Waldmann, H., Characterization of the CAMPATH-1 (CDw52) antigen: biochemical analysis and cDNA cloning reveal an unusually small peptide backbone, *Eur. J. Immunol.*, 21, 1677, 1991.
74. Hale, G., Bright, S., Chumbley, G., Hoang, T., Metcalf, D., Munro, A., and Waldmann, H., Removal of T cells from bone marrow for transplantation: a monoclonal antilymphocyte antibody that fixes human complement, *Blood*, 62, 873, 1983.
75. Riechmann, L., Clark, M., Waldmann, H., and Winter, G., Reshaping human antibodies for therapy, *Nature*, 332, 323, 1988.
76. Weinblatt, M. E., Coblyn, J., Maier, A., Anderson, R., Helfgott, S., Thurmond, L., Spreen, W., and Johnston, J., Continued lymphocyte suppression following single dose Mab therapy with CAMPATH®-1H: A 20 month followup, *Arthritis Rheum.*, 37, S420, 1994.
77. Isaacs, J. D., Watts, R. A., Hazleman, B. L., Hale, G., Keogan, M. T., Cobbold, S. P., and Waldmann, H., Humanised monoclonal antibody therapy for rheumatoid arthritis, *Lancet*, 340, 748, 1992.
78. Moreau, T., Thorpe, J., Miller, D., Moseley, L., Hale, G., Waldmann, H., Clayton, D., Wing, M., Scolding, N., and Compston, A., Preliminary evidence from magnetic resonance imaging for reduction in disease activity after lymphocyte depletion in multiple sclerosis, *Lancet*, 344, 298, 1994. [Published erratum appears in Lancet 1994 344,486, 1994.]
79. Weiner, H. L., Zhang, Z. J., Khoury, S. J., Miller, A., AlSabbagh, A., Brod, S. A., Lider, O., Higgins, P., Sobel, R, Nussenblat, R. B., and Haffler, D., Antigen driven peripheral tolerance. Suppression of organ specific autoimmune diseases by oral administration of autoantigens, *Ann. N. Y. Acad. Sci.*, 636, 227, 1991.
80. Bach, J. F., Insulin-dependent diabetes mellitus as an autoimmune disease, *Endocrine Rev.*, 15, 516, 1994.
81. Makino, S., Kunimoto, K., Muraoka, Y., Mizushima, Y., Katagiri, K., and Tochino, Y., Breeding of a non-obese diabetic strain, *Exp. Anim.*, 29, 1, 1980.
82. Ogawa, M., Maruyama, T., and Hasegawa, T., The inhibitory effect of neonatal thymectomy on the incidence of insulitis in NOD mice, *Biomed. Res.*, 6, 103, 1985.
83. Yagi, H., Matsumoto, M., Kunimoto, K., Kawagushi, J., Makino, S., and Harada, M., Analysis of the roles of CD4+ and CD8+ T cells in autoimmune diabetes of NOD mice using transfer to NOD athymic nude mice, *Eur. J. Immunol.*, 22, 2387, 1992.
84. Wicker, L. S., Miller, B. J., and Mullen, Y., Transfer of autoimmune diabetes mellitus with splenocytes from non-obese diabetic (NOD) mice, *Diabetes*, 35, 855, 1986.
85. Mori, Y., Suko, M., Okudiara, H., Matsuba, I., Tsuruoka, S., Sasaki, A., Yokoyama, H., Tanase, T., Shida, T., Nishimura, M., Terada, E., and Ikeda Y., Preventive effect of cyclosporin on diabetes in NOD mice, *Diabetologia*, 29, 244, 1986.
86. Hayward, A. R., and Shreiber, M., Neonatal injection of CD3 antibody into non-obese diabetic mice reduces the incidence of insulitis and diabetes, *J. Immunol.*, 143, 1555, 1989.
87. Shizuru, J. A., Taylor-Edwards, C., Banks, B. A., Gregory, A. K., and Fathman, C. G., Immunotherapy of the nonobese diabetic mouse: treatment with an antibody to helper T cells, *Science*, 240, 659, 1988.
88. Sempé, P., Bédossa, P., Richard, M. F., Villà, M. C., Bach, J. F., and Boitard, C., Anti α/β(T-cell receptor monoclonal antibody provides an efficient therapy for autoimmune diabetes in nonobese diabetic (NOD) mice, *Eur. J. Immunol.*, 21, 1163, 1991.
89. Maki, T., Ichikwa, T., Blanco, R., and Porter, J., Long-term abrogation of autoimmune diabetes in nonobese diabetic mice by immunotherapy with anti-lymphocyte serum, *Proc. Natl. Acad. Sci. U.S.A.*, 89, 3434,1992.

90. Hirsch, R., Eckhaus, M., Auchincloss, H., Jr., Sachs, D. H., and Bluestone, J. A., Effect of *in vivo* administration of anti-T3 monoclonal antibody on T cell function in mice. I. Immunosuppression of transplantation responses, *J. Immunol.*, 140, 3766, 1988.
91. Chatenoud, L., and Bach, J. F., Antigenic modulation — a major mechanism of antibody action, *Immunol Today*, 5, 20, 1984.
92. Chatenoud, L., Baudrihaye, M. F., Kreis, H., Goldstein, G., Schindler, J., and Bach, J. F., Human *in vivo* antigenic modulation induced by the anti-T cell OKT3 monoclonal antibody, *Eur. J. Immunol.*, 12, 979, 1982.
93. Ferran, C., Dy, M., Sheehan, K., Merite, S., Schreiber, R., Landais, P., Grau, G., Bluestone, J., Bach, J. F., and Chatenoud, L., Inter-mouse strain differences in the *in vivo* anti-CD3 induced cytokine release, *Clin. Exp. Immunol.*, 86, 537, 1991.

Chapter 7

MONOCLONAL ANTIBODIES IN TRANSPLANTATION

Maria-Luisa Alegre

CONTENTS

0-8493-8547-4/97/$0.00+$.50

7.1 ORGAN ALLOGRAFT REJECTION

7.1.1 Mechanisms of Graft Recognition and Rejection

Rejection of organ allografts involves the participation of multiple cell types, including CD4+ and CD8+ T lymphocytes and antigen presenting cells (APCs). The alloantigen can be recognized by T cells either directly on graft APCs or indirectly on APCs from the host, for example, after phagocytosis of debris of the graft. Recognition of alloantigen depends on the interaction between an antigenic peptide bound to the major histocompatibility complex (MHC) molecules expressed on APCs and the T-cell receptor (TCR) complex on T cells. The TCR is composed of a disulfide-linked heterodimer (α and β or γ and δ) noncovalently associated with a group of low molecular weight proteins designated CD3. The CD3 molecules are responsible for the transduction of a signal (signal 1) to the T cell upon binding of the TCR to its ligand,[1] whereas the CD4 or CD8 molecules are coreceptor proteins that are specialized in the recognition of class II or class I MHC molecules, respectively. In addition to the interaction of the TCR with the MHC-peptide complex, other surface molecules on T cells and APCs have been identified that deliver a second signal (signal 2) to the T lymphocyte. These surface glycoproteins have been termed costimulatory molecules (Figure 1). The interactions most studied are those of CD28 on T cells with members of the B7 family on APCs.[2-4] In the absence of signal 2, ligation of the TCR on T lymphocytes results in T-cell anergy, a state in which T cells are unable to produce IL-2 and to proliferate upon restimulation.[5] In contrast, when host CD4+ T lymphocytes receive both signal 1 and 2 from graft or host APCs that express costimulatory molecules, they are induced to secrete IL-2[2] which acts, in part, as an autocrine growth factor through its binding to IL-2 receptor (IL-2R, of which CD25 is one of the chains). CD4+ T lymphocytes therefore proliferate, differentiate, and in turn activate other cell types including CD8+ cytolytic T cells and natural killer cells (NK cells) that also directly participate in graft rejection.[6] Finally, other surface glycoproteins play an important role in allograft rejection, as they are involved in lymphocyte migration into the allograft, as well as in stabilization of the interaction between T cells and APCs and intracellular signaling. Leukocyte function-associated molecule-1 (LFA-1) and intercellular adhesion molecule-1 (ICAM-1) participate in such critical combinations.[7]

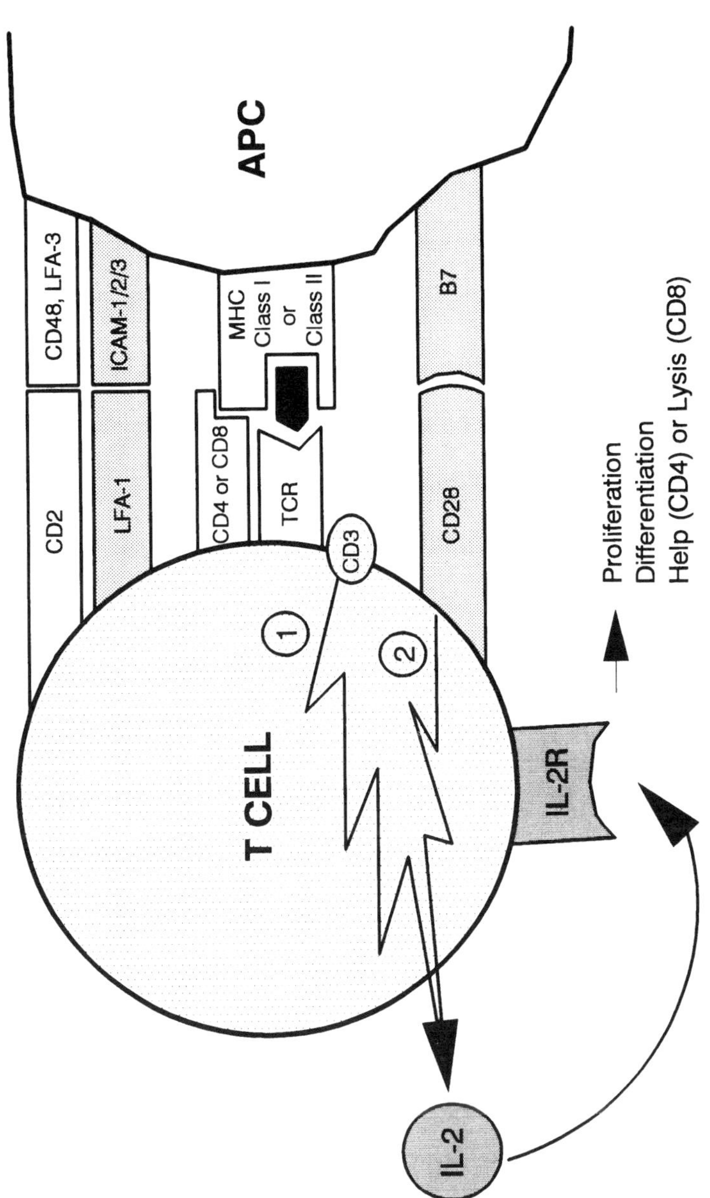

FIGURE 1
Molecular interactions involved in T-cell allorecognition. Schematic illustration of molecules used as targets of MAbs to achieve immunosuppression. 1 and 2 represent the two signals involved in T-cell activation and IL-2 production.

The efforts toward developing immunosuppressive MAbs have been aimed, consequently, at interrupting these essential interactions for the initial process of T-cell activation, and surface molecules such as the TCR, CD3, CD2, CD4, CD8, CD25, MHC, LFA-I, ICAM-1, and B7 have been targeted (Figure 1). Thus, existing MAbs can be divided into three categories: those directed at a surface molecule expressed on all T cells, such as the TCR, CD3 or CDw52 molecules; those reaching a subset of T cells such as CD4+ or CD8+ T cells, or activated T lymphocytes expressing CD25; and those targeting adhesion or costimulatory molecules such as CD2, LFA-1, ICAM-1, or B7. Treatment with pan-T-cell MAbs may result in depressed immune responses not only against the grafted organ but also against viruses or tumor antigens. Therefore, research efforts are aimed toward the development of MAbs that will induce indefinite graft-specific tolerance, while respecting immune responses against all other antigens.

MAbs have been used both for preventing and treating allograft rejection, but some MAbs (such as anti-LFA-1) seem to be effective only for prophylaxis of rejection rather than to treat an ongoing rejection episode. The initial combination therapies that included an immunosuppressive MAb started with OKT3 in 1980. The first generation MAbs, still administered to patients today, are of mouse or rat origin. These MAbs are of limited utility inasmuch as they can induce a strong humoral response (HAMA) upon repeated injections, preventing their long-term administration in patients. The second generation reagents are "humanized" MAbs that are less immunogenic, although anti-idiotypic antibodies can still arise. Clinical trials using these MAbs in transplantation started in 1993. A third line of investigation has generated humanized MAbs, the use of which is still experimental, that contain point mutations in their Fc portion aimed at reducing side effects dependent on Fc receptor (FcR) binding.

7.1.2 The Importance of Binding to Fc Receptors (FcRs)

The great majority of the MAbs currently in use, whether of murine, rat, or human origin are of the IgG isotype and therefore react potentially not only with their ligand through the Fab portion, but also with FcγRs on APCs or FcγR-bearing cells, through their Fc portion. This interaction has been shown in certain circumstances to activate FcγR+ cells to produce cytokines, or to result in antibody-dependent-cellular cytotoxicity (ADCC).[8-10] Three types of FcγRs react with IgG: FcγRI (CD64, 72 kDa) is a high-affinity receptor that binds IgG monomers and FcγRII (CD32, 40 kDa) and FcγRIII (CD16) are low-affinity receptors that bind to IgG immune complexes. The three types of FcγR are members of the immunoglobulin supergene family. FcγRI is expressed on macrophages, monocytes, and interferon-γ (IFN-γ)-stimulated neutrophils, whereas FcγRII is present on B lymphocytes, macrophages, monocytes, polymorphonuclear cells, and platelets. FcγRIII is found on granulocytes, NK cells, macrophages, and activated monocytes. Human FcγRI reacts preferentially with human IgG1 and IgG3 and mouse IgG2a and IgG3, whereas human FcγRII interacts with human IgG1 and IgG3 and mouse IgG2a, IgG2b, and IgG1. The affinity of Ig isotypes for each subtype of FcγRs varies across species. This reduces the predictability of animal models, because an antibody isotype that proves certain properties in mouse because of its murine FcγR-binding affinity might behave very differently in human patients after binding human FcγRs.[10]

The region comprised of amino acids 234–238 in the C_H2 portion of IgGs has been shown to mediate binding to FcγRs.[11-13] Ollo et al. have demonstrated that the mutation of a single amino acid in the FcγR-binding domain of a murine IgG2b, converting the sequence to that found in murine IgG2a, results in a 100-fold enhancement of the binding to mouse FcγRs.[14] Because FcR-binding is required for crosslinking of ligands by MAbs, mutations performed to reduce their binding capacity to FcRs would be expected to decrease their activating potential. In addition, the glycosylation site at amino acid 297 is also necessary for the binding of IgG to FcγRs to occur, as nonglycosylated antibodies are unable to bind FcγR-bearing cells or to activate complement.[15]

7.1.3 Pan-T-Cell Immunosuppressive MAbs

7.1.3.1 Anti-CD3 MAbs

The injection into transplanted patients of OKT3, a murine IgG2a MAb directed against a conformational epitope expressed by the association of the CD3-ε chain of the TCR complex with CD3-δ or CD3-γ,[16] induces an efficient and rapid immunosuppression by preventing allorecognition as a result of modulation of the TCR from the surface of T lymphocytes and clearance of T cells from the circulation.[17] OKT3 was first used in 1980 by Cosimi et al. to treat renal graft rejection.[18] Since then, OKT3 has been widely administered to treat corticosteroid-resistant organ graft rejection,[19-21] and more recently, as prophylaxis of rejection.[22-25] Its use has allowed prolongation of graft survival as compared with other immunosuppressive therapies. In particular, kidney graft survival has been significantly enhanced in patients receiving OKT3 during the first 14 days after transplantation, as compared with cyclosporin A (CsA).[26] Despite the efficacy of OKT3 therapy as an immunosuppressive agent, major limitations to its administration remain, including a massive cellular activation resulting in severe side effects,[27-29] and the generation of anti-OKT3 MAbs that preclude subsequent treatments with the drug.[30-32] Indeed, the first and sometimes the second administration of OKT3 often induce, within 24 h of the injection, an array of adverse reactions such as high fever, chills, hypotension, headaches, gastrointestinal symptoms, pulmonary edema, transient acute tubular necrosis, hypercoagulability, aseptic meningitis, and even seizures.[27-29,33] This so-called "first-dose reaction" syndrome immediately follows the systemic release of cytokines produced by T cells and FcγR-bearing cells, such as tumor necrosis factor α (TNF-α), interleukin-2 (IL-2), granulocyte-macrophage colony-stimulating factor (GM-CSF), and IFN-γ, that occurs 1 to 3 h after the administration of the MAb.[34-36] The correlation between the release of cytokines and the first-dose reaction syndrome observed after the injection of anti-CD3 MAbs has been hypothesized on the basis of an established role of TNF-α in the toxicity of septic shock in patients, and after lipopolysaccharide (LPS) administration in different animal models.[37,38] Further evidence supporting this correlation has emerged from the reports of side effects induced by recombinant cytokines (IL-2, IFN-γ, and TNF-α) in cancer patients[39-43] that are similar to the adverse reactions observed in transplanted patients receiving OKT3, whose serum contains some of the same cytokines. Indeed, the administration of drugs that reduce the production, or neutralize the activity of some cytokines, such as corticosteroids[44,45] or anti-TNF-α antibodies,[46] has been proven to markedly diminish the severity of the acute toxicity of OKT3. Several pieces of evidence strongly suggest that the cross-linking between T cells and FcγR-bearing cells mediated by OKT3 is responsible for the cellular activation observed after OKT3 therapy (Figure 2).[47-49] In particular, blocking of murine FcγR with the MAb 2.4G2 *in vitro* prevents T-cell proliferation induced by a hamster anti-murine CD3 MAb, 145-2C11,[50] that shares many properties with OKT3 (J. Bluestone and M-L. Alegre, unpublished observations).

The second problem associated with the administration of OKT3 is the fact that multiple injections of OKT3 lead to the appearance of both anti-xenotypic and anti-idiotypic antibodies in about 20% of the patients, despite concomitant treatment with other immunosuppressive agents capable of inhibiting B-cell function, such as corticosteroids or azathioprine.[30-32] This humoral response neutralizes the MAb, thus preventing its efficacy following readministration of the drug. In fact, the activating properties of OKT3 might enhance the humoral response against the MAb by non-specifically activating T cells to produce cytokines, some of which promote B-cell differentiation. Indeed the administration to mice of $F(ab')_2$ fragments of 145-2C11 (anti-CD3),[51] or of a fusion molecule composed of the $F(ab')_2$ fragments of 145-2C11 fused to the low FcγR-affinity murine IgG3 Fc portion, has been shown to

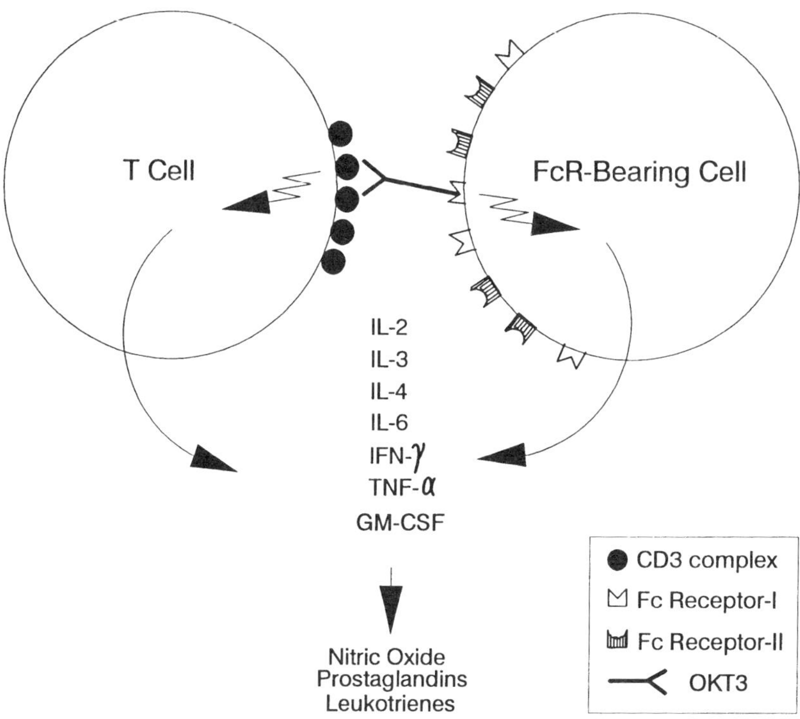

FIGURE 2
Cross-linking triggered by OKT3. Schematic representation of the cross-linking mediated by OKT3 between T cells and FcR-bearing cells, which results in the production of cytokines and other soluble factors.

result in a reduced anti-idiotypic humoral response when compared with that of whole Mab.[52]

To circumvent these problems, humanized OKT3 MAbs have been generated on human IgG4 (the gOKT3-5 MAb) and IgG1 frameworks,[53] the Fc portions of which were subsequently mutated in their C_H2 regions to generate MAbs with a very low affinity for FcγRs.[54] Specifically, the sequence phenylalanine-leucine-glycine-glycine-proline at amino acids 234–238 of the Fc region was transformed into phenylalanine-glutamic acid-glycine-glycine-proline (the Glu-235 MAb) and into alanine-alanine-glycine-glycine-proline (the Ala-Ala-IgG4 MAb). We have confirmed, using *in vitro* binding assays, the reduced capacity of these mutant MAbs to bind to FcγRs+ cell lines. In addition, human peripheral blood leukocytes (PBLs) stimulated by these MAbs *in vitro* were almost completely unable to produce the cytokines TNF-α, IFN-γ, or GM-CSF, or to proliferate. However, we observed similar TCR modulation in PBLs incubated with OKT3, humanized FcγR-binding anti-CD3 MAbs, and mutant humanized MAbs, suggesting that at least some immunosuppressive potential was intact despite lack of FcR binding.[54] We have performed *in vivo* preclinical experiments on SCID mice that are devoid of T and B cells as a result of a rearrangement defect. These animals were first injected intraperitoneally with a suspension of human splenocytes from cadaveric organ donors. Human leukocytes, and in particular T cells, were found to migrate out of the peritoneal cavity and to colonize the blood and the spleen of these animals, which become capable of rejecting allogeneic human foreskin grafts.[55] The administration of OKT3 to these mice was able to impede rejection of the human foreskin. Interestingly, both mitogenic (the 209-IgG1 MAb) and nonmitogenic (the Ala-Ala-IgG4 MAb) humanized anti-CD3 MAbs also prevented allograft rejection in a similar fashion to OKT3, suggesting comparable immunosuppressive properties in this model. In addition, both MAbs achieved a similar level of TCR modulation as OKT3 *in vivo* (Table 1).[56] In contrast, T-cell depletion was more complete after the injection of OKT3 or 209-IgG1 than after that of Ala-Aa-IgG4 (Table 1). Another nonmitogenic humanized anti-CD3 (the Ala-Ala-IgG1) seemed to induce better clearance of T lymphocytes (unpublished observations), suggesting that effector functions triggered by the Fc isotype are responsible for these differences. The use of nonmitogenic, mutated, humanized anti-CD3 MAbs in a clinical setting would be expected, therefore, to result in a strong immunosuppressive state, while causing less toxicity, as a consequence of a weaker activating potential. In addition, these MAbs are anticipated to be less immunogenic *in vivo* because of their humanized state and of their reduced aptitude to induce cytokine production.

Another immunosuppressive anti-CD3 MAb, the rat anti-human CD3 Mab YTH 12.5, has also been re-engineered to contain a human Fc region. In an attempt to reduce its affinity to human FcγRs, an aglycosylated form of an IgG1 isotype was produced by site-directed mutagenesis of amino acid 297 (asparagine to alanine).[57] This mutated MAb was non-mitogenic *in vitro* for human PBLs, unless incubated in IgG-free medium, and induced a 16-fold lower quantity of TNF-α than the parental IgG1 form, while still being able to promote ADCC and to inhibit mixed lymphocyte reactions of both naive and primed T cells. The aglycosyl IgG1 MAb is also a promising candidate for immunosuppressive use in patients while avoiding first-dose reactions and acute toxicity of cytokine-inducing anti-CD3 MAbs. Clinical trials will determine whether its immunosuppressive properties will remain potent enough to revert allograft rejection.

WT32 is a murine IgG2a anti-human CD3-ε MAb with very similar properties to OKT3. Its administration to renal graft recipients also results in first-dose reactions, depletion of T cells from the peripheral blood, and the occurrence of a humoral response.[58] This agent has been

TABLE 1

Immunosuppressive Properties of Murine and Humanized Anti-CD3 MAbs *In Vivo*

Treatment	%T Cells at 24 h[a]	%T Cells at 48 h[a]	%Modulated TCR[b]	%Graft Survival[c]
PBS	62	59	0	0–25
OKT3	8	2	63	75–100
209-IgG1	6	3	62	75–80
Ala-Ala-IgG4	40	17	60	75

[a] Percent T cells of initial engraftment. SCID mice received an i.p. injection of 10^8 human splenocytes on day 0 and initial engraftment in the peripheral blood was assessed on day 11 by flow cytometry, using phycoerythrine-coupled anti-mouse MHC class I and FITC-coupled anti-human CD45 MAbs. Data shown were determined on days 12 and 13, 24 and 48 h after the administration of PBS or anti-CD3 MAbs (100 μg i.p.).

[b] Surface expression of CD3 was assessed in the peripheral blood 6 h after injection of PBS or anti-CD3 MAbs to SCID mice, 12 days after having received the human inoculum. Flow cytometry determinations using FITC-coupled OKT3 allowed calculations of free and modulated (internalized + coated) CD3.

[c] Data show the ranges of survival of allogeneic human foreskin obtained in 3 independent experiments of SCID mice transplanted 12 days after the injection of human splenocytes and treated with PBS or anti-CD3 MAbs (50 μg/day for 5 days, followed by 10 μg/day for 10 days). No significant difference was found between the three MAb-treated groups (Fisher's exact test).

found to be very effective at both reversing[58] and preventing [59] renal allograft rejection. However, there is much less clinical and experimental experience with its use than with that of OKT3.

7.1.3.2 Anti-TCR MAbs

MAbs directed at the αβ chains of the TCR have also been generated and found to exert immunosuppressive effects. Both T10B9.1A-31 (a mouse IgM) and BMA 031 (a mouse IgG2b) have reduced affinity for FcRs, are less mitogenic *in vitro,* and result in the secretion of fewer cytokines and demonstrate fewer side effects *in vivo,* as compared with OKT3.[60,61] The injection of BMA 031 into patients is followed by the systemic release of TNF-α, but not of other cytokines, suggesting that TNF alone might not be sufficient for the induction of the first-dose reaction syndrome.[61] However, the efficacy of BMA 031 at preventing graft rejection seems diminished also with respect to OKT3. T10B9.1A031 might be more promising, as a randomized trial comparing it to OKT3 for treatment of acute rejection showed similar 95% reversal of rejection.[60] Importantly, some patients failing to respond to the initially administered anti-T-cell MAb had their rejection episode reversed by the other MAb. This suggests the potential for improved efficacy by combining several MAbs. Despite their weaker activating potential, both MAbs led to a human anti-mouse antibody response. It is important to note, however, that T10B9.1A-31 has the disadvantage over OKT3 of having a shorter half-life, so that intravenous injections are required two to three times a day, as opposed to once daily with OKT3.

7.1.3.3 Anti-CDw52 MAbs (CAMPATH-1)

CAMPATH-1 is a rat IgM or IgG2b MAb directed at the phosphatidylinositol-anchored CDw52 molecule, that is expressed on the surface of all peripheral T cells, B cells, NK cells, monocytes, and macrophages. Its administration results in pan-T-cell depletion as a consequence of antibody-dependent cell-mediated cytotoxicity as well as complement-mediated cell lysis. This MAb has been shown to be effective at preventing kidney, liver, and pancreas allograft rejection.[62-64] In particular, in a randomized trial comparing high doses of CsA to the combination of high doses CsA and CAMPATH-1 in renal allograft recipients, the group receiving the MAb displayed a longer graft survival than the CsA alone group.[64] However, the incidence of major infections was also significantly higher. In addition, despite the concomitant use of CsA, strong humoral responses against the MAb were detected in those patients. Since those studies, humanized CAMPATH-1 MAbs have been generated, using a human IgG1 framework. This humanized MAb has been shown to induce peripheral blood lymphocyte depletion and to successfully reverse allograft rejection in kidney recipients. Nevertheless, all patients experienced first-dose reactions and most of them also developed mild to severe infections.[65]

7.1.4 MAbs Directed at a Subset of T Lymphocytes

Most pan-T-cell immunosuppressive agents predispose toward the emergence of major viral infections and virus-derived malignant transformations. An area of active research is therefore the attempt to develop therapies capable of inducing allograft-specific tolerance, while preserving a competent immune system against all other T-dependent antigens. Several MAbs have been generated to try and inactivate specific subsets of T cells.

7.1.4.1 Anti-CD4 and Anti-CD8 MAbs

CD4+ T cells play a central role in the initiation of the process of allograft rejection. This property has made the CD4 molecule a particular target of immunotherapeutic strategies for prophylaxis of rejection. Anti-CD4 MAbs of rodent origin have proven very effective at preventing rejection in several rat, mouse, and primate models. In rodents, anti-CD4 MAbs have been able to achieve donor-specific unresponsiveness;

second grafts of the same donor were accepted, whereas third party allografts were found to be rejected.[66-68] The mechanisms by which anti-CD4 MAbs might induce tolerance are still uncertain. Depleting antibodies at the time of transplant might give time for alloantigen to migrate into the thymus and induce apoptosis or tolerance of newly arising alloreactive thymocytes, although it is unclear why depleting anti-CD3 MAbs would not achieve the same results. A second hypothesis derives from extensive *in vitro* work showing that specific T-cell death, or in some cases unresponsiveness, results when anti-CD4 MAbs bind to CD4 molecules before TCR ligation,[69-71] suggesting that the CD4 glycoprotein might be capable of transducing a negative signal to the triggered T cells.[72,73]

A murine anti-human CD4 IgG2a MAb, OKT4A, has been used successfully in non-human primates to prevent kidney allograft rejection.[74,75] However, most monkeys developed anti-mouse antibodies despite the concomitant treatment with CsA or total-lymphoid irradiation.[75] Murine OKT4A has also been used in pilot studies in humans, and was well tolerated both in renal and cardiac transplantation settings,[76,77] but most of the patients generated human anti-mouse antibodies, and the immunosuppressive potential of this drug in humans remains to be proven.

Humanized depleting and non-depleting anti-CD4 MAbs have been engineered over the past few years. Humanized OKT4A MAbs transferred onto human IgG1 and IgG4 frameworks both retained immunosuppressive efficacy in nonhuman primates, although the IgG1 isotype induced more prolonged renal allograft survival than the IgG4 one, in correlation with CD4+ T-cell depletion, probably because of complement binding by IgG1 but not by IgG4.[78] Treatment of cynomolgus monkeys with chimeric or CDR-grafted humanized OKT4A still gave rise to a strong humoral response against the remaining murine determinants of the MAbs.[75] A chimeric anti-CD4 MAb, MT412, has been used recently in patients grafted with cardiac or heart-lung transplants, in addition to classical triple immunosuppressive therapy with more encouraging results than in the previous studies using murine anti-CD4 MAbs. Indeed, patients receiving the humanized MAb had fewer and delayed rejection episodes than anti-thymocyte globulin (ATG) treated control patients.[79] More extensive trials testing the efficacy of this MAb are on their way and might allow an assessment of the immunogenicity of the molecule and whether treated patients can develop graft-specific tolerance.

CD8+ T lymphocytes are major effectors in the process of graft destruction and could be, therefore, an important specific target for MAbs to revert allograft rejection, although other cell types, such as NK cells, might also be involved in this process. However, experimental models to study reversal of ongoing rejection are more difficult to establish than those aimed at testing prophylactic agents, which might account for the scarcity of publications on the subject. Nevertheless, a clinical trial using anti-CD8 MAbs to treat steroid-resistant renal allograft rejection was able to show successful graft survival in four out of six patients.[80]

The combination of both anti-CD4 and anti-CD8 MAbs requires a special mention. Indeed, not only does an association of non-depleting rat antibodies induce permanent specific skin graft acceptance in a murine model of weak mismatches, but it also introduces the concept of "infectious" tolerance, demonstrating that CD4+ T cells that have become tolerant to a graft are capable of passing on this state of unresponsiveness to naive T cells *in vivo*, when an interaction sufficiently long between them is allowed.[81] It has been more difficult to induce tolerance to stronger MHC differences. However, a combination of depleting anti-CD4 and anti-CD8 MAbs followed by a nondepleting pair of antibodies was able to achieve graft-specific unresponsiveness.[82]

7.1.4.2 Anti-IL-2 Receptor MAbs

Fully stimulated T cells produce IL-2 and can use this cytokine both as an autocrine growth factor and as a paracrine hormone to help growth and differentiation of effector cells. IL-2-mediated signaling depends upon binding to the IL-2R, that itself relies on other activation steps for its expression. Another pathway of immunosuppression targets only these activated T cells, that, in a setting of organ transplantation and in the absence of another antigenic stimulation such as a simultaneous infection, would be selectively allograft specific. IL-2R consists of a low-affinity p55 α chain (the Tac antigen), an intermediate affinity p75 β chain,[83] required to internalize IL-2, and the γ chain, shared by several other cytokine receptors (IL-4, IL-7, IL-9, and IL-15)[84] and involved in the final conformation of the receptor. Expression of the α chain is increased upon activation, and its association with the constitutive β and γ chains forms the high-affinity IL-2R. In a mouse model, treatment with an anti-Tac MAb induced permanent survival of heart allografts in 50% of the animals.[85] A randomized prospective clinical trial has compared a nondepleting rat IgG2a MAb (33B3.1) to ATG in prophylaxis of cadaveric renal transplant recipients also treated with corticosteroids and azathioprine. More early rejection episodes were observed in the 33B3.1 than in the ATG group, but the total incidence of rejections at one year was 5% in both groups, with fewer infections occurring when the MAb was used.[86] Similar results were obtained in another clinical trial involving recipients of kidney transplants treated in this case with CsA, corticosteroids, and azathioprine with or without a murine IgG2a anti-Tac MAb. The group receiving the MAb had fewer early rejection episodes than the control group

(12.5% vs. 52.5%, $p < 0.001$) and delayed onset of the first rejection event also was observed.[87] There was no increase in the incidence of infections. In both studies most patients mounted a strong humoral response against the MAb. Less impressive results were obtained in a pilot study that tested the efficacy of 33B3.1 at reversing rejection in first kidney graft recipients. Only six out of ten episodes of rejection partially responded to the injection of the MAb and four required rescue treatments,[88] suggesting that effector cells have already differentiated in an ongoing rejection episode and therefore targeting of IL-2R-expressing cells is no longer sufficient.

The murine anti-IL-2R MAb has been engineered into a human IgG1 framework. Administration to cynomolgus monkeys of this humanized version resulted in delayed humoral response and further prolongation of heart allograft survival, when compared to that of the parental murine MAb.[89] A MAb directed at the β chain of the IL-2R (the murine Mikβ1 MAb) has been used also in experimental models. Mikβ1 acts synergistically with anti-Tac to prevent IL-2-induced T-cell proliferation of activated T cells, and inhibits IL-2-induction of efficient NK and lymphokine-activated killer (LAK) cell activity.[90] Humanized Mikβ1 IgG1 MAb prolonged primate cardiac allograft survival as compared with murine Mikβ1-treated and control animals, probably as a result of ADCC that was detected only in animals receiving the human IgG1 isotype.[91] Interestingly, one of the animals retained its graft for over 300 days, suggesting that specific tolerance might be attainable. No further survival was observed when the combination of humanized Mikβ1 and anti-Tac MAb was used. Again, most of the animals did develop a humoral response against the humanized MAbs.

The failure to induce prolonged acceptance of the grafted organs might be due to the absence of complete depletion of activated T cells. Another approach has been, therefore, to molecularly combine either these MAbs or IL-2 directly to radionuclides[92,93] or cytolytic toxins, such as *Pseudomonas* exotoxin,[94] *diphtheria* toxin,[95] etc. that have the potential to destroy specifically the cells expressing IL-2Rs that would bind the MAb or the cytokine. Such treatments could be dangerous, however, as the toxin might recirculate, either because of molecular dissociation or of shedding of the bound receptor. In addition, humoral responses could induce ligation of the complex to FcR-bearing cells and thus result in lysis of untargeted cells.

7.1.5 Anti-Adhesion and Costimulatory Molecule MAbs

7.1.5.1 Anti-CD2 MAbs

CD2 is a 50–55-kDa surface molecule expressed on all T lymphocytes and NK cells that contributes to intercellular stability by adhesion to its ligands CD48 and LFA-3. This interaction seems to enhance the signal transduced following antigen-specific TCR recognition.[96] Anti-CD2 MAbs have proven very promising in experimental models of organ transplantation. Indeed, the administration of anti-CD2 MAbs has induced not only prolongation of cardiac allo- and xenografts,[97] but also permanent transplantation tolerance when given in association with other immunosuppressive agents such as FK506,[98] anti-CD48 MAbs,[99] or anti-CD3 MAbs.[100] In addition, anti-CD2 MAbs have been shown to reduce anti-CD3-mediated toxicity.[101] More recently, some anti-CD2 MAbs have been capable of promoting permanent cardiac allograft survival, even when injected alone, if appropriate timing around the surgical procedure was respected.[102] As a consequence of these exciting data, some clinical trials using anti-CD2 MAbs in transplanted patients are ongoing. Results from these human studies are awaited impatiently.

7.1.5.2 Anti-LFA-1 and Anti-ICAM-1 MAbs

LFA-1 is a member of the integrin family of molecules involved both in specific T-cell activation and nonspecific intercellular adhesion, through its binding to ICAM-1 (CD54), ICAM-2, and ICAM-3. LFA-1 is expressed on T cells, NK cells, polymorphonuclear cells, macrophages, and monocytes, whereas the ICAM molecules are found on endothelial vascular cells, macrophages, monocytes, and activated B lymphocytes, and can be induced on fibroblasts, keratinocytes, and epithelial cells.[7] LFA-1 is composed of two non-covalently associated polypeptide chains, an α chain (CD11a), and a β chain (CD18).

In patients, anti-LFA-1 MAbs have not been successful in treating ongoing rejection.[103] However, much more encouraging results have been published when used in prophylactic therapy. A randomized clinical trial has compared the efficacy of a mouse IgG1 anti-human CD11a with that of ATG, at preventing rejection of kidney allografts, in addition to corticosteroids and azathioprine. Three-month graft survival was similar in both groups, as were the number of rejection episodes, although their occurrence seemed to happen sooner after transplantation in the MAb-treated group.[104] Similar infectious episodes were reported in both groups. Recent results seem to indicate that anti-LFA-1 MAbs might be effective at reducing acute tubular necrosis and delayed graft function in human kidney recipients.[105]

A mouse IgG2a anti-ICAM-1 MAb was tested in human recipients of kidney grafts at high risk for delayed graft function (prolonged renal ischemia or highly sensitized patients) along with standard induction immunosuppressive therapy and was found to be associated with better allograft survival than the contralateral kidneys grafted in control patients treated with standard therapy only, suggesting that this MAb might be useful at limiting reperfusion injury.[106]

Combinations of anti-ICAM 1, 2, and 3 MAbs or the association of anti-ICAM-1 with anti-LFA-1 MAb might be needed to obtain permanent graft tolerance, as was seen in a murine model of heart allograft rejection,[107] inasmuch as multiple ligands for LFA-1 are available and functionally redundant.

7.1.5.3 CTLA4Ig

An exciting variation of molecular engineering using MAbs is the generation of fusion molecules, comprising the Fc portion of an Ig, that can specifically block interactions that are important for T-cell activation. CTLA4Ig, one of such molecules, is composed of the human IgG1 constant domains and of the human CTLA4 protein, that binds with high affinity to both human and murine B7 family members. Administration of CTLA4Ig during allograft recognition would prevent costimulation, while allowing TCR recognition to proceed, theoretically generating anergy only of allospecific T cells. In a model of human pancreatic islets transplanted under the kidney capsule of mice previously rendered diabetic by an injection of streptozotocin, treatment with CTLA4Ig for 2 weeks immediately post-transplant totally prevented islet rejection.[108] In addition, when these mice were nephrectomized to remove the human graft and retransplanted with human islets under the remaining kidney capsule, only second party islets were rejected, whereas first party donor islets were permanently accepted, indicating that CTLA4Ig had induced long-term, donor-specific T-cell unresponsiveness in this xenogeneic model. Treatment with CTLA4Ig was able to achieve transplantation tolerance also in two allogeneic models of rat and mouse heart grafts.[109,110]

7.1.5.4 Anti-CD45 MAbs

Finally, as direct presentation of alloantigen by graft APCs to host T cells may represent an important trigger for transplant rejection, MAbs have been used also to deplete graft passenger leukocytes and interstitial dendritic cells *ex vivo* prior to transplantation. CD45 (leukocyte common antigen) is a ubiquitous glycoprotein existing in six differently spliced isoforms and expressed on all leukocytes. The cytotoxic combination of two rat IgG2b, complement-fixing, anti-human CD45 MAbs (YTH54.12 and YTH24.5) has been used to perfuse human renal allografts *in vitro*. Transplantation of these leukocyte-depleted kidneys led to a decrease in allograft rejection without adverse effects to the hosts.[111]

7.2 GRAFT-VERSUS-HOST DISEASE (GVHD)

Bone marrow transplantation has the potential to cure a variety of diseases ranging from genetic abnormalities, such as thalassemia major and immune deficiencies, to aplastic anemia and leukemia. In addition, injections of bone marrow have been used experimentally as adjunctive therapy to induce tolerance in organ transplantation. However, there are several limitations to this procedure, that derive from the existence of two mutually aggressive sets of cells. First, the immunocompetent system of the host can recognize and reject the donor bone marrow-derived cells, resulting in host-versus-graft disease (HVGD). Conversely, donor marrow T cells can react against a variety of host alloantigens and cause GVHD, that can manifest as gastrointestinal dysfunction (diarrhea), hepatic dysfunction (jaundice) and skin rash that can lead to desquamation.[112] HVGD can be prevented in the majority of patients by conditioning the host with different cytotoxic chemotherapeutic agents and/or with body irradiation, that will disable their immune system. GVHD poses a more serious problem, as purging the donor bone marrow from mature T cells indeed reduces the incidence of GVHD, but also decreases both the engraftment of the transplant and the lymphocyte-mediated destruction of remaining host malignant cells. A considerable amount of work is being performed to try and distinguish the specific T cells that will promote engraftment and have anti-leukemic effects from the ones that will induce GVHD, in order to perform selective depletion before transplantation, but no conclusively applicable rules are yet available. Similar issues overcast newer transplantation techniques of transfusion of peripheral blood CD34+ progenitor cells.[113]

7.2.1 Anti-T-Cell MAbs

Anti-T-cell MAbs such as T10B9.1A-31[114] or CAMPATH-1[115] have been used to purge T cells from human bone marrow *in vitro* with good prevention of GVHD. However, *in vivo* administration of CAMPATH -1G to the recipients to deplete residual T cells was more efficient than *in vitro* treatment, with almost complete absence of GVHD and reduction of graft failure from 21 to 9%.[116] Murine studies suggest that anti-TCR MAbs have to be given at day zero of the transplant to prevent severe GVHD, whereas delayed rescue treatment can still be effective for milder forms of the disease.[117]

Anti-CD3 MAbs have been used also to treat GVHD *in vivo*. In two murine models of bone marrow transplantation, 145-2C11, or a rat IgG2b anti-mouse CD3 MAb, were more effective at preventing GVHD when administered *in vivo*, than when bone marrow was depleted of T cells by incubation with the MAb *in vitro*.[118,119] However, acute toxicity due to the cytokine release induced by the 145-2C11 MAb was severe, leading to cachexia and mortality.[118] Nonmitogenic F(ab')$_2$ fragments of 145-2C11 have been used, therefore, without evidence of toxicity and with high efficacy at preventing GVHD.[120] Interestingly, CD3+CD4–CD8– cells, that may have the property of suppressing the onset of GVHD[121] were present in higher numbers in anti-CD3-treated mice than in animals having received the combination of anti-murine T-cell anti-Thy-1.2 MAb and complement. Similarly, patients experiencing GVHD despite administration of CsA and corticosteroids were treated with a mouse anti-human CD3 IgG2b, with low FcγR-binding-affinity and T-cell-activation ability. Most of the patients had complete or partial reversion of GVHD.[122] Further studies will be necessary to determine whether survival is improved in MAb-treated patients.

The combination of anti-CD4 and anti-CD8 MAbs also has been shown to promote engraftment and reduce GVHD when given to murine recipients of allogeneic bone marrow.[123-125]

Finally, an anti-human CD5 MAb conjugated to ricin A-toxin (XomaZyme H65) has been used recently in a clinical trial, in association with anti-T-cell MAb as a conditioning regimen of bone marrow before transplantation. Patients also received the immunotoxin as GVHD prophylaxis. Although quite effective at preventing GVHD, this treatment led to increased incidence of severe and sometimes lethal viral infections during the first year after transplantation.[126]

7.2.2 Anti-IL-2R MAbs

Humanized anti-Tac with the IgG1 isotype has been used in patients suffering from corticosteroid-resistant GVHD, in an attempt to deplete activated T cells, thus removing only GVHD reactive cells without globally impairing T-cell function. Improvement of GVHD occurred to various degrees in 40% of the patients.[127] Surprisingly, given results obtained in solid organ transplant recipients, no humoral response was mounted against the humanized MAb in this group of patients. However, recent data using the rat IgG2a MAb, 33B3.1, in a randomized prospective trial in post-transplantation leukemic patients, showed only a delay in the onset of GVHD in the MAb-treated group, as compared with a control group receiving only CsA and methotrexate.[128] Furthermore, the MAb-treated group had a significantly reduced leukemic-free survival, with a higher rate of relapses.

7.2.3 Anti-Cytokine MAbs

It has been shown that mice undergoing chronic GVHD spontaneously produce IL-4 and IL-10, that could be responsible for the hyperactivity of B cells in this disease.[129] Moreover, GVHD has been correlated with high circulating levels of antibodies of the IL-4-associated IgE and IgG1 isotypes.[130] Treatment with anti-IL-4 MAb prevented liver disease and splenomegaly, and led to reduced titers of IgE and IgG1 in a murine GVHD model,[130] confirming that IL-4 plays an important role in the pathogenesis of this disease.

In addition, an anti-human TNF-α MAb has induced modest improvement in patients with severe refractory GVHD.[131] Rapid relapse was observed, however, when administration of the antibody was stopped.

7.2.4 Anti-Adhesion and Costimulatory Molecule MAbs

Modest delays in GVHD mortality have been achieved in mice using anti-LFA-1 or anti-ICAM-1 MAbs.[132] GVHD also has been reduced when marrow was treated *in vitro* with a ricin A-conjugated anti-LFA-1 Mab.[133]

Very promising results have been obtained by Soiffer et al.,[134] using anti-human CD6 MAb (the T12 MAb) and rabbit complement to deplete mature T cells from bone marrow before transplantation in a retrospective study of patients with hematological malignancies. Indeed, 96% of patients had stable hematological reconstitution after marrow infusion and only 15% developed acute GVHD.[134] A prospective study comparing this prophylactic regimen to standard therapy is awaited to confirm these exciting results.

Treatment of recipient mice with human or murine CTLA4Ig prolonged the survival of the animals, even when the administration of the fusion molecule was delayed up to six days after transplantation.[135,136] However, some signs of GVHD such as pancytopenia and abnormal spleen cell composition were still present in CTAL4Ig-treated animals, suggesting that this mouse CTLA4IgG2a can block some, but not all aspects of murine GVHD. Whether this is the consequence of costimulatory-independent pathways or is the result of some unknown mechanism triggered by FcγR-binding of the high-affinity murine IgG2a Fc portion, remains to be determined.

7.3 CONCLUSION

The use of monoclonal antibodies has opened a field of new possibilities in the prevention and treatment of GVHD and of solid organ rejection. It is important to remember that results obtained with MAbs can vary widely depending on the epitope targeted (different epitopes on the same surface molecule may trigger separate effects), the affinity with which a MAb binds to FcRs inducing accessory cell function, and whether the MAb is cell depleting or only ligand blocking. Immune responses may also vary across species, sometimes rendering uncertain the predictability of experimental models. In addition, the associated immunosuppressive regimen given to transplanted patients may modify immune responses. Genetic engineering of MAbs allows for careful selection of the Ig isotype, depending on the expected effect, and for specific mutations if a property is to be avoided. Humanization techniques also have the theoretical advantage of reducing the immunogenicity of xenogeneic MAbs. However, all but one study[127] using humanized MAbs in human or non-human primate trials have demonstrated the onset of an anti-idiotypic response, although MAb-neutralization generally occurs later than with parental MAbs. A better understanding of mechanisms leading to both T- and B-cell unresponsiveness will enable us to generate better MAbs that might induce specific long-term antibody and graft tolerance.

7.4 ACKNOWLEDGMENTS

I wish to acknowledge Thomas F. Gajewski and Michel Goldman for their critical reading of this manuscript. I am indebted to Jeffrey A. Bluestone for making this review possible.

REFERENCES

1. Weiss, A., Imboden, J. B., Hardy, K., Manger, B., Terhorst, C., and Stobo, J., The role of the T3/antigen receptor complex in T-cell activation, *Annu. Rev. Immunol.*, 4, 593, 1986.
2. Jenkins, M. K., Taylor, P. S., Norton, S. D., and Urdahl, K. B., CD28 delivers a costimulatory signal involved in antigen-specific IL-2 production by human T cells, *J. Immunol.*, 147, 2461, 1991.
3. Harding, F. A., McArthur, J. G., Gross, J. A., Raulet, D. H., and Allison, J. P., CD28-mediated signalling co-stimulates murine T cells and prevents induction of anergy in T cell clones, *Nature*, 356, 607, 1992.
4. Norton, S. D., Zuckerman, L., Urdahl, K. B., Shefner, R., Miller, J., and Jenkins, M. K., The CD28 ligand, B7, enhances IL-2 production by providing a costimulatory signal to T cells, *J. Immunol.*, 149, 1556, 1992.
5. Jenkins, M. J., Ashwell, J. D., and Schwartz, R. H., Allogeneic non-T spleen cells restore the responsiveness of normal T cell clones stimulated with antigen and chemically modified antigen-presenting cells, *J. Immunol.*, 140, 3324, 1988.
6. Wecker, H. and Auchincloss, H., Cellular mechanisms of rejection, *Curr. Opin. Immunol.*, 4, 561, 1992.
7. Springer, T. A., Adhesion receptors of the immune system, *Nature*, 346, 425, 1990.

8. Debets, J. M., Van de Winkel, J. G., Cueppens, I. E., Dieteren, M., and Buurman, W. A., Cross-linking of both FcγRI and FcγRII induces secretion of tumor necrosis factor by human monocytes, requiring high affinity Fc-FcγR interactions: functional activation of FcγRII by treatment with proteases or neuraminidase, *J. Immunol.*, 144, 1304, 1990.
9. Krutmann, J., Kirnbauer, R., Kock, A., Schwarz, T., Schopf, E., May, T., Sehgal, P. B., and Luger, T. A., Cross-linking Fc receptors on monocytes triggers IL-6 production. Role in anti-CD3 induced T cell activation, *J. Immunol.*, 145, 1337, 1990.
10. Ravetch, J. V. and Anderson, C. L., Fcgamma-receptor family: proteins, transcripts and genes, *Fc Receptors and the Action of Antibodies*, Metzger H. American Society for Microbiology, Washington, D.C., 1990, 211.
11. Burton, D. R., Immunoglobulin G: functional sites, *Mol. Immunol.*, 22, 161, 1985.
12. Duncan, A. R., Woof, J. M., Partridge, L. J., Burton, D. R., and Winter, G., Localization of the binding site for the human high affinity Fc receptor on IgG, *Nature*, 332, 563, 1988.
13. Gergely, J. and Sarmay, G., The two binding-site models of human IgG binding Fc-amma receptors, *FASEB J.*, 4, 3275, 1990.
14. Ollo, R. and Rougeon, F., Gene conversion and polymorphism: generation of mouse immunoglobulin gamma2a chain alleles by differential gene conversion by gamma2b chain gene, *Cell*, 32, 515, 1983.
15. Jefferis, R., Lund, J., and Pound, J., Molecular definition of interaction sites on human IgG for Fc receptors (huFcR), *Mol. Immunol.*, 27, 1237, 1990.
16. Salmeron, A., Sanchez-Madrid, F., Ursa, M. A., Fresno, M., and Alarcon, B., A conformational epitope expressed upon association of CD3-ε with either CD3-γ or CD3-δ is the main target for recognition by anti-CD3 monoclonal antibodies, *J. Immunol.*, 147, 3047, 1991.
17. Chatenoud, L., Baudrihaye, M. F., Kreis, H., Goldstein, G., Schindler, J., and Bach, J. F., Human *in vivo* antigenic modulation induced by the anti-T cell OKT3 monoclonal antibody, *Eur. J. Immunol.*, 12, 979, 1982.
18. Cosimi, A. B., Burton, R. C., and Colvin, B., Treatment of acute renal allograft rejection with OKT3 monoclonal antibody, *Transplantation*, 32, 535, 1981.
19. Cosimi, A. B., Burton, R. C., Colvin, R. B., Goldstein, G., Delmonico, F. L., LaQuaglia, M. P., Tolkoff-Rubin, N., Rubin, R. H., Herrin, J. T., and Russell, P. S., Treatment of acute renal allograft rejection with OKT3 monoclonal antibody, *Transplantation*, 32, 535, 1985.
20. Ortho Multicenter Transplant Study Group, A randomized clinical trial of OKT3 monoclonal antibody for acute rejection of cadaveric renal transplants, *N. Engl. J. Med.*, 313, 337, 1985.
21. Thistlethwaite, J. R., Gaber, A. O., Haag, B. W., Aronson, A. J., Broelsch, C. E., Stuart, J. K., and Stuart, F. P., OKT3 treatment of steroid-resistant renal allograft rejection, *Transplantation*, 43, 176, 1987.
22. Debure, A., Chkoff, N., Chatenoud, L., Lacombe, M., Campos, H., Noel, L. H., Goldstein, G., Bach, J. F., and Kreis, H., One-month prophylactic use of OKT3 in cadaver kidney transplant recipients, *Transplantation*, 45, 546, 1988.
23. Kreis, H., Chkoff, N., Chatenoud, L., Debure, A., Lacombe, M., Chrëtien, Y., Legendre, C., Caillat, S., and Bach, J. F., A randomized trial comparing the efficacy of OKT3 used to prevent or to treat rejection, *Transplant. Proc.*, 21, 1741, 1989.
24. Vigeral, P., Chkoff, N., Chatenoud, L., Campo, S. H., Lacombe, M., Droz, D., Goldstein, G., Bach, J. F., and Kreis H., Prophylactic use of OKT3 monoclonal antibody in cadaver kidney recipients. Utilization of OKT3 as the sole immunosuppressive agent, *Transplantation*, 41, 730, 1986.

25. Norman, D. J., Kahana, L., Stuart, F. P., Thistlethwaite, J. R., Shield, C. F., Monaco, A., Dehlinger, J., Wu, S. C., Van Horn, A., and Haverty, T. P., A randomized clinical trial of induction therapy with OKT3 in kidney transplantation, *Transplantation*, 55, 44, 1993.
26. De Pauw, L., Abramowicz, D., Goldman, M., Vereerstraeten, P., Kinnaert, P., and Toussaint, C., Comparison between prophylactic use of OKT3 and cyclosporine in cadaveric renal transplantation, *Transplant. Proc.*, 22, 1759, 1990.
27. Thistlethwaite, J. R., Stuart, J. K., Mayes, J. T., Gaber, A. O., Woodle, S., Buckingham, M. R., and Stuart, F. P., Complications and monitoring of OKT3 therapy, *Am. J. Kidney Dis.*, 11, 112, 1988.
28. Toussaint, C., De Pauw, L., Vereerstraeten, P., Kinnaert, P., Abramowicz, D., and Goldman, M., Possible nephrotoxicity of the prophylactic use of OKT3 monoclonal antibody after cadaveric renal transplantation, *Transplantation*, 48, 524, 1989.
29. Abramowicz, D., Pradier, O., Marchant, A., Florquin, S., De Pauw, L., Vereerstraeten, P., Kinnaert, P., Vanherweghem, J. L., and Goldman, M., Induction of thromboses within renal grafts by high-dose prophylactic OKT3, *Lancet*, 339, 777, 1992.
30. Jaffers, G. J., Colvin, R. B., Cosimi, A. B., Giorgi, J. V., Goldstein, G., Fuller, T. C., Kurnick, J. T., Lillehei, C., and Russell, P. S., The human immune response to murine OKT3 monoclonal antibody, *Transplant. Proc.*, 15, 646, 1983.
31. Chatenoud, L., Jonker, M., Villemain, F., Goldstein, G., and Bach, J.-F., The human immune response to the OKT3 monclonal antibody is oligoclonal, *Science*, 232, 1406, 1986.
32. Chatenoud, L., Humoral immune response against OKT3, *Transplant. Proc.*, 25, 68, 1993.
33. Richards, J. M., Vogelzang, N. J., and Bluestone, J. A., Neurotoxicity after treatment with muromonab-CD3, *N. Engl. J. Med.*, 323, 487, 1990.
34. Abramowicz, D., Schandene, L., Goldman, M., Crusiaux, A., Vereerstraeten, P., De Pauw, L., Wybran, J., Kinnaert, P., Dupont, E., and Toussaint, C., Release of tumor necrosis factor-alpha and interferon-gamma in serum after injection of OKT3 monoclonal antibody in kidney transplant recipients, *Transplantation*, 47, 606, 1989.
35. Chatenoud, L., Ferran, C., Reuter, A., Legendre, C., Gevaert, Y., Kreis, H., Franchimont, P., and Bach, J. F., Systemic reaction to the anti-T cell monoclonal antibody OKT3 in relation to serum levels of tumor necrosis factor and interferon-gamma, *N. Engl. J. Med.*, 320, 1420, 1989.
36. Chatenoud, L., Ferran, C., Reuter, A., and Bach, J. F., Clinical use of OKT3: the role of cytokine release and xenosensitization, *J. Autoimmun.*, 1, 631, 1988.
37. Mannel, D. N., Northoff, H., Bauss, F., and Falk, W., Tumor necrosis factor: a cytokine involved in toxic effects of endotoxin, *Rev. Infect. Dis.*, 5, S602, 1987.
38. Bauss, F., Droge, W., and Mannel, D. N., Tumor necrosis factor mediates endotoxic effects in mice, *Infect. Immun.*, 55, 1622, 1987.
39. Hoffman, M., Mittelman, A., Dworkin, B., Rosenthal, W., Beneck, D., Gafney, E., Arlin, Z., Levitt, D., and Podack, E., Severe intrahepatic cholestasis in patients treated with recombinant interleukin 2 and lymphokine-activated killer cells, *J. Cancer Res. Clin. Oncol.*, 115, 175, 1989.
40. Tracey, K. J., Beutler, B., Lowry, S. F., Merryweather, J., Wolpe, S., Milsark, I. W., Hariri, R. J., Fahey, III, T. J., Zentel, A., Albert, J. D., Shires, T., and Cerami, A., Shock and tissue injury induced by recombinant human cachectin, *Science*, 234, 470, 1986.
41. Creaven, P. J., Plager, J. E., Dupere, S., Huben, R. P., Takita, H., Mittelman, A., and Proefrock, A., Phase I trial of recombinant human tumor necrosis factor, *Cancer Chemother. Pharmacol.*, 20, 137, 1987.
42. Kimura, K., Tagushi, T., Urushizaki, R., Ohno, R., Abe, O., Furue, H., Hattori, T., Ichihashi, H., Inogushi, K., and Majima, H., Phase I study of recombinant tumor necrosis factor, *Cancer Chemother. Pharmacol.*, 20, 223, 1987.

43. Quesada, J. R., Talpaz, M., Rios, A., Kurzrock, R., and Gutterman, J. U., Clinical toxicity of interferons in cancer patients: a review, *J. Clin. Oncol.*, 4, 234, 1986.
44. Goldman, M., Abramowicz, D., De Pauw, L., Alegre, M. L., Widera, I., Vereerstraeten, P., and Kinnaert, P., OKT3-induced cytokine release attenuation by high dose methylprednisolone, *Lancet*, 2, 802, 1989.
45. Chatenoud, L., Ferran, C., Legendre, C., Thouard, I., Merite, S., Reuter, A., Gevaert, Y., Kreis, H., Franchimont, P., and Bach, J. F., *In vivo* cell activation following OKT3 administration. Systemic cytokine release and modulation by corticosteroids, *Transplantation*, 49, 697, 1990.
46. Charpentier, B., Hiesse, C., Lantz, O., Ferran, C., Stephens, S., O'Shaugnessy, D., Bodmer, M., Benoit, G., Bach, J. F., and Chatenoud, L., Evidence that antihuman tumor necrosis factor monoclonal antibody prevents OKT3-induced acute syndrome, *Transplantation*, 54, 997, 1992.
47. van Lier, R. A., Brouwer, M., Rebel, V. I., van Noesel, C. J., and Aarden, L. A., Immobilized anti-CD3 monoclonal antibodies induce accessory cell-independent lymphokine production, proliferation and helper activity in human T lymphocytes, *Immunology*, 68, 45, 1989.
48. van Lier, R. A., Boot, J. H., Verhoeven, A. J., de Groot, E. R., Brouwer, M., and Aarden, L. A., Functional studies with anti-CD3 heavy chain switch variant monoclonal antibodies. Accessory-cell independent induction of IL-2 responsiveness in T cells by epsilon-anti-CD3, *J. Immunol.*, 139, 2873, 1987.
49. Parleviet, K. J., Jonker, M., ten Berge, R. J., van Lier, R. A., Wilmink, J. M., Strengers, P. F., and Aarden, L. A., Anti-CD3 murine monoclonal isotype switch variants tested for toxicity and immunologic monitoring in four chimpanzees, *Transplantation*, 50, 889, 1990.
50. Leo, O., Foo, M., Sachs, D. H., Samelson, L. E., and Bluestone, J. A., Identification of a monoclonal antibody specific for murine T3 polypeptide, *Proc. Natl. Acad. Sci. U.S.A.*, 84, 1374, 1987.
51. Hirsch, R., Bluestone, J. A., DeNenno, L., and Gress, R. E., Anti-CD3 F(ab')2 fragments are immunosuppressive in vivo without evoking either the strong humoral response or morbidity associated with whole MAb, *Transplantation*, 49, 1117, 1990.
52. Alegre, M. L., Tso, J. Y., Sattar, H. A., Smith, J., Desalle, F., Cole, M., and Bluestone, J. A., An anti-murine CD3 monoclonal antibody with a low affinity for Fc-gamma receptors suppresses transplantation responses while minimizing acute toxicity and immunogenicity, *J. Immunol.*, 155, 1544, 1995.
53. Adair, J. R., Athwal, D. S., Bodmer, M. W., Bright, S. M., Collins, A. M., Pulito, V. L., Rao, P. E., Reedman, R., Rothermel, A. L., Xu, D., Zivin, R. A., and Jolliffe, L. K., Humanization of the murine anti-human CD3 monoclonal antibody OKT3, *Hum. Antibod. Hybridomas*, 5, 41, 1994.
54. Alegre, M. L., Collins, A. M., Pulito, V. L., Brosius, R. A., Olson, W. C., Zivin, R. A., Knowles, R., Thistlethwaite, J. R., Jolliffe, L. K., and Bluestone, J. A., Effect of a single amino acid mutation on the activating and immunosuppressive properties of a "humanized" OKT3 monoclonal antibody, *J. Immunol.*, 148, 3461, 1992.
55. Alegre, M. L., Peterson, L. J., Jeyarajah, R. D., Kowalkowski, K., Thistlethwaite, J. R., and Bluestone, J. A., Severe combined immunodeficient mice engrafted with human splenocytes have functional human T cells and reject human allografts, *J. Immunol.*, 153, 2738, 1994.
56. Alegre, M. L., Peterson, L. J., Xu, D., Sattar, H. A., Jeyarajah, D. R., Kowalkowski, K., Zivin, R. A., Knowles, R., Jolliffe, L. K., Thistlethwaite, J. R., and Bluestone, J. A., A non-activating "humanized" anti-CD3 monoclonal antibody retains immunosuppressive properties *in vivo*, *Transplantation*, 57, 1537, 1994.

57. Bolt, S., Routledge, E., Lloyd, I., Chatenoud, L., Pope, H., Gorman, S. D., Clark, M., and Waldmann, H., The generation of a humanized, non-mitogenic CD3 monoclonal antibody which retains in vitro immunosuppressive properties, *Eur. J. Immunol.*, 23, 403, 1993.
58. Tax, W. J. M., van de Heijden, H. M. W., Willems, H. W., Hoitsma, A. J., Berden, J. H. M., Capel, P. J. A., and Koene, R. A. P., Immunosuppression with monoclonal anti-T3 antibody (WT32) in renal transplantation, *Transplant. Proc.*, 19, 1905, 1987.
59. Frenken, L. A. M., Hoitsma, A. J., Tax, W. J. M., and Koene, R. A. P., Prophylactic use of anti-CD3 monoclonal antibody WT32 in kidney transplantation, *Transplant. Proc.*, 23, 1072, 1991.
60. Waid, T. H., Lucas, B. A., Thompson, J. S., Brown, S. A., Munch, L., Prebeck, R. J., and Jezek, D., Treatment of acute cellular rejection with T10B9.1A-31 or OKT3 in renal allograft recipients, *Transplantation*, 53, 80, 1992.
61. Chatenoud, L., Legendre, C., Kurrle, R., Kreis, H., and Bach, J. F., Absence of clinical symptoms following the first injection of anti-T cell receptor monoclonal antibody (BMA 031) despite isolated TNF release, *Transplantation*, 55, 443, 1993.
62. Hale, G., Waldmann, H., Friend, P., and Calne, R., Pilot study of Campath-1, a rat monoclonal antibody that fixes human complement, as an immunosuppressant in organ transplantation, *Transplantation*, 42, 308, 1986.
63. Friend, P. J., Calne, R. Y., Hale, H., Waldmann, H., Evans, D. B., Rolles, K., Thiru, S., and Gore, S., Prophylactic use of an anti-lymphocyte monoclonal antibody following renal transplantation: a randomized controlled trial, *Transplant. Proc.*, 19, 1898, 1987.
64. Friend, P. J., Hale, G., Waldmann, H., Gore, S., Thiru, S., Joysey, V., Evans, D. B., and Calne, R. Y., Campath-1 M prophylactic use after kidney transplantation. A randomized controlled trial, *Transplantation*, 48, 248, 1989.
65. Friend, P. J., Rebello, P., Oliveira, D., Manna, V., Cobbold, S. P., Hale, G., Jamieson, N. V., Jamieson, I., Calne, R. Y., Harris, D. T., and Waldmann, H., Successful treatment of renal allograft rejection with a humanized antilymphocyte monoclonal antibody, *Transplant. Proc.*, 27, 869, 1995.
66. Shizuru, J. A., Seydel, K. B., Flavin, T. F., Wu, A. P., Kong, C. C., Hoyt, E. G., Fugimoto, N., Billingham, M. E., Starnes, V. A., and Fathman, C. G., Induction of donor specific unresponsiveness to cardiac allografts in rats by pretransplant anti CD4 monoclonal antibody therapy, *Transplantation*, 50, 366, 1990.
67. Alters, S. E., Shizuru, J. A., Ackerman, J., Grossman, D., Seydel, K. B., and Fathman, C. G., Anti CD4 mediates clonal anergy during transplantation tolerance induction, *J. Exp. Med.*, 173, 491, 1991.
68. Pearson, T. C., Darby, C. R., Bushell, A. R., West, L. J., Morris, P. J., and Wood, K. J., The assessment of transplantation tolerance induced by anti-CD4 monoclonal antibody in the murine model, *Transplantation*, 55, 361, 1993.
69. Julius, M., Newell, K., Maroun, C., and Haughn, L., Functional consequences of CD4-TCR/CD3 interactions, *Semin. Immunol.*, 3, 161, 1991.
70. Newell, M. K., Haughn, L. J., Maroun, C. R., and Julius, M. H., Death of mature T cells by separate ligation of CD4 and the T-cell receptor for antigen, *Nature*, 347, 286, 1990.
71. Haughn, L., Gratton, S., Caron, L., Sékaly, R.-P., Veillette, A., and Julius, M., Association of tyrosine kinase $p56^{lck}$ with CD4 inhibits the induction of growth through the αβ T-cell receptor, *Nature*, 358, 328, 1992.
72. Bank, I. and Chess, L., Perturbation of the T4 molecule transmits a negative signal to T cells, *J. Exp. Med.*, 162, 1294, 1985.
73. Tite, J. P., Sloan, A., and Janeway, C. A., The role of L3T4 in T cell activation: L3T4 may be both an Ia-binding protein and a receptor that transduces a negative signal, *J. Mol. Cell. Immunol.*, 2, 179, 1986.

74. Wee, S. L., Stroka, D. M., Preffer, F. I., Jolliffe, L. K., Colvin, R. B., and Cosimi, A. B., The effects of OKT4A monoclonal antibody on cellular immunity of nonhuman primate renal allograft recipients, *Transplantation*, 53, 501, 1992.
75. Delmonico, F. L., Cosimi, A. B., Kawai, T., Cavender, D., Lee, W. H., Jolliffe, L. K., and Knowles, R. W., Nonhuman primate responses to murine and humanized OKT4A, *Transplantation*, 55, 722, 1993.
76. Cooperative Clinical Trials in Transplantation (CCTT) Research Group, Murine OKT4A immunosuppression in cadaver renal allograft recipients: a cooperative pilot study (report 1), *Transplant. Proc.*, 27, 863, 1995.
77. Norman, D. J., Bennett, W. M., Cobanoglu, A., Hershberger, R., Hosenpud, J. D., Meyer, M. M., Misiti, J., Ott, G., Ratkovec, R., Shihab, F., Vitow, C., and Barry, J. M., Use of OKT4A (a murine monoclonal anti-CD4 antibody) in human organ transplantation: initial clinical experience, *Transplant. Proc.*, 25, 802, 1993.
78. Powelson, J. A., Knowles, R. W., Delmonico, F. L., Kawai, T., Mourad, G., Preffer, F. I., Colvin, R. B., and Cosimi, A. B., CDR-grafted OKT4A monoclonal antibody in cynomolgus renal allograft recipients, *Transplanation*, 57, 788, 1994.
79. Reichart, B., Meiser, B. M., Reiter, C. H., Wene, K., Reichenspurner, H., Kreizer, E., Rietmuller, G., and Uberfuhr, P., A new chimeric monoclonal CD4 antibody for heart and heart-lung transplantation, *Transplantation*, in press.
80. Wee, S. L., Colvin, R. B., Phelan, J. M., Preffer, F. I., Reichert, T. A., Berd, D., and Cosimi, A. B., Fc-receptor for mouse IgG1 (Fc-gamma-RII) and antibody-mediated cell clearance in patients treated with Leu2a antibody, *Transplantation*, 48, 1012, 1989.
81. Qin, S., Cobbold, S. P., Pope, H., Elliott, J., Kioussis, D., Davies, J., and Waldmann, H., "Infectious" transplantation tolerance, *Science*, 259, 974, 1993.
82. Cobbold, S. P., Martin, G., and Waldmann, H., The induction of skin graft tolerance in major histocompatibility complex-mismatched or primed recipients: primed T cells can be tolerized in the periphery with anti-CD4 and anti-CD8 antibodies, *Eur. J. Immunol.*, 20, 2747, 1990.
83. Wang, H. M. and Smith, K. A., The interleukin-2 receptor: functional consequences of its bimolecular structure, *J. Exp. Med.*, 166, 1055, 1987.
84. Kimura, Y., Takeshita, T., Kondo, M., Ishii, N., Nakamura, M., Van Snick, J., and Sugamura, K., Sharing of the IL-2 receptor gamma chain with the functional IL-9 receptor complex, *Int. Immunol.*, 7, 115, 1995.
85. Kupiec-Weglinski, J. W., Diamantstein, T., and Tilney, N. L., Interleukin-2 receptor-targeted therapy: rationale and applications in organ transplantation, *Transplantation*, 46, 785, 1988.
86. Soulillou, J. P., Peyronnet, P., Le Mauff, B., Hourmant, M., Olive, D., Mawas, C., Delaage, M., and Jacques, Y., Randomized trial of an anti-interleukin-2 receptor monoclonal antibody (33B3.1) vs. rabbit anti-thymocyte globulin (ATG) in prophylaxis of early rejection in human renal transplantation, *N. Engl. J. Med.*, 322, 1175, 1990.
87. Kirkman, R. L., Shapiro, M. E., Carpenter, C. B., McKay, D. B., Milfored, E. L., Ramos, E. L., Tilney, N. L., Waldmann, T. A., Zimmerman, C. E., and Strom, T. B., A randomized prospective trial of anti-Tac monoclonal antibody in human renal transplantation, *Transplantation*, 51, 107, 1991.
88. Cantarovitch, D., Le Mauff, B., Hourmant, M., Giral, M., Denis, M., Hirn, M., Jacques, Y., and Soulillou, J. P., Anti-interleukin-2 receptor monoclonal antibody in the treatment of on-going acute rejection episodes of human kidney graft. A pilot study, *Transplantation*, 47, 454, 1989.
89. Brown, P. S., Parenteau, G. L., Dirbas, F. M., Garsia, R. J., Goldman, C. K., Bukowski, M. A., Junghans, R. P., Queen, C., Hakimi, J., Benjamin, W. R., Clark, R. E., and Waldmann, T. A., Anti-Tac-H, a humanized antibody to the interleukin-2 receptor, prolongs primate cardiac allograft survival, *Proc. Natl. Acad. Sci. U.S.A.*, 88, 2663, 1991.

90. Grant, A. J., Roessler, E., Ju, G., Tsudo, M., Sugamura, K., and Waldmann, T. A., The interleukin 2 receptor (IL-2R): the IL-2R alpha subunit alters the function of the IL-2R beta subunit to enhance IL-2R binding and signaling by mechanisms that do not require binding of IL-2 to IL-2R alpha subunit, *Proc. Natl. Acad. Sci. U.S.A.*, 89, 2165, 1992.
91. Tinubu, S. A., Hakimi, J., Kondas, J. A., Bailon, P., Familletti, P. C., Spence, C., Crittenden, M. D., Parenteau, G. L., Dirbas, F. M., Tsudo, M., Bacher, J. D., Kasten-Sportes, C., Martinucci, J. L., Goldman, C. K., Clark, R. E., and Waldmann, T. A., Humanized antibody directed to the IL-2 receptor beta-chain prolongs primate cardiac allograft survival, *J. Immunol.*, 153, 4330, 1994.
92. Kozak, R. W., Atcher, R. W., Gansow, O. A., Friedman, A. M., Hines, J. J., and Waldmann, T. A., Bismuth-212-labelled anti-TAC monoclonal antibody: Alpha-particle emitting radionuclides as modalities for radioimmunotherapy, *Proc. Natl. Acad. Sci. U.S.A.*, 83, 474, 1986.
93. Kozak, R. W., Raubitschek, A., Mirzadeh, S., Brechbriel, M. W., Junghans, R., Gansow, O. A., and Waldmann, T. A., Nature of the bifunctional chelating agent used for radioimmunotherapy with yttrium-90 monoclonal antibodies: critical factors in determining *in vivo* survival and organ toxicity, *Cancer Res.*, 49, 2639, 1989.
94. Fitzgerald, D. J. P., Waldmann, T. A., Willingham, M. C., and Pastan, I., Pseudomonas-exotoxin-anti-Tac: cell-specific immunotoxin active against cells expressing human T cell growth factor receptor, *J. Clin. Invest.*, 74, 966, 1984.
95. Kirkman, R. L., Bacha, P., Barrett, L. V., Forte, S., Murphy, J. R., and Strom, T. B., Prolongation of cardiac allograft survival in murine recipients treated with a diphtheria toxin-related interleukin-2 fusion protein, *Transplantation*, 47, 327, 1989.
96. Meuer, S. C., Hussey, R. E., Fabbi, M., Fox, D., Acuto, O., Fitzgerald, K. A., Hodgdon, J. C., Protentis, J. P., Schlossman, S. F., and Rienherz, E. I., An alternative pathway of T-cell activation: a functional role for the 50 kd sheep erythrocyte receptor protein, *Cell*, 36, 897, 1984.
97. Chavin, K. D., Lau, H. T., and Bromberg, J. S., Prolongation of allograft and xenograft survival in mice by anti-CD2 monoclonal antibody treatment, *Transplantation*, 54, 1098, 1992.
98. Chavin, K. D., Qin, L., Woodward, J. E., Lin, J., and Bromberg, J. S., Anti-CD2 monoclonal antibodies synergize with FK506 but not with cyclosporin or rapamycin to induce tolerance, *Transplantation*, 57, 736, 1994.
99. Qin, L., Chavin, K. D., Lin, J., Yagita, H., and Bromberg, J. S., Anti-CD2 receptor and anti-CD2 ligand (CD48) antibodies synergize to prolong allograft survival, *J. Exp. Med.*, 179, 341, 1994.
100. Chavin, K. D., Qin, L., Lin, J., Yagita, H., and Bromberg, J. S., Combined anti-CD2 and anti-CD3 receptor monoclonal antibodies induce donor-specific tolerance in a cardiac transplant model, *J. Immunol.*, 151, 7249, 1993.
101. Chavin, K. D., Qin, L., Lin, J., Kaplan, A. J., and Bromberg, J. S., Anti-CD2 and anti-CD3 monoclonal antibodies synergize to prolong allograft survival with decreased side effects, *Transplantation*, 55, 901, 1993.
102. Hirahara, H., Tsuchida, M., Watanabe, T., Haga, M., Matsumoto, Y., Abo, T., and Egushi, S., Long-term survival of cardiac allografts in rats treated before and after surgery with monoclonal antibody to CD2, *Transplantation*, 59, 85, 1995.
103. Le Mauff, B., Hourmant, M., Rougier, J. P., Hirn, M., Dantal, J., Baatard, R., Cantarovich, D., Jacques, Y., and Soulillou, J. P., Effect of anti-LFA-1 (CD11a) monoclonal antibodies in acute rejection in human kidney transplantation, *Transplantation*, 52, 291, 1991.
104. Hourmant, M., Bedrossian, J., Durand D., Kessler, M., Le Branchu, Y., Caudrelier, P., Simi B., and Soulillou, J. P., Multicenter comparative study of an anti-LFA-1 adhesion molecule monoclonal antibody and antithymocyte globulin in prophylaxis of acute rejection in kidney transplantation, *Transplant. Proc.*, 27, 864, 1995.

105. Le Mauff, B., Le Meur, Y., Scherrmann, J. M., Hourmant M., Dantal, J., Cantarovich, D., Giral M., Alberici, G., and Soulillou, J. P., Interest of anti-LFA1 MAb in prophylaxis of rejection in human kidney transplantation, *The 9th International Congress of Immunology Abstract Book*, 860, 1995.
106. Haug, C. E., Colvin, R. B., Delmonico, F. L., Auchincloss, H., Tolkoff-Rubin, N., Preffer, F. I., Rothlein, R., Norris, S., Scharschmidt, L., and Cosimi, A. B., A phase I trial of immunosuppression with anti-ICAM-1 (CD54) MAb in renal allograft recipients, *Transplantation*, 55, 766, 1993.
107. Isobe, M., Yagita, H., Okumura, K., and Ihara, A., Specific acceptance of cardiac allografts after treatment with antibodies to ICAM-1 and LFA-1, *Science*, 255, 1125, 1992.
108. Lenschow, D. J., Zeng, Y., Thistlethwaite, J. R., Montag, A., Brady, W., Gibson, M. G., Linsley, P. S., and Bluestone, J. A., Long-term survival of xenogeneic pancreatic islet grafts induced by CTLA4lg [see comments], *Science*, 257, 789, 1992.
109. Lin, H., Bolling, S. F., Linsley, P. S., Wei, R. Q., Gordon, D., Thompson, C. B., and Turka, L. A., Long-term acceptance of major histocompatibility complex mismatched cardiac allografts induced by CTLA4Ig plus donor-specific transfusion, *J. Exp. Med.*, 178, 1801, 1993.
110. Pearson, T. C., Alexander, D. Z., Winn, K. J., Linsley, P. S., Lowry, R. P., and Larsen, C. P., Transplantation tolerance induced by CTLA4-Ig, *Transplantation*, 57, 1701, 1994.
111. Brewer, Y., Palmer, A., Taube, D., Welsh, K., Bewick, M., Bindon, C., Hale, G., Waldmann, H., Dische, F., Parsons, V., and Snowden, S., Effect of graft perfusion with two CD45 monoclonal antibodies on incidence of kidney allograft rejection, *Lancet*, 2, 935, 1989.
112. Graze, P. R. and Gale, R. P., Chronic graft vs. host disease: a syndrome of disordered immunity, *Am. J. Med.*, 66, 611, 1979.
113. Dreger, P., Viehmann, K., Steinmann, J., Eckstein, V., Muller-Ruchholtz, W., Loffler, H., and Schmitz, N., G-CSF-mobilized peripheral blood progenitor cells for allogeneic transplantation: comparison of T cell depletion strategies using different $CD34^+$ selection systems or Campath-1, *Exp. Hematol.*, 23, 147, 1995.
114. Drobyski, W. R., Ash, R. C., Casper, J. T., McAuliffe, T., Horowitz, M. M., Lawton, C., Keever, C., Baxter-Lowe, L. A., Camitta, B., Garbrecht, F., Pietryga, D., Hansen, R., Chitambar, C. R., Anderson, T., and Flomenberg, N., Effect of T-cell depletion as graft-versus-host disease prophylaxis on engraftment, relapse, and disease-free survival in unrelated marrow transplantation for chronic myelogenous leukemia, *Blood*, 7, 1980, 1994.
115. Jacobs, P., Wood, L., Fullard, L., Waldmann, H., and Hale, G., T cell depletion by exposure to Campath-1G *in vitro* prevents graft-versus-host disease, *Bone Marrow Transplant.*, 13, 763, 1994.
116. Hale, G. and Waldmann, H., Control of graft-versus-host disease and graft rejection by T cell depletion of donor and recipient with Campath-1 antibodies. Results of matched sibling transplants for malignant diseases, *Bone Marrow Transplant.*, 13, 597, 1994.
117. Maeda, T., Eto, M., Lin, T., Nishimura, Y., Kong, Y. Y., and Nomoto, K., Amelioration of acute graft-versus-host disease and re-establishment of tolerance by short-term treatment with an anti-TCR antibody, *J. Immunol.*, 153, 4311, 1994.
118. Blazar, B. R., Taylor, P. A., and Vallera, D. A., *In vivo* or *in vitro* anti-CD3-epsilon chain monoclonal antibody therapy for the prevention of lethal murine graft-versus-host disease across the major histocompatibility barrier in mice, *J. Immunol.*, 152, 3665, 1994.
119. Mysliwietz, J. and Thierfelder, S., Antilymphocytic antibodies and marrow transplantation. XII. Suppression of graft-versus-host disease by T-cell-modulating and depleting antimouse CD3 antibody is most effective when preinjected in the marrow recipient, *Blood*, 10, 2661, 1992.

120. Blazar, B. R., Taylor, P. A., Snover, D. C., Bluestone, J. A., and Vallera, D. A., Nonmitogenic anti-CD3F(ab')2 fragments inhibit lethal murine graft-versus-host disease induced across the major histocompatibility barrier, *J. Immunol.*, 150, 265, 1993.
121. Palathumpat, V., Dejbakhsh-Jones, S., Holm, B., and Strober, S., Different subsets of T cells in the adult mouse bone marrow and spleen induce or suppress acute graft-versus-host disease, *J. Immunol.*, 149, 808, 1992.
122. Anasetti, C., Martin P. J., Storb, R., Appelbaum, F. R., Beatty, P. G., Davis, J., Doney, K., Hill, H. F., Stewart, P., Sullivan, K. M., Witherspoon, R. P., Thomas, E. D., and Hansen, J. A., Treatment of acute graft-versus-host disease with a nonmitogenic anti-CD3 monoclonal antibody, *Transplantation*, 54, 844, 1992.
123. Cobbold, S. P., Martin, G., Qin, S., and Waldmann, H., Monoclonal antibodies to promote marrow engraftment and tissue graft tolerance, *Nature*, 323, 164, 1986.
124. Cobbold, S., Martin, G., and Waldmann, H., Monoclonal antibodies for the prevention of graft-versus-host disease and marrow graft rejection, *Transplantation*, 42, 239, 1986.
125. Reinecke, K., Mysliwietz, J., and Thierfelder, S., Single as well as pairs of synergistic anti-CD4 + CD8 antibodies prevent graft-versus-host disease in fully mismatched mice, *Transplantation*, 57, 458, 1994.
126. Koehler, M., Hurwitz, C. A., Krance, R. A., Coustan-Smith, E., Williams, L. L., Santana, V., Rieiro, R. C., Brenner, M. K., and Heslop, H. E., XomaZyme-CD5 immunotoxin in conjunction with partial T cell depletion for prevention of graft rejection and graft-versus-host disease after bone marrow transplantation from matched unrelated donors, *Bone Marrow Transplant.*, 13, 571, 1994.
127. Anasetti, C., Hansen, J. A., Waldmann, T. A., Appelbaum, F. R., Davis, J., Deeg, H. J., Doney, K., Martin, P. J., Nash, R., Storb, R., Sullivan, K. M., Witherspoon, R. P., Binger, M. H., Chizzonite, R., Hakimi, J., Mould, D., Satoh, H., and Light, S. E., Treatment of acute graft-versus-host disease with humanized anti-Tac: An antibody that binds to the interleukin-2 receptor, *Blood*, 4, 1320, 1994.
128. Blaise, D., Olive, D., Michallet, M., Marit, G., Leblond, V., and Maraninchi, D., Impairment of leukemia-free survival by addition of interleukin-2-receptor antibody to standard graft-versus-host prophylaxis, *Lancet*, 345, 1144, 1995.
129. De Wit, D., Van Mechelen, M., Zanin, C., Doutrelepont, J. M., Velu, T., Gerard, C., Abramowicz, D., Scheerlinck, J. P., De Baetselier, P., Urbain, J., Leo, O., Goldman, M., and Moser, M., Preferential activation of Th2 cells in chronic graft-versus-host reaction, *J. Immunol.*, 150, 361, 1993.
130. Ushiyama, C., Hirano, T., Miyajima, H., Okumura, K., Ovary, Z., and Hashimoto, H., Anti-IL-4 antibody prevents graft-versus-host disease in mice after bone marrow transplantation. The IgE allotype is an important marker of graft-versus-host disease, *J. Immunol.*, 154, 2687, 1995.
131. Herve, P., Flesh, M., Tiberghien, P., Wijdenes, J., Racadot, E., Bordigoni, P., Plouvier, E., Stephan, J. L., Bordeau, H., and Holler, E., Phase I-II trial of a monoclonal antitumor necrosis factor alpha antibody for the treatment of refractory severe acute graft-versus-host disease, *Blood*, 79, 3362, 1992.
132. Harning, R., Pelletier, J., Lubbe, K., Takei, F., and Merluzzi, V. J., Reduction in the severity of graft-versus-host disease and increased survival in allogeneic mice by treatment with monoclonal antibodies to cell adhesion antigens LFA-1 alpha and Mala-2, *Transplantation*, 52, 842, 1991.
133. Blazar, B. R., Carroll, S. F., and Vallera, D. A., Prevention of murine graft-versus-host disease and bone marrow alloengraftment across the major histocompatibility barrier after donor graft preincubation with anti-LFA-1 immunotoxin, *Blood*, 78, 1915, 1991.
134. Soiffer, R. J. and Ritz, J., Selective T cell depletion of donor allogeneic marrow with anti-CD6 monoclonal antibody: rationale and results, *Bone Marrow Transplant.*, 12, S7, 1993.

135. Wallace, P. M., Johnson, J. S., MacMaster, J. F., Kennedy, K. A., Gladstone, P., and Linsley, P. S., CTLA4Ig treatment ameliorates the lethality of murine graft-versus-host disease across major histocompatibility complex barriers, *Transplantation*, 58, 602, 1994.
136. Blazar, B. R., Taylor, P. A., Linsley, P. S., and Vallera, D. A., *In vivo* blockade of CD28/CTLA4: B7/BB1 interaction with CTLA4-Ig reduces lethal murine graft-versus-host disease across the major histocompatibility complex barrier in mice, *Blood*, 12, 3815, 1994.

Part III

Development of Antibody Therapeutics

Chapter **8**

Regulatory Issues for the Development of Antibody Therapeutics

Kathy J. Lambert

CONTENTS

0-8493-8547-4/97/$0.00+$.50

8.1 INTRODUCTION

This chapter reviews regulatory issues for clinical trials and registration of murine, human, and engineered therapeutic monoclonal antibodies (MAbs) in the U.S. and the European Community (EC).

Following an outline of the regulatory background, examples of manufacturing/control, preclinical and clinical regulatory concerns for MAbs are discussed, with particular emphasis on potential unintended immunological cross-reactivity of the antibody product with human tissue antigens other than those desired and the possible presence of virus contaminants. Finally, strategies for management of MAbs regulatory concerns are proposed and future regulatory opportunities suggested.

8.2 REGULATORY BACKGROUND

8.2.1 Legislative Framework

In the U.S. the Food and Drug Administration (FDA), through the administration of the Code of Federal Regulations, regulates the manufacture and licensing of pharmaceuticals; MAb therapeutics are therefore subject to the relevant sections of these regulations.[1] In common with other biological products many MAb therapeutics are regulated by the FDA Center for Biologics Evaluation and Research (CBER). However, certain MAbs may be designated for review by the Center for Devices and Radiological Health (CDRH) or Center for Drug Evaluation and Research (CDER), with center jurisdiction being allocated on a product basis according to the October 1991 intercenter agreements.[2,3] All biological products sold for human use in the U.S. or sold for export or import must be licensed by the FDA, with different rules and constraints applying for each FDA center. For products regulated by CBER, both the manufacturing process and the facility must currently be covered by a license (product license and establishment license, respectively). Prior to commencing clinical trials of a new drug or biological, sponsors must submit an investigational new drug (IND) application dossier to the FDA. Key elements of the FDA's regulatory approach are that no new procedures or systems are needed for biotechnology since existing regulations are sufficiently broad in scope and also that review responsibilities are assigned on a product rather than a manufacturing process basis.

The EC currently comprises the original six member states (Belgium, France, Germany, Italy, Luxembourg, and The Netherlands) from 1957 together with Austria, Denmark, Finland, Germany, Greece, Ireland, Spain, Switzerland, and the U.K. In the EC, regulation of MAb therapeutics and other medicinal products developed by means of biotechnology operates at a national level (with independent procedures for each country) national for clinical trials but at a supranational level for registration.

The EC supranational regulatory framework is defined in EC regulations and directives issued by the Council of Ministers or the Commission of the European Communities. At the registration (marketing authorization) stage, use of the Centralized Procedure, established through EC Regulation 2309/93[4] and effective from January 1, 1995, is obligatory for medicinal products developed by recombinant DNA technology, hybridoma, and MAb methods or controlled expression of genes coding for biologically active proteins in prokaryotes and eukaryotes. The Centralized Procedure allows a single application, evaluation, and authorization to be made, with the final decision being binding for all the EC member states. Applications are submitted to the European Agency for Evaluation of Medicinal Products (EMEA) within which the Committee on Proprietary Medicinal Products (CPMP), comprised of two delegates per member state, is responsible for formulating EMEA opinion for referral to the commission and Council of Ministers for final adoption or rejection. A key feature of the EC regulatory framework in addition to a specific procedure for biotechnology-derived products is that the registration dossier (marketing authorization application) requires a very specific format, including three expert reports.[5]

8.2.2 Regulatory Experience

Three MAb products (Orthoclone OKT3 and ReoPro for therapy and the immunoconjugate OncoScint CR/OV for *in vivo* diagnosis) were approved for marketing in the U.S. from 1986 to 1994. These three products have also been licensed in the EC together with Panorex, and the imaging agent MyoScint. At least four immunopurification MAbs have been assessed as part of the manufacturing process for licensed therapeutic proteins.

Over the same period a number of "Points to Consider" documents relevant to manufacture and testing of hybridoma-derived and recombinant DNA-based MAbs have been published by FDA CBER.[6-9] Guidelines have also been published by the CPMP ad hoc Working Party on Biotechnology[10-14] and by the World Health Organization.[15] General biotechnology guidelines useful in formulating regulatory strategy for a MAb product include those on virus validation,[16] EC dossier format,[17] product stability,[18] and genetic stability.[19] Guidelines are statements of procedures or standards of general applicability which are not legal requirements. They are designed to cover development to licensing stage and not all of the information discussed in the guidelines is required at the initial clinical trial stage.

8.3 MANUFACTURING AND CONTROL ISSUES

8.3.1 Generation of the Clone

Sources of parental and immune cells, materials, and procedures for generation of the cell line should be thoroughly documented. For recombinant (rDNA) MAbs, details of the source, and construction of the expression vector also the method for its introduction into the host cell line are required.[14] Source cells and reagents of biological origin (e.g., medium proteins, trypsin, fetal calf serum[12]) should be free of microbial and exogenous virus contamination. Early assessment of the MAb product specificity and cross-reactivity are important as a basis for clinical and manufacturing control development.

8.3.2 Cell Line Qualification

FDA recommendations for qualification of murine and human cell lines producing MAbs for phase I trials were proposed by Kozak.[20] For clinical development from phase II through to licensing, a master cell bank (MCB) and manufacturers working cell bank (MWCB) system is required.[8,14] For validation of this system, a cell bank of cells from the end of production (EPC) for cell culture production[9] and/or a post-production cell bank (PPCB)[14] should be prepared.

Stabilization of the production cell line is important for lot-to-lot consistency and can best be achieved through repeated recloning or other selection procedures prior to creation of an MCB. Where cells are adapted from serum-containing to serum-free medium, they should be recloned.[9] For rDNA MAbs, cell line qualification should include assessment of genetic stability.[14,19] The MCB, MWCB, and EPC/PPCB all should be qualified on a one-time basis for the presence of biological contaminants, including:

1. Absence of mycoplasma using the assays described in the FDA cell lines PTC[8] and bacterial/fungal sterility
2. Screening for adventitious viruses by *in vitro* culture on at least three appropriate indicator cell lines[8,14] and hemadsorbing virus assay
3. Screening for adventitious viruses by *in vivo* testing[8,14]
4. Screening for retroviruses, with the analytical approach depending on the cell line species[9]
5. Screening for other species-specific viruses[9,14]

Cell lines containing LCMV, reovirus, rotavirus, sendai virus, or Hantaan virus are not suitable for production. Murine hybridomas, however, may be assumed to contain potentially infectious retrovirus particles; the levels in bulk harvest must be quantified and linked to the design and validation of the purification process.

Qualification of the cell line for authenticity (confirmation of species and typical phenotypic characteristics) is required for the MCB, MWCB, and ECB/PPCB.

8.3.3 Production

The FDA and EC guidelines offer advice on both *in vivo* (ascites) and *in vitro* cell culture methods of generating crude MAb.[9,14] Although the first licensed MAb Orthoclone OKT3 was produced using *in vivo* methods,[21] the current EC guideline notes that *in vitro* production offers important safety and consistency advantages over *in vivo* production (including the feasibility of using serum free medium) and that the choice of the *in vivo* route should be justified.[14]

Purification processes for MAb therapeutics should prevent the introduction of and eliminate contaminants such as cellular DNA, pyrogens, animal proteins, medium components, column process materials, as well as viruses, also cell-derived immune mediators such as interferon and other cytokines.[14] Purification design should be linked to a measurement of bulk harvest virus bioburden and include one or more robust steps known to remove or inactivate retroviruses; for example, solvent/detergent treatment and exposure to low pH or filtration. Whatever process is chosen it must allow clear and unambiguous definition of a batch.

8.3.4 Validation

The overall aim of validation studies is to show that a process, when carried out according to standard operating procedures, will reliably give a certain result. At phase I it is usual to have carried out laboratory spiking experiments involving scaled down models of the purification process to demonstrate clearance of potential virus contaminants, also cell-derived DNA.

These studies should be linked to testing for viral contaminants; for example, it is recommended that retrovirus in rodent cell MAb bulk harvests is quantified by transmission electron microscopy and that the purification process is shown to be capable of removing at least 3 logs more than the initial level of contamination.[9] FDA allows the use of abbreviated virus validation studies after prior consultation with CBER and in certain circumstances for rodent cells, and in phase I studies in life-threatening illness or severely debilitating disease and where full testing for cell line adventitious agents has been completed.[9]

For the registration dossier, process validation studies should be modeled on the final manufacturing process. The virus validation studies should involve a carefully selected group of viruses exhibiting a relevant range of physicochemical features. These studies are technically demanding and much useful guidance is available on selection of viruses, experimental design and interpretation of log reduction or inactivation kinetics data.[8,16]

Other critical purification process validation studies include demonstration of intermediate product stability and demonstration from analysis of in-process production samples of the consistency of removal of impurities (medium, process reagent, and cell derived). It should also be shown that any proposed reuse of columns has no effect on product quality, removal of impurities, or ligand leakage and that column regeneration/sanitization procedures are effective.[17]

8.3.5 Quality Control and Quality Assurance

The FDA Points to Consider and EC guideline on MAbs[9,14] include recommendations on lot-to-lot quality control monitoring of unprocessed harvest, purified bulk, and final container product. Unpurified harvest lots should be routinely tested for sterility, cultivable and noncultivable mycoplasma, virus detectable *in vitro* using at least three indicator cell lines, and retroviruses (which should be quantified for murine MAbs). Ascites-derived harvests should be tested for species-specific virus. Quality control testing of the purified bulk MAb should include confirmation of identity by isoelectric focusing (IEF) spectrotype, biological activity, immunoglobulin class, and, for rDNA MAbs, peptide mapping. Limits should be set for product purity (analyzed by reduced and nonreduced SDS-PAGE) and the levels of contaminants such as residual medium components and affinity chromatography ligands (assays capable of detecting 1 ppm contaminant levels are required). Levels of DNA of host cell and, for rDNA MAbs, vector origin should not exceed the equivalent of 100 pg per dose. Molecular integrity, including the presence of aggregated, denatured or fragmented product should be determined (e.g., by gel permeation high performance liquid chromatography; HPLC). The purified bulk specification may also include presentation details such as appearance, protein concentration, pH, and osmolarity. Virus testing of the purified bulk may be necessary if virus contamination was detected in the bulk harvest. Quality control testing on the contents of final containers from each filling of product should include the following: sterility (to 21 CFR 610.12 and/or European pharmacopeial monograph), potency, purity by reduced and non-reduced SDS-PAGE, protein concentration, general safety (to 21 CFR 610.11 and/or European abnormal toxicity pharmacopeial monograph), endotoxin, or pyrogens, and an identity test.

The MAbs guidelines[9,14] include statements on the requirement for Good Manufacturing Practices (GMPs) and an FDA guideline on the preparation of investigational new products is available.[22] Important GMP controls even for the earliest stages of clinical trial supplies manufacture are pharmaceutical grade equipment and utilities, maintenance of complete records, control of raw materials, availability of an independent QA unit, and retention of samples of each lot. Compliance of non-clinical laboratory safety studies such as cell bank validation, viral removal/inactivation, and analytical methods validation with Good Laboratory Practice (GLP) requirements[1,4] should also be considered. Early establishment of a well-characterized in-house reference standard derived from a production lot is fundamental for product characterization, validation of analytical methods, stability studies, and development of product quality specifications.

8.3.6 Characterization

Thorough characterization of the MAb product should be carried out prior to the start of clinical trials using sensitive reproducible and reliable methods. Such characterization is necessary on an ongoing basis as a foundation for the selection of routine quality control tests also for the purpose of demonstrating product equivalence when process changes are required. The extent of product heterogeneity is particularly relevant when other agents exhibiting heterogeneity (such as immunotoxins) are used to modify the protein since a range of products with different toxic and therapeutic properties could be present.

Characterization of the MAb product should include biochemical/physiochemical, biological/immunological, and specificity/cross-reactivity parameters. The FDA Points to Consider on MAbs[9] discusses structural integrity, specificity, and potency characterization issues for purified unmodified MAbs. The EC guideline[14] lists immunological characterization parameters and also requirements for rDNA MAbs such as terminal amino acid sequencing and secondary and tertiary structure studies. Peptide mapping technology capable of detecting a single amino acid variant in an rDNA MAb has been described.[23]

8.3.7 Stability

As a minimum, sponsors require sufficient data to justify product stability for the duration of the proposed clinical trial. MAb stability studies should include monitoring of structural integrity (for example, by IEF, SDS-PAGE, and GP-HPLC analysis) and potency/biological activity. Real time stability studies on at least three lots in the container/closure intended for distribution are required for marketing authorization applications.[18]

8.3.8 Immunoconjugates

Additional manufacturing and control issues for immunoconjugates include the details of construction (including the source, specification, and toxicity profile of all components) and the purity, immunoreactivity, potency, and stability of the immunoconjugate. Detailed recommendations on these issues are available in the FDA Points to Consider on MAbs.[9] This document together with the EC guideline on MAb radiopharmaceuticals[11] also provides advice on the specific manufacturing, animal testing (dose estimation and biodistribution), and stability requirements for MAbs coupled to radionuclides.

8.4 PRECLINICAL ISSUES

8.4.1 Cross-Reactivity

A major concern for MAb therapeutics is that of unintentional product reactivity with human cells or tissues other than the intended target tissue. Laboratory tests to screen for potential cross-reactivity are required prior to phase I clinical trials. Such studies should be carried out using the finished product intended for clinical use since coupling to a radiolabel, drug, or toxin may alter the specificity of the MAb for the desired antigen. The current FDA and EC guidelines [9,14] provide reference lists from which an appropriate range of human tissues for cross-reactivity studies may be selected. Recommendations on immunohistochemical procedures, acquisition of samples, and assessment of cross-reactivity are provided in the FDA document.[9] If *in vitro* MAb cross-reactivity is detected, a comprehensive *in vivo* evaluation of its physiological significance will be required, initially in animals and later in human trials. Studies in more than one animal species or repeat dose animal studies may be necessary.[9]

8.4.2 Toxicology, Pharmacology, and Pharmacokinetics

Products used in preclinical studies should be manufactured using the same procedures as the batch intended for clinical trials. Preclinical study protocols should parallel those intended for the clinical trials as closely as possible with respect to dose, concentration, route, and dosing regimen. At least one dose equivalent to and one that is a multiple of the highest proposed clinical dose should be studied. Preclinical testing concerns in addition to cross-reactivity include immunogenicity, stability, and effector functions. Species differences may complicate the design and evaluation of preclinical studies.

The extent of preclinical toxicology studies necessary to support initiation of clinical trials will be specific to each new MAb product.[9,10] At one extreme, for an unmodified MAb with no demonstrable cross-reactivity *in vitro* for human tissues and no animal model of disease activity or animal that carries the relevant antigen, testing may be as limited as the General Safety Test (21 CFR 610.11).[9] In contrast, immunoconjugates containing radionuclides, toxins, or drugs will require detailed animal toxicity studies linked to studies of conjugate stability. The toxicity and target organs of the individual immunoconjugate components including free toxin, drug, or nuclide, should also be examined. Immunoconjugate toxicology testing should be performed in a species possessing the relevant target antigen or disease model, if feasible. Toxicity testing of the free toxin or nuclide may be performed in a different species.[9]

Where an animal model is available, pharmacological studies to investigate dose dependence of biological effects and provide a rationale for the proposed clinical use should be undertaken. For determination of pharmacokinetics and biodistribution, an animal species that shares a cross-reactive or identical target antigen with humans is preferable. Pharmacokinetic experiments should involve more than one measurement method for the presence of the product: for immunoconjugates, levels of the intact conjugate, the free MAb, and the free ligand should all be measured. The presence of antibodies to the product may alter biodistribution, metabolism, and clearance particularly on repeat dosing.[9]

8.5 CLINICAL TRIAL ISSUES

The FDA Points to Consider on MAbs[9] includes general recommendations on the design of clinical studies. MAb therapeutics administered to humans have usually been well tolerated. The rare cases of serious or fatal adverse events have generally resulted from unintended MAb cross-reactivity. Phase I studies are intended to obtain information on the safety and pharmacology of a new compound in human subjects. For MAb therapeutics phase I aims should include: definition of common toxicities and also the relation between dose and toxicity, determination of pharmacokinetics in a human population with the appropriate antigen, and collection of data on immunogenicity. Healthy volunteers are not usually appropriate for phase I trials of MAb therapeutics due to the risks of product immunogenicity and lack of relevant toxicity data. The selection of the phase I starting dose should be based on safety and toxicity information from a relevant animal model wherever possible.

Phase II studies are intended to provide preliminary evidence of efficacy in a specific disease condition, also additional safety information. Aims should include establishment of the most reliable clinical endpoint for determination of MAb clinical efficacy and identification of an active dose range which has an acceptable toxicity profile. Phase III trials should generate the definitive efficacy and safety database for licensing. Design considerations include defined endpoint, defined target population, adequate statistical power, and a detailed analytical plan. Major manufacturing changes should be addressed prior to phase III trials.

Monitoring of patient immune response to MAb therapeutics is critical since host antibodies can affect biodistribution and efficacy of administered MAbs. The FDA Points to Consider on MAbs provides detailed recommendations on such monitoring.[9] Assays to detect human anti-mouse antibodies (HAMA), human anti-rat antibodies (HARA), human antibodies directed against chimeric or humanized antibodies, immunonuclides, or immunotoxins may be required, according to the MAb source and design, and should be carefully standardized. Skin testing is now not generally recommended as it is a poor predictor of sensitivity to mouse proteins and can cause sensitization.[9] Where immune response to a MAb occurs, adverse events should be anticipated and appropriate precautions taken during clinical trials.

Regulatory concerns on MAbs coupled to radionuclides (for diagnosis or therapy) include the absorbed radiation dose distribution, also the excretion and kinetics of the radioimmunoconjugate.[11] Sufficient data from animal or human studies should be available to allow a reasonable calculation of radiation-absorbed dose to the whole body and critical organs upon administration to a human subject. Detailed advice on radiation dosimetry estimates are provided in the EC guideline on MAb radiopharmaceuticals[11] and the FDA Points to Consider on MAbs.[9] These documents also discuss clinical trial requirements for radiopharmaceuticals and cancer imaging agents.

8.6 MANAGEMENT OF REGULATORY ISSUES

8.6.1 General Principles

Effective management of regulatory issues starts with awareness of the relevant regulations, biologicals GMPs, guidelines, and pharmacopeial monographs. The onus is then on the sponsor to customize a regulatory strategy for their specific product and situation. For Europe, the appropriate experts (for the expert reports) should be involved in developing this strategy. Regulatory objectives should then be integrated into long term multidisciplinary project plans. Investment in robust and scalable purification procedures, validated analytical methods, and product characterization/stability studies are pivotal.

Early interaction with regulatory agencies to discuss the regulatory strategy, available data, special concerns, and clinical development plans is crucial. The FDA specifically encourages such meetings at the pre-IND and end of phase II stages of clinical development and on specific topics such as design of virus removal/inactivation procedures and process validation for Mab therapeutics.[9] Such contact is also possible with national institutions in Europe such as the National Institute for Biological Standards and Control in England and the Paul Ehrlich Institut in Germany. The methods for making EMEA, CPMP Biotech Working Party, or rapporteur advice available to sponsors prior to submission of centralized registration are dossiers currently being evaluated in the light of industry comment.

8.6.2 Influence of Phase of Development

A major complication with interpretation of regulatory guidelines is that they do not usually differentiate between manufacturing and control requirements for clinical trial supplies and those for licensed product. Minimum product characterization and process validation expectations from the regulatory perspective at the various stages of development may, however, be outlined as follows.[24]

For phase I studies, the cell line should be qualified and a detailed product structure available. Acceptance criteria for raw materials should be established, also a product stability estimate preferably based on biological activity. Identification and measure of indigenous virus load in supernatants together with validated procedures for virus removal are needed. Expectations for phase II supplies include the establishment of master and working cell banks, full written production and test procedures, and establishment of lot-to-lot yield analyses. Quality control (QC) in-process, release, and stability assays together with supporting validation and a qualified product standard should be established.

Pivotal phase III supplies should be manufactured in the facilities and by the process and scale intended for commercial supply. Equipment and process validation, including the effects of any scale up carried out during process development should be completed. The product specification can be refined on the basis of full-scale lot-to-lot experience and also multiple lots placed on stability. In practice commercial pressures to maintain a competitive lead together with the need for only limited numbers of batches to provide the overall clinical study product demand usually lead to the initial GMP batch being required to meet both the phase I and II standards. The phase I standards are of course appropriate where only a short term clinical goal is involved.

8.6.3 Manufacturing Changes

An important issue for MAb manufacture is the impact of process changes on the stability, safety, and potency of the product. Examples of changes which can lead to an altered form of the product are: transition from *in vivo* to *in vitro* manufacture, modified cell culture or purification procedure, or additional modifications to the MAb molecule. The impurity profile may also be altered, the level of retrovirus load at harvest being a particular concern for murine MAbs.

Product equivalence studies to support such process changes should include rigorous *in vitro* biochemical and functional characterization studies.[9,14] Where cell culture is modified without changes to the MCB, relevant characteristics such as cell growth and stability of production should be compared.[14] *In vivo* equivalence of MAb pharmacokinetics, biodistribution, and half-life should also be determined. Where both MAbs are demonstrated to have identical biochemical, functional, and pharmacological characteristics, clinical equivalence studies should not be necessary. However, if differences are seen or a different MCB is to be used for production, or product equivalence cannot be adequately characterized by analytical testing, then clinical evaluation of the MAb produced by the new process is likely to be required. Where changes in manufacturing occur during early clinical development, evaluations of clinical equivalence can be included in ongoing clinical trials. For licensed products, such changes would require submission of a license amendment with supporting data such as repetition of adventitious agent testing and virus removal validation.[9]

8.6.4 Contract Manufacture

The specialized nature of MAb manufacture and the increasing number of products being developed for niche markets have led to widespread use of contract suppliers for bulk MAbs.

Regulatory issues when purchasing bulk intermediate MAb for further processing include consistency in QC assessment across the interface between the supplier release and the recipient acceptance. Provision for GMP audit of the supplier and explicit definition of the respective long term GMP compliance responsibilities of the supplier and recipient are also essential. Finally, provision for release of R & D data by the supplier and full knowledge of relevant product licensing conditions by both parties are required. In the U.S., the supplier of bulk active biological ingredient requires a product license in addition to that held by the final manufacturer placing the dosage form product on the market. The FDA's policy allowing shared manufacturing of licensed biologicals was introduced in 1983 and updated in 1992.[25] The first licensed product under this procedure was an *in vitro* MAb; more recently a MAb therapeutic has been licensed under the system.

Strategies for successful management of the issues involved in contract manufacture include effective collaboration between the parties concerned on analytical method development, bulk product regulatory strategy, and stability studies. A pre-contract audit to establish agreement on GMP approach can then be followed by audits to monitor supplier compliance. Written agreements listing respective routine manufacture and control responsibilities for the supplier and receiving manufacturer should be available (at the registration stage, this can be filed as part of the U.S. PLA submission). Effective handling of confidential information and commitment to long term partnership by both parties are fundamental to the relationship.

8.7 CONCLUSIONS AND FUTURE OPPORTUNITIES

The current FDA and EC guidelines on MAb therapeutics are comprehensive, complementary, and based on extensive experience (at least

74 MAbs are currently in clinical trials[26]). Continuation of case-by-case regulatory assessment of MAb products is essential. This depends upon industry customizing regulatory strategies for specific products through current and specific interpretation of the guidelines and interaction with the regulatory agencies both for advice on regulatory approach and to influence guideline development. The regulatory philosophy for MAbs has been through characterization of the cell substrate, detailed process control, and process validation, as well as quality of the finished product. However, in recent years enhanced technology for assessing lot-to-lot variation and stability of the final MAb product has been developed.

Future opportunities for effective management of regulatory issues for MAb therapeutics include development in the EC of the EMEA and CPMP mechanisms for early interaction and provision of advice to sponsors using the centralized procedure. In the U.S. the FDA has recently confirmed that pilot manufacturing facilities can be used for production of licensed product.[27] The current FDA reform proposals offer opportunities for streamlining approvals of well-characterized MAb therapeutics and recombinant DNA products.[28] Separation of FDA establishment and product licensing for such products could provide sponsors with greatly increased flexibility over investment in manufacturing plant, since it could become possible to manufacture phase III supplies in a different facility to that intended for commercial supply.

REFERENCES

1. Code of Federal Regulations Title 21, U.S. Printing Office, Washington (updated annually): Parts 58, 200–211, 312, 314, 600–680, 800.
2. Food and Drug Administration, Intercenter agreement between the Center for Biologics Evaluation and Research and the Center for Devices and Radiological Health, 1991.
3. Food and Drug Administration, Intercenter agreement between the Center for Drug Evaluation and Research and the Center for Biologics Evaluation Research, 1991.
4. European Commission, *The Rules Governing Medicinal Products in the European Union*, Volume 1, Office for Official Publications of the European Communities, Luxembourg, 1994, 3.
5. European Commission, *The Rules Governing Medicinal Products in the European Community*, Volume II, Office for Official Publications of the European Communities, Luxembourg, 1989, 48.

FDA CENTER FOR BIOLOGICS EVALUATION AND RESEARCH, 1401 ROCKVILLE PIKE, ROCKVILLE, MD 20852-1448 U.S.

6. Points to Consider in the production and testing of new drugs and biologicals produced by recombinant DNA technology, 1985.

7. Supplement to the Points to Consider in the production and testing of new drugs and biologicals produced by recombinant DNA technology: nucleic acid characterization and genetic stability, 1992.
8. Points to Consider in the characterization of cell lines used to produce biologicals, 1993.
9. Points to Consider in the manufacture and testing of monoclonal antibody products for human use, 1994.

EUROPEAN COMMISSION, *THE RULES GOVERNING MEDICINAL PRODUCTS IN THE EUROPEAN COMMUNITY,* VOLUME III, OFFICE FOR OFFICIAL PUBLICATIONS OF THE EUROPEAN COMMUNITIES, LUXEMBOURG:

10. Preclinical biological safety testing of medicinal products derived from biotechnology, 1988 (in original volume, 1989, 73).
11. Radiopharmaceuticals based on monoclonal antibodies, Doc III/3487/89 (in Addendum 2, 1992, 15).
12. Minimising the risk of transmission from animals to man of agents causing spongiform encephalopathies via medicinal products Doc III/3298/91 (in Addendum 2, 1992, 117).
13. Production and quality control of medicinal products derived by recombinant DNA technology, Revision 1994, Doc III/3477/92 (in Addendum 3, 1995, 47).
14. Production and quality control of monoclonal antibodies, Doc III/5271/94 (in Addendum 3, 1995, 57).
15. World Health Organisation, Guidelines for assuring the quality of monoclonal antibodies, Technical Report Series 822, Annex 3, 1992, 47.

EUROPEAN AGENCY FOR THE EVALUATION OF MEDICINAL PRODUCTS CPMP BIOTECH WORKING PARTY GUIDELINES:

16. Revised CPMP guideline on virus validation studies, Doc CPMP/268/95.
17. Note for guidance on biotech headings for Notice to Applicants Part II Doc III/3153/91.
18. Quality of biotechnological products: stability testing of biotechnological/biological products (previously numbered ICH7), Doc CPMP/138/95.
19. Quality of biotechnological products: genetic stability (previously numbered ICH6), Doc CPMP/139/95.

20. Kozak, R. W., Current FDA recommendations for Phase I studies, presented at FDA/NIH Preclinical Safety Testing of Monoclonal Antibodies Workshop, Bethesda, January 9–10, 1992.
21. Lime, W. W., Regulatory issues concerning Orthoclone OKT®3 (Muromonab CD3) monoclonal antibody, in *Regulatory Practice for Biopharmaceutical Production*, Lubiniecki, A.S. and Vargo, S.A., Eds., Wiley-Liss, New York, 1994, 235.
22. FDA Center for Biologics Evaluation and Research, Guideline on the preparation of investigational new drug products (human and animal), 1991.
23. Harris, R. J., Murnane, A. A., Utter, S. L., Wagner, K. L., Cox, E. T., Polastri, G. D., Helder, J. C., and Sliwkowski, M. B., Assessing genetic heterogeneity in production lines: detection by peptide mapping of a low level Tyr to Gln sequence variant in a recombinant antibody, *Bio/Technology*, 11, 1293, 1993.
24. Risso, S. T., Licensing a biological: GMP Issues presented at Biopharm Conference Cambridge Mass, June 21-23, 1993.

25. FDA's policy statement concerning cooperative manufacturing arrangements for licensed biologics, *Fed. Reg.*, 57, 55544, 1992.
26. Pharmaceutical Research and Manufacturers of America, Biotechnology medicines and vaccines approved and under development, *Genetic Eng. News*, August 12, 1995.
27. Food and Drug Administration, FDA guidance document concerning the use of pilot manufacturing facilities for the development and manufacture of biological products: availability, 1995.
28. FDA readies reform package, *BioCentury*, 3, A1, 1995.

Chapter 9

Manufacture of Antibodies by Large-Scale Mammalian Cell Culture

David K. Robinson, Vijay Yabannavar, and Yashwant Deo

CONTENTS

0-8493-8547-4/97/$0.00+$.50

9.1 INTRODUCTION

The *in vivo* dosages of therapeutic monoclonal antibodies (MAbs) used in many experimental clinical protocols are quite high, approaching 1 g in some trials.[1] To reach a reasonable market sizes of one hundred thousand to one million doses per year, such MAbs must be produced at rates of tens to hundreds of kilograms per year. In addition, these large dosages require that these MAbs be produced as economically as possible. Cell culture reactors and downstream processes must be prepared to process many thousands of liters of crude culture broth. As described below, large-scale production of therapeutic MAbs requires high productivity cell lines and processes, coupled with reliable operations and a high assurance of product safety, efficacy, and consistency.

9.2 CELL LINE DEVELOPMENT

9.2.1 Development and Selection of High Producing Cell Lines

MAbs have traditionally been produced in continuous cell lines created via fusion of activated rodent B-cell lymphocytes with myeloma tumor cells (see Reference 2 for review). Due, however, to the potential elicitation of human antimouse antibodies (HAMA)[3] by murine or other nonhuman MAbs, future therapeutic applications will rely on chimeric, humanized, or human MAbs. Human MAbs can be expressed as recombinant gene products or in human-human hybridoma cell lines, heterohybridoma cell lines, or Epstein-Barr virus (EBV) transformed lymphocytes (see Reference 4 for review). The rates of MAb production by hybridoma and heterohybridoma cell lines is quite variable, ranging from as little as 2 pg/cell/day, yielding less than 10 mg/l in batch culture, up to 80 pg/cell/day, yielding over 100 mg/l (see Reference 5 for review). Repeated single-cell cloning can be used, at times, to isolate and select higher producing cells from even a low producing parental population.[6,7] In some cases, recloning after subjecting cells to "stress", e.g., serum-free medium or suspension culture, can be used to isolate higher producers when simple recloning has failed.[4]

In addition to isolation of human B lymphocytes expressing MAbs to the correct target, human MAbs of the appropriate specificity can be selected by screening of human combinatorial libraries.[8,9] Alternatively, the non-binding domains of nonhuman MAbs can be changed to corresponding human sequences to minimize potential HAMA responses[10] (see Reference 11 for review). Expression of these MAbs requires transfection of the antibody genes into host cells, most typically Chinese hamster ovary (CHO) cells[12-14] or two different murine cell lines, SP2/0 and NS0 (for review see References 14 and 15). Early efforts to express MAbs in transfected cells resulted in relatively low antibody production, less than 5 pg/cell/day with batch yields less than 50 mg/l. However, the use of improved vectors incorporating selectable markers, highly active promoters, and the heavy and light chain genes on a single plasmid have resulted in cell lines that express MAb at up to 15 pg/cell/day in non-amplified cell lines.[16] Cells that express antibody at even greater rates can be selected after gene amplification; cells transfected with a selectable marker are grown in a deficient medium and exposed to increasing concentrations of an otherwise toxic drug, e.g., methionine sulfoximine (MSX) for vectors containing the glutamine synthetase (GS) gene[17] or methotrexate (MTX) for vectors containing the dihydrofolate reductase (DHFR) gene.[18] Amplification has resulted in NS0 cell lines that express antibody at up to 50 pg/cell/day[15] and in CHO cell lines that express antibody at up to 100 pg/cell/day.[12-14] Although selection and amplification of these cell lines requires addition of selective agents, e.g., MSX or MTX, to the culture medium, careful screening can result in the isolation of cell lines that are reasonably stable (e.g., >20 generations) in the absence of selective agents. Given the cost of these selective agents, as well as the potential risk to product safety and of occupational exposure during large-scale culture, the effort required to develop such stable cell lines is well justified.

Experience to date suggests that the common host cell lines, SP2/0, NS/0, and CHO, can secrete antibody at maximum rates of 50 to 100 pg/cell/day. Further increases in antibody gene transcription via use of more active promoters or gene amplification are unlikely to further increase the secretion rate.[19] Mosser and Massie describe a number of genes that could be expressed as recombinant gene products in cell lines to either increase the secretion rate or delay the onset of apoptotic cell death, resulting in improved cell lines that could further increase antibody yields.[20] Assembly of heavy and light chain genes has been identified as a potentially rate-limiting step, suggesting that elevated levels of ER chaperones or PDI could increase further MAb secretion rates.[21] However, overexpression of such chaperones has yet to result in increased antibody secretion rates.[20] As described below, yields in batch and fed-batch culture are a function of both the specific rate of antibody secretion and cell culture longevity.[5] Cell death for a number of cell lines appears to occur via apoptosis (for review see References 22 and 23). Overexpression of one gene involved in the apoptotic pathway, bcl-2, was recently shown to increase hybridoma cell culture longevity and antibody yields,[24] demonstrating that genetic intervention in the apoptotic pathway can increase culture productivity.

9.2.2 Biosafety and Product Consistency

A variety of stringent regulations related to product quality, safety, consistency, efficacy, and purity need to be satisfied for diagnostic and therapeutic MAbs.[25] These regulations are discussed at length elsewhere in this volume (Chapter 8). Here we briefly describe the regulatory considerations related to cell line characterization, cell stability, and process validation for product consistency and safety. This involves addressing the following key issues: (1) origin and history of the cell substrate; (2) cell banking or seed lot system; (3) examination of seed lots for endogenous and adventitious microbial contaminants as well as inherent traits; (4) examination of cell and product stability during the production process; and (5) validation of purification process steps for reduction of viral contaminants. Several guidelines have been published by the U.S. Food and Drug Administration (FDA)[26,27] and the European Committee on Proprietary Medicinal Products (CPMP)[28] as well as Japan's and other countries' regulatory agencies. The recent efforts to harmonize regulations between Europe, North America, and Japan may result in only one set of rules in the near future. Until that point, the above documents provide useful guiding principles.

9.2.2.1 Origin and Seed Lot System

A variety of cell substrates including murine and human hybridoma cells, recombinant mammalian cells, e.g., myeloma or CHO, and microbial cells are used to produce MAbs. The origin of the cell substrate must be traced as far back as possible. For a hybridoma, the origin and cultivation history of the fusion partners as well as further manipulations of the hybridoma must be fully documented. All biological components including feeder layers, erythrocytes used for isolation of B cells, EBV used to immortalize B cells, animal-derived nutrients such as serum and growth factors as well as animal or human donors of B cells, and the operators handling the cells may introduce a variety of adventitious agents in the final production cell line. These contaminants may remain as permanent intracellular parasites, raising concerns for product safety. The presence of mycoplasma, a known pathogen, or an unknown prion or virus may preclude the use of a cell line. The origin and history of all steps involved in preparation of the ultimate cell line are important for two reasons: (1) to develop a strategy for cell line characterization and (2) to select model virus strains for purification process validation. Current state-of-the-art cell testing methods are not adequate to detect all the potential known and unknown adventitious agents from various animal species. Therefore, detailed documentation in support of the cell substrate origin and cultivation history minimizes concerns about animal species that were not used for a given cell substrate. If one is starting preparation of a new hybridoma or recombinant cell line, the golden rule for the use of animal- and human-derived products may be "less is better."

For recombinant cell substrates, e.g., chimeric, humanized or primatized antibodies, and antibody fragments, the origin and cultivation history becomes relatively less complex. Selection of a well characterized host cell substrate minimizes concern of introducing contaminants. Generally, the genes or sections of genes coding for the recombinant antibody or antibody fragments are obtained from a hybridoma cell line with a potentially complex history. It is assumed that the phenol extraction and ethanol precipitation steps used for DNA purification are adequate to minimize or eliminate the possibility of microbial or prion contaminant carryover to the recombinant cell substrate. In spite of this assumption, careful documentation on the origin and history of the DNA donor is advisable.

The use of combinatorial libraries and microbial cell substrates for generating "human" MAbs almost totally eliminates the possibility of animal-derived contaminants, but introduces new concerns regarding the viral vectors, the purity and homogeneity of the microbial host, and any animal-derived media components used in microbial fermentations. Therefore, use of a well-characterized host strain, bacteriophage strain, and simple cultivation conditions is advisable.

9.2.2.2 Seed Lot System and Characterization

The most commonly used seed lot system involves one 100-200 vial master cell bank (MCB) and one or more 400-500 vial manufacturer's working cell banks (MWCBs or WCBs) derived from the MCB. It is useful to prepare a preliminary cell bank before the MCB, which serves as an intermediate step to examine the production levels, nutrient requirements, growth characteristics, product quality, etc. before the MCB is established. This initial cell bank is variously termed as a pre-MCB, research cell bank (RCB), or security cell bank (SCB). However, only the MCB and MWCBs constitute the main seed lot system for a product. The MCB generally acts as the "queen bee" in that it is not directly used for production, while the MWCBs are "worker bees" and one or more vials of a MWCB are used to begin each production lot. The MCB is expected to maintain continuity and product consistency throughout the life of the product. The MCB and MWCBs should be thoroughly characterized as described below. When a microbial host is used to produce a recombinant antibody or antibody fragment, it is possible to maintain the recombinant vector and host strain as two separate components of the MCB. New transfectants can then be obtained when a new MWCB is required. However, this practice may require significantly greater characterization of the new transfectants than required for a standard MWCB.

The characterization of either an MCB or MWCB can be divided in three categories: (1) detection and classification of endogenous agents; (2) detection and classification of adventitious agents; and (3) determination of inherent characteristics. The endogenous contaminants include mostly the endogenous retroviruses found in rodent cells, e.g., murine or hamster cell lines, and rarely an EBV genome. Several *in vitro* tests have been developed for detection, characterization, and quantification of endogenous retroviruses.[29,30] However, it is well established that all murine cell lines have endogenous retroviral genomes and frequently these cells produce large numbers of viral particles. Therefore, detailed characterization of such endogenous retroviruses in murine cell lines and cell banks is not critical. Such characterization may be important for hamster or human heterohybridomas, since human cells contain highly mutated retroviral genomes and a theoretical possibility of generating "new" recombinant retroviruses should be considered. Thorough process validation demonstrating >15–20 log reduction of retroviruses may alleviate such a theoretical concern. EBV genomes and live virus particles can be detected by the *in vitro* tests described below.

Adventitious agents include prions, viruses, mycoplasma, bacteria, and fungi. These contaminants are either contributed by the parental cells and animal-derived nutrients or introduced during handling. Various tests used for detection and characterization of adventitious agents have been reviewed by Lees and Darling.[29] These tests can be classified in the following categories.

Sterility and Mycoplasma Tests — Bacterial and fungal contaminants are detected by inoculation of the cell substrate in appropriate microbial media, incubation for 2–4 weeks followed by microscopic examination or biochemical tests. Mycoplasma are detected by DNA staining, immunological tests, and cultivation on indicator cells such as Vero or NIH-2-T3.

In vitro virus tests — Live cells, cell lysate, or culture supernatant from an MCB/MWCB are inoculated or co-cultivated with appropriate indicator cell lines. The indicator cell lines are selected on the basis of the origin and history of the MCB/MWCB to be tested. For example, if sheep erythrocytes and EBV derived from a monkey cell line were used to obtain the hybridoma and fetal calf serum was used in its cultivation, the *in vitro* test should include ovine, simian, and bovine indicator cell lines susceptible to adventitious agents from these animal species. Human indicator cells are almost always used because of human handling. The inoculated indicator cells are typically incubated for 2-4 weeks and then examined for evidence of contamination by microscopy, and biochemical, immunological, or hematological tests. Similar *in vitro* tests can be used to detect the presence of adventitious bacteriophage or fungal viruses in microbial hosts.

In vivo tests — In these tests the cells or lysate are injected into animals by various routes of administration, e.g., oral, intravenous, or intraperitoneal. The animals are then observed for any overt signs of sickness, weight loss, death, etc., for a period of 2-4 weeks. The animals may be examined by immunological, hematological, and biochemical tests or sacrificed and examined for systemic growth of any potential contaminants. For detection of prions the *in vivo* test is the only reliable one available today. Mouse is the animal of choice for these tests due to supply and cost considerations. However, depending upon the history of the MCB, other animal species may be required.

Genetic, immunological, and biochemical tests — Recently a variety of genetic and immunological probes have been developed for detection of specific viral and prion contaminants employing standard immunohistology and hybridization methods. These probes can be most useful when the potential presence of a defined contaminant, e.g., EBV, HIV, hepatitis, or papilloma virus, is suspected. The biochemical tests include assays for specific enzymatic activity, such as reverse transcriptase since murine and human retroviruses possess two distinct classes of reverse transcriptase enzymes. Biochemical tests are also used to confirm identity and stability of a microbial host.

Electron microscopy — Since the biological and immunological tests require growth and multiplication of the contaminant under selected conditions, dormant, defective, or latent contaminants could defy detection. Therefore, direct physical examination by electron microscopy (transmission or scanning) is recommended to detect virus- or prion-like particles. This test is also used to quantify total viral contaminants in the MCB/MWCB.

Tests for inherent traits — To establish the identity of cell, specific inherent characteristics such as the isoenzyme patterns of well-defined enzymes (e.g., lactate dehydrogenate, nucleoside phosphorylase, or glutamine synthetase), or the chromosomal composition (e.g., ploidy, structures, and total number) can be monitored. Isoenzyme analysis is useful to confirm the species of origin, but chromosomal analysis has very little utility since most continuous cell lines are transformed and therefore their chromosomal composition varies significantly. For recombinant cells, genetic analysis of the vector and specific antibody genes by *in situ* hybridization could serve as a useful identification tool.

In summary, several tests are available to examine the presence of numerous adventitious agents which may compromise safety of the final product. Although some "rescue" methods have been described, the presence of an intracellular adventitious agent such as mycoplasma, virus, or prion would generally preclude use of the cell line. Unless absolutely necessary, it is advisable to discard the contaminated cell bank and begin with fresh cells. It is most prudent to use a well-characterized host strain and the most stringent techniques while developing a new cell substrate. Otherwise, a very exciting new product may be significantly delayed by a contaminated cell substrate.

9.2.2.3 In-Process Testing

In spite of thorough testing of the MCB and MWCBs, it is possible that some unknown adventitious agents may have escaped detection: new contaminants may be introduced during the cultivation process;

expression of endogenous agents (such as murine retroviruses) may be induced; or a latent endogenous agent may be activated in high cell density culture or during long term continuous cultivation. In-process testing of samples collected at the pre-culture (inoculum) step, at specific intervals during the large-scale cultivation process, and at the end of the bioreactor run is necessary to detect new or activated adventitious agents. The sterility, mycoplasma, *in vitro* virus, immunological, or electron microscopy tests described above are used for in-process samples. These tests also facilitate quantification of endogenous retrovirus particles in the culture supernatant before further processing to yield purified product. If mycoplasma or a new viral or prion adventitious agent is found in any of the in-process samples, the bioreactor run should be terminated and all the product obtained from the contaminated culture should be discarded. A thorough investigation to determine the source of contaminant must be launched and extensive decontamination of the bioreactor and all the affected areas should be performed. Again, complete documentation to support the investigation and decontamination activities should be maintained.

In conclusion, a three-pronged approach comprising of cell bank characterization, in-process testing, and purification process validation should be used to ensure product safety. The final step in dealing with endogenous retroviruses and potential adventitious agents is purification process validation as described in Section 9.5.2.6.

9.2.3 Cell Line Stability

As described above, large-scale production of antibody involves storage of cells as an MCB and MWCB for up to several years as well as expansion of cells from an MWCB vial to large volumes for the production of each antibody lot. Thus, cell line stability should be demonstrated at three levels: during the storage of cell banks, through several cell divisions in each production batch, and during various production batches.[31]

Cell bank stability during storage is determined by detailed characterization of each MWCB prior to use in production and of the MCB at defined intervals (e.g., once every 3-5 years), as described in the previous section. In addition, the equivalence of the MCB and MWCB is examined by clonality (fraction of producer cells in the cell bank), kinetics of cell growth, and specific productivity (pg/cell/day). For genetic stability of recombinant cell lines, specific guidelines have been suggested by the U.S. regulatory agencies[32] as described below. Finally, antibody purified from the new MWCB and the reference standard are compared by biochemical, immunological and bioactivity tests (see Section 9.5.3) to demonstrate that the product produced by the two cell banks is equivalent.

The next level of cell line stability tests are carried out during the production process. For this purpose, cells are collected from the beginning, middle, and terminal phases ("end of production") of the cultivation cycle. For example, in a batch process, cells are collected from the pre-culture, inoculum, and three times during the production — the lag phase, the exponential growth phase, and at the end of production. The pre-culture and inoculum samples are optional if MWCB cells are used as a reference standard. For a continuous perfusion process, cells are collected just after inoculation of the production reactor — in the middle of the run after reaching steady levels of perfusion rate, cell density and specific productivity — and just prior to the termination of the run. Along with cells, antibody is also collected at these time points and examined by biochemical, immunological, and bioactivity tests. It is recommended that cell and product samples be collected from at least three different, preferably consecutive, bioreactor runs to show lot-to-lot consistency.

The following types of tests are recommended for cells collected at the various stages of the production process. For hybridoma cell lines, inherent characteristics and endogenous murine retrovirus expression levels are examined by isoenzyme analysis, karyology, and murine retrovirus tests. In addition, the fraction of producer cells, cell doubling time, and specific productivity can be examined to demonstrate physiological stability with respect to antibody production. For recombinant cell lines, it is required to demonstrate genetic stability. This can be accomplished by examination of (1) the coding sequence of the antibody gene; (2) MAb-specific mRNA levels per cell; and (3) sequence analysis of cDNA derived from the antibody-specific mRNA. These tests are not intended to detect low levels of variant sequences, but rather to demonstrate that the predominant protein species prior to purification will have the correct amino acid sequence throughout full-scale production. If the recombinant vector is integrated in the cellular genome, it may be of value to examine the stability of insertion sites by restriction analysis of the flanking sequences. This relatively gross analysis indicates if significant variation has occurred in the location of vector insertion, although low level variants may not be detected.

In summary, the cell banks, cells from the production train, and the end of production cells should be examined by morphological, physiological, biochemical, and genetic tests to confirm that no significant variation occurred during the manufacture of various lots of the antibody. Finally, the examination of the antibody by biochemical, immunological, and bioactivity tests (see Section 9.5.3) demonstrates product consistency.

9.3 CELL CULTIVATION METHODS

In vitro production of MAbs is the norm for large-scale manufacturing. Suspension systems, such as stirred tank or airlift reactors, and entrapped systems, such as fluidized bed or hollow fiber reactors, are commonly used for antibody production.[34] Stirred tank and airlift reactors can operate in batch, fed-batch, or perfusion mode and are the reactors of choice for producing kilogram quantities of MAbs, while hollow fiber reactors are more frequently employed for smaller, gram-scale, operations.

9.3.1 Suspension Reactors (Stirred Tank and Airlift)

Suspension culture allows for homogenous mixing, direct sampling of the cell mass, and precise monitoring and control of temperature, dissolved oxygen, and pH. Stirred tank and airlift reactors have been used in a variety of microbial fermentations and the design and operation of these microbial reactors is well understood. Consequently, by the 1960s suspension culture was applied for large-scale production of veterinary vaccines, such as the foot and mouth disease (FMD) vaccine, in animal cells.[35] As described below, the design basis of stirred tank and airlift reactors for the animal cultivation is well developed. The design of cell retention devices for perfusion culture of suspended cells, as described in the next section, is still under development.

9.3.1.1 Stirred Tank Reactors

Vessels of 3000 l working volume are used for FMD vaccine production[36] and vessels up to 8000 l capacity are used for the production of interferon.[37-38] Recently, stirred tank reactors have been used for the culture of CHO cells for the production of recombinant proteins and of hybridoma cells for antibody production.[39] Cells are grown in stainless steel vessels with height-to-diameter ratios of 1:1 to about 3:1. Mixing is accomplished with one or more agitators based on bladed-disk (Rushton) or marine-propeller patterns. Agitation systems may be driven directly or indirectly by magnetically coupled drives. Indirect drives reduce the risk of microbial contamination through the seals that must be used on direct-drive stirrer shafts. Both top- and bottom-drive systems have been used successfully.

Various techniques have been developed to provide adequate oxygen supply to cultures. The most common method is to sparge air or oxygen directly into the culture. Under some circumstances, sparging may damage cells, but in general, conditions have been established empirically which are not harmful.[40] Alternative methods of oxygen supply exist. For example, Wagner and Lehmann developed a bubble-free aeration system using hollow fiber membrane aerators.[41]

9.3.1.2 Airlift Reactors

This type of reactor relies on a gas stream to both mix and aerate the culture. As shown in Figure 1, the gas stream enters the riser section of the fermentor driving circulation.[42] Gas disengages at the culture surface, causing the denser liquid free of gas bubbles to travel downward in the downcomer section of the vessel toward the sparger region. A draught tube is typically used to separate riser and downcomer sections. The height-to-diameter ratio of airlift reactors (typically 10:1) is greater than that of stirred vessels. The design principles are described in reviews by Onken and Weiland,[43] Merchuk and Seigel,[44] and Smart.[45] The advantage of this type of reactor is that it uses no motors or agitators. However, the requirement for a draught tube limits the volumes that can be used in a given reactor to a narrow range, e.g., 70–80% of the tank volume. The airlift reactor is quite efficient in oxygen transfer and produces less shear stress than a stirred tank reactor.[46,47] This type of reactor has been operated at scales up to 2000 l for the production of MAbs (Figure 1).[42]

9.3.2 Cell Retention in Suspension Reactors for Perfusion Operation

Perfusion refers to a continuous flow of medium through a population of cells that are retained within the culture unit.[48] To increase cell densities beyond 2–4 × 10^6/ml, the medium has to be constantly replaced in order to supply fresh nutrients and remove inhibitory byproducts. Volumetric scaleup has been more readily achieved for suspension perfusion reactors. Cell retention in these systems is based on filtration or sedimentation techniques which support densities up to 5 × 10^7/ml. This chapter discusses the systems used for suspension cells.

9.3.2.1 Spin Filter Technology

A spin filter is a filter device (usually fabricated of stainless steel, although porcelain or sintered glass have also been used) attached to a rotating shaft inside the bioreactor.[49] Tolbert and co-workers describe the history of the spin filter development,[50] while Avgerinos and co-workers describe a spin filter system used for CHO cells.[51] Spin filters reduce fouling because they have a large surface area and as they rotate, the boundary effect at the surface of the filter prevents cells and microcarriers from attaching to the filter surface. Deo et al. have shown that high cell concentrations and high perfusion rates contribute to fouling.

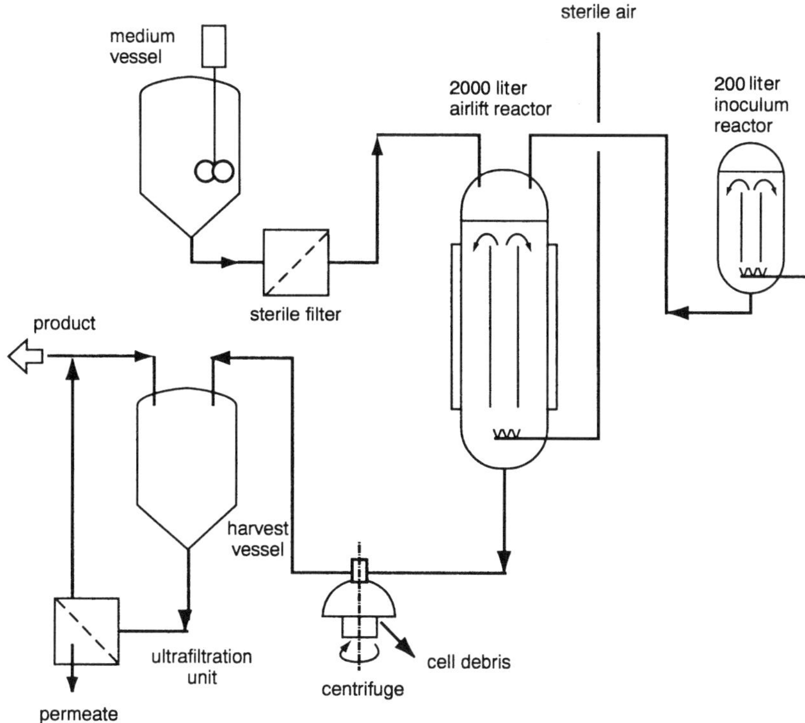

FIGURE 1
Schematic of a 2000 l airlift reactor. (From Rhodes M. and Birch J., *Biotechnology*, 6, 518, 1988. With permission, courtesy of Celltech Ltd.)

Increases in the spin filter mesh area (relative to the reactor volumes and the tangential velocity of the spin filter) reduce fouling.[52] For microcarrier culture, a filter mesh of 60–100 μm can be used which allows high perfusion rates (at least up to 2 vol/h) without blockage. Filter screens with openings (25 μm) slightly larger than the average cell size have been used to retain single cells in suspension over a long period of operation without clogging.[53,54] Using the concept of similarity between the spin filter and crossflow microfilter, scaleup of the spin filter from a 12 l working volume to 175 l[55] and from 7 to 500 l[52] has been accomplished.

9.3.2.2 Gravity Method

Early perfusion reactors used a vertical sedimentation column that was sufficiently long to allow suspended cells to settle back into the bioreactor before they could be washed out.[56-57] Batt et al.[58] have used an inclined settler, which is a long and narrow tube or channel inclined from the vertical. Larger viable cells are removed from suspension by settling onto the upward-facing surfaces of the settler, forming a thin sediment layer that slides down to be collected at the bottom of the vessel. Smaller cells, mostly dead, do not settle as rapidly and are collected from the top. At high dilution rates over 95% of the viable cells partitioned to the bottom of the settler while over 50% of the nonviable cells were removed through the top of the settler. Using such a device, a stable viable concentration of 1×10^7 cells/ml was achieved as well as a sixfold increase in the antibody titer compared to that in a chemostat culture without cell retention.[58]

9.3.3 Entrapped Cell Reactors (Fluidized Bed and Hollow Fiber)

Entrapped cell reactors can culture cells to high cell densities in confined volume, minimizing the size requirements of the central bioreactor system. Furthermore, the production can be maintained for extended periods as long as the nutritional needs of the cells are met. Fluidized bed and hollow fiber reactors are the most popular of these kind of production systems.

9.3.3.1 Fluidized Bed Bioreactors

Continuous culture with macroporous microcarriers in a fluidized bed system was popularized by Verax.[59,60] The basic element of this technology is the use of porous microcarriers that are weighted so as to be retained within a fluidized bed. The macroporous microspheres allow cells to enter and populate the internal volume of each sphere. These microspheres are fluidized by the reconditioned culture medium which provides oxygen and carbon dioxide mass transfer. High rates of mass transfer can be achieved at relatively low hydrodynamic shear. Fluidized bed reactors were scaled up to 24 l bed volumes with perfusion rates of over 500 l/day, designed to produce kilogram quantities per year of therapeutic proteins. Such large-scale reactors are no longer readily available commercially.

9.3.3.2 Hollow Fiber Bioreactors

Herschel and Gruenberg have discussed the use of hollow fiber systems for large-scale production.[61] Hollow fiber systems maintain viable cells at high densities (10^7 to 5×10^8/ml) and allow concentrated product harvest. Cells are grown outside the fibers in the extracapillary space (ECS). Media nutrient and oxygen are delivered via the fiber lumen and pass to the ECS by simple diffusion. One of the problems which prevents scaleup beyond the liter volume size is that the pressure drop along the reactor leads to severe nutrient gradients along the cartridge.[62] Various modifications have been used to overcome this problem. One, as described below, is to alternate the fluid cycling processes from within the lumen to an extracapillary expansion chamber (Acusyst technology, Endotronics).

The ACUSYST-P contains 10,000 individual cuprophane fibers (220 μm inner diameter, 265 μm outer diameter, 20 cm length) that have a nominal cutoff of 6000 kDa. Cultures within these cartridges reach densities of 5×10^8 to 10^9 cells/ml. Each unit can support 10^{11} to 10^{12} viable cells for a period of months. For example, six cartridges each were inoculated with 3.3×10^7 mouse-mouse hybridoma cells expressing an IgG2a MAb. The culture was maintained for 71 days, during which the total antibody yield was 54 g in 39 liters of supernatant.[63] This system reduces the scaleup problems of gradient formation, anoxia, and microenvironment toxicity. Difficulties that remain are associated with cells and cellular debris in the product harvest after long term culture.

Other modifications for scaleup purposes include mixing aeration and medium supply fibers, using filtration grade rather than ultrafiltration grade membranes, and using radial flow techniques which give a short flow path. One such reactor design is the Static Maintenance Reactor (Invitron, SMR), which has cells immobilized in a bulk matrix through which porous tubes perfuse either fresh medium or oxygen.[64] In spite of the efficient production capability, hollow fiber reactors have inherent heterogeneity disadvantages and limitations of scale due to diffusion problems, nonsteam sterilization, possibility of fiber blockage and membrane leakage, complexity of process control, and monitoring growth.

9.4 PROCESS DEVELOPMENT AND SCALEUP

9.4.1 Cell Line Adaptation

As discussed above, large-scale cultivation of cells for the production of MAbs increasingly occurs in stirred tank or airlift reactors, requiring that cells grow in suspension culture. In addition, large-scale production is increasingly driven toward the use of low protein, serum-free medium (SFM) due to the high cost, potential variability, and risk of adventitious agent contamination associated with the use of serum and serum-derived proteins. Most cell lines must, however, be adapted to grow as suspended cells in low protein SFM. Some cell lines are particularly shear sensitive and must be adapted further. Regulatory authorities suggest that all such adaptation occurs prior to establishment of the MCB.[26]

In very few cases, growth of a cell line in a particular SFM will require little or no adaptation. This will be dependent on the requirements of the cell line for particular nutrients and growth factors and the ability of the SFM to supply these requirements. In the majority of other cases, some period of adaptation is necessary. Cells can be gradually adapted to a particular SFM by sequential passaging in media with decreasing serum content. Shinmoto and Dosako[65] describe such an adaptation of mouse-human hybridoma cells to a protein-free medium (PFM). Cells were first cultured in PFM containing 0.1% serum for one week. They were then seeded into PFM supplemented with insulin, transferrin, ethanolamine, and selenium and cultured for two weeks by serial dilution. Finally, cells were passaged in PFM by serial dilution for an additional two weeks. Four out of six cell lines could be adapted for growth in PFM in this manner.[65] Alternatively, cells can be adapted by resuspending a washed cell pellet from a serum-containing culture directly into SFM, the "sink-or-swim" approach. Finally, serum-independent cells can be selected by dilution cloning in SFM. The success of these different methods will depend both on the cell line and the SFM.

Most cell lines require additional adaptation to growth in suspension culture and the high shear environment of a stirred tank reactor. A general protocol for suspension adaptation has been described by Mather.[66] Cells are removed from the surface, using proteases if necessary, and resuspended in a gently agitated environment, e.g., shake flasks on a reciprocating shaker with a moderate throw. As the rate and extent of cell growth increases in a set environment, the degree of agitation is gradually increased, e.g., by increasing the rate of shaking for cells in a shake flask. Figure 2 illustrates the gradual adaptation of transfected NS0 cells to growth in spinner flasks.[67] Cells were initially adapted to grow in suspension culture in shake flasks in SFM. Once cell growth was reproducibly established at a moderate shaker speed, cells were transferred to a spinner flask (Bellco Microcarrier spinner flask). Initially cells grew at a very slow rate with doubling times of approximately 200 h. Cells were sequentially passaged by dilution into fresh medium. As cell growth increased, e.g., doubling time less than 72 h, the agitation rate was gradually increased to 40 rpm and then 45 rpm. Once the cell growth rate was reproducible with a doubling time less than 72 h, the cells were considered "adapted" and a cell bank established. As shown in Figure 3, cells adapted in this manner could be cryopreserved, thawed, retain their phenotype, and readily scaled to growth in large stirred tank reactors (about 200 l) with no further adaptation.[16] The requirement for such "agitation-adaptation" is dependent on both the cell line and medium composition. Although techniques are being developed to measure the "shear-sensitivity" of cells (e.g., see References 68 and 69), the extent of process adaptation

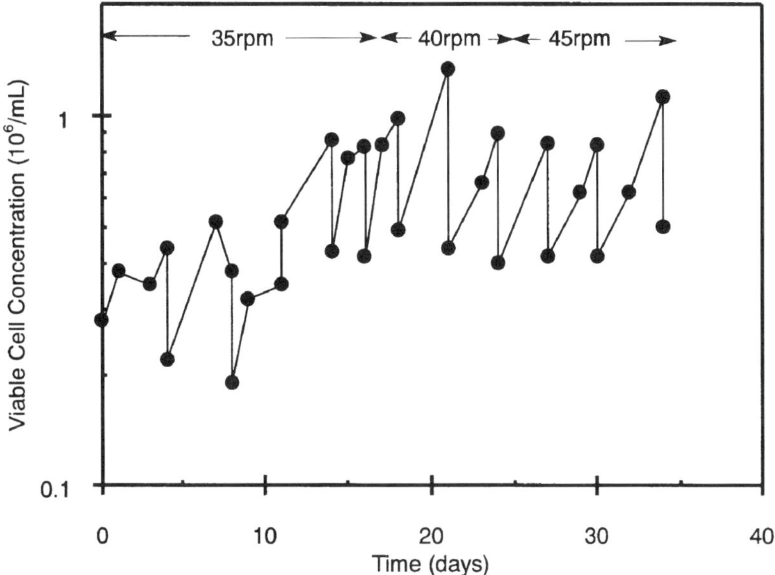

FIGURE 2
Shear adaptation. Viable cell concentration of a recombinant NS0 cell line during sequential passaging in spinner flasks with gradual increases in the agitation rate.

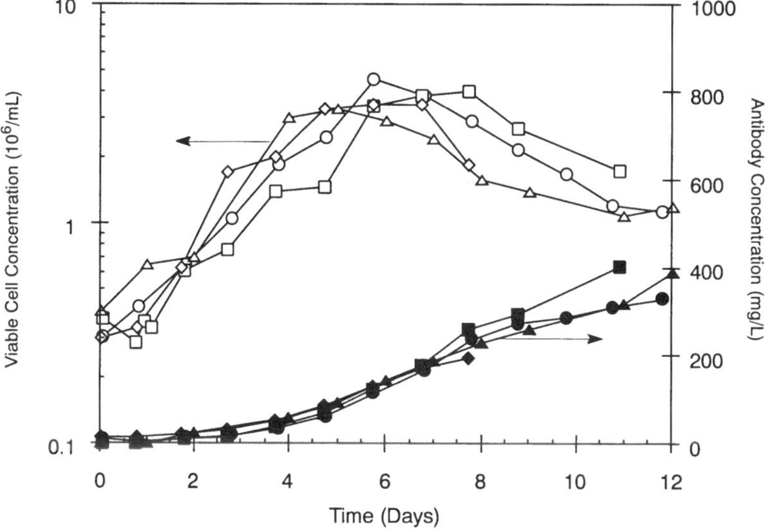

FIGURE 3
Scaleup of an NS0 Fed-batch process. Profiles of the viable cell (open symbols) and antibody concentrations (filled symbols) in an 8 l spinner flask (triangles), 150 l (circles), and 200 l (squares) stirred tank bioreactors.

required for large-scale cultivation of different cell lines must currently be empirically determined.

Birch et al. discuss a number of other desirable adaptations that could improve cell characteristics for production.[70] For example, cells can be adapted or selected for growth in a cholesterol-free medium. This greatly simplifies the design and preparation of low protein media. Similarly, cells can be adapted to grow in glutamine-free medium, reducing the problems associated with controlling the levels of ammonia buildup in culture.[71] Alternatively, cells can be selected for or adapted to growth in the presence of high levels of lactate or ammonia.[72,73] Cells can also be selected for other desirable characteristics such as increased stability to freezing and thawing.[7] At a minimum, cells must be adapted to the process conditions required for large-scale production, typically growth in SFM and agitated suspension culture.

9.4.2 Development of High Productivity Processes

Reactor volumetric productivities are determined by the number of cells secreting antibody and the rate at which they secrete it. As described above, the major goal of cell line development is to construct or isolate high producing cell lines. The goal of process development is then to create a reactor environment that maximizes the rate of antibody secretion and the cell number while maintaining process simplicity, robustness, and fidelity upon scaleup to production levels. As detailed below, most large-scale processes concentrate on either extending culture longevity in batch and fed-batch operations or increasing cell concentrations via perfusion in cell-retention reactors.

9.4.2.1 Batch and Fed-Batch Processes

Cell concentrations in batch and fed-batch operations are determined by the balance between nutrient limitations, growth inhibition, and cell death. In addition, antibody secretion rates can vary as a function of the medium environment, e.g., osmolarity and presence of specific inducers[74] (see Reference 5 for review). As such, optimization of batch and fed-batch processes requires a detailed study of the nutritional requirements for cell growth and antibody production. Antibody yields in batch culture have been increased by nearly eightfold, reaching final titers of nearly 0.5 g/l, by increasing the concentration of the more readily consumed nutrients, glucose and glutamine, together with the amino acids and other nutrients, to severalfold their common basal concentration (see Reference 5 for review). Volumetric productivities were increased up to twofold using a repeated batch culture with complete cell recycle.[75]

However, some nutrients are growth inhibitory at relatively low concentrations or rapidly lead to the buildup of byproducts, e.g., lactate and ammonia, to inhibitory levels. Furthermore, the pattern of nutrient consumption can vary during batch culture, suggesting that a different profile of nutrients are required to sustain antibody production late in culture.[76] As such, further improvement in cell yields require the addition of nutrients during the course of culture, i.e., a fed-batch culture.

Fed-batch processes have been developed that allow antibody production to greater than 1 g/l from hybridoma,[77-78] CHO,[19] and NS0 cells.[79] Each of these processes required detailed analysis of the nutritional requirements of the cell line. These nutritional requirements can be determined by analyzing the composition of the depleted medium and calculating the rate at which nutrients must be added back to the culture to maintain nutrients at near their initial basal levels. For nutrients that are not readily assayed, the rates of feeding must be determined empirically by adding these nutrients back to the medium.[5,15,79] Alternatively, the nutritional requirements of the cells can be determined based on a stoichiometric analysis of cell and product composition and a model of cellular metabolism.[78] Both approaches have resulted in fed-batch processes that yield more than 1 g/l of MAb.[5,15,77,79] As shown in Figure 3, fed-batch processes developed at the spinner flask scale have been successfully scaled up to 200 l stirred tank bioreactors.[16] A simpler approach to fed-batch process design is to merely add back all medium components, except for the salts, in concentrated form. This minimizes the extent of analysis required and has resulted in antibody yields approaching 0.5 g/l.[80]

For cells that require glutamine as a nutrition source, the rate of glutamine addition must be carefully adjusted to minimize the accumulation of ammonia, often by limiting the rate of glutamine addition to a point where the cell growth rate is limited (e.g., Reference 78). Simultaneous control of glucose and glutamine concentrations at 0.2 and 0.1 g/l, respectively, resulted in a twofold increase in antibody yields.[81] Fed-batch process development is much simpler for cell lines, arising either from selection[71] or transfection with glutamine synthetase,[70] that do not require glutamine for growth and antibody production, since glutamine need not be added and the rate of glucose does not need to be carefully controlled.[5,82]

9.4.2.2 Perfusion

The cell densities achieved in perfusion culture (10^7–10^8 cells/ml) are typically 1 to 2 orders of magnitude higher than those reached in fed-batch cultures (1–5 × 10^6 cells/ml). In general, volumetric productivities are tenfold higher in perfusion processes as compared to fed-batch cultures. On the other hand, perfusion culture titers are in most cases lower than those obtained in fed-batch culture.[5] Rigorous process optimization is required for successful perfusion operation.[53-54,83-84]

In a perfusion bioreactor, the medium flow rate is typically increased in response to the increasing cell density. The medium perfusion helps to provide nutrients for cell growth and wash away waste metabolites. Since perfusion systems do not always have complete cell retention, cell growth occurs with new cells replacing the cells lost in the perfusate even under steady-state conditions. As the perfusion rate is increased in a stepwise fashion, new steady states are achieved. Dilution rates (typically five- to tenfold) higher than the maximum specific growth rates are possible because of the cell retention.

Optimization of antibody production in perfusion systems typically seeks to maximize total production rate while keeping the antibody concentration reasonably high. This optimization depends a great deal on the inherent kinetics of antibody production by the cell line. There are three different kinetic patterns reported in literature: (1) specific productivity increases with the specific growth rate; (2) specific productivity is almost unchanged as a function of specific growth rate; and (3) specific productivity decreases with the increasing specific growth rate.

Robinson et al.[84] described a SP2/0 myeloma cell line producing a chimeric antibody where the specific rate of antibody production increased linearly as the specific growth rate increased. Interestingly, with such kinetics, product titers were independent of both the degree of cell retention and the total dilution rates.[84] However, since the cell retention bioreactors can be operated at dilution rates in excess of the maximum specific growth rate, higher volumetric productivities are possible.

Reddy and Miller[85] reported that the specific productivity of a hybridoma was fairly constant over a range of specific growth rates. In an open (no cell retention) system, they observed a slight decline in the product concentration at high dilution rates because the viable cell density increased linearly with increasing dilution rate.[85] In a closed perfusion system with cell retention, where the cell density increases with increasing media flow rate, the product concentration would have been maintained constant. Owing to the high flow rates, higher volumetric productivities would have been reached.

Miller et al. reported that a different hybridoma cell line which exhibited different kinetics of antibody production, the specific productivity declined with increasing specific growth rate.[86] In such a case, the product concentration in a perfusion reactor would decrease as the flow rates increase. An optimal flow rate exists where the volumetric productivity is high and the product concentration still reasonable.

9.4.3 Process Monitoring and Control

Numerous advanced monitoring and control strategies (e.g., the use of flow injection analysis, *in situ* optical density probes, or *ex situ* image analysis coupled to an adaptive control or expert control system) have been applied in small-scale cell culture process (see References 87 and 88 for reviews). However, these advanced strategies are at most sparingly applied in large-scale cell culture processes. Production processes typically utilize on-line control for pH, temperature, and dissolved oxygen only. Batch cultures often require little to no additional monitoring and control other than frequent off-line measurements of cell density and viability. Fed-batch cultures require control of nutrient feed rates as described above. Control strategies based on cell growth estimates,[78] on-line oxygen utilization rates (OUR),[89] or glucose and lactate measurements[81] have been applied. In large-scale cultures, however, nutrient addition rates are more frequently based on time-triggered events and less frequently employ feedback control. Model simulations by Hansen et al. suggest that more frequent control of nutrient feeding in fed-batch cultures lead to low and variable antibody titers.[90] However, experimental evidence shows that increased frequency of nutrient addition either has no effect[5] or improves antibody yields.[91] Large-scale perfusion cultures often rely solely on setpoint control of perfusion flow rates with simple feedback control to adjust the setpoint based on off-line measurements. As the reliability of on-line sensors and the sophistication of fed-batch and perfusion processes increase, increasingly sophisticated control procedures will be implemented for reliable large-scale production of MAbs.

9.5 RECOVERY, PURIFICATION, AND FORMULATION

Therapeutic MAbs should be prepared so as to pose a very low risk of containing potentially harmful substances such as pyrogens, viruses, fragments of DNA, and immunogenic protein contaminants, while retaining activity and specificity.[92] Such preparation typically requires a primary recovery or cell operation step, followed by one or more column chromatographic operations.

9.5.1 Primary Recovery Operations

Centrifugation and filtration have been used for clarification of cell broth. For large fermentations, continuous flow centrifuges are available wherein solids build up in the bowl, and the centrifuge must be stopped to empty the bowl when filled.[93] For very large-scale industrial processes with fermentation volumes of many hundreds or thousands of liters, intermittent discharge centrifuges are available that periodically eject the solids accumulated in the centrifuge bowl without interrupting operation.[94-95] Typically, complete clarification is not achieved through centrifugation and further clarification, often by means of depth filters, is required.[96]

Clarification by filtration, either with conventional dead-end filters or with cross-flow filters, is an alternative to centrifugation.[97,98] Cross-flow filtration, in which the liquid is continuously recirculated through a channel whose walls are composed of filtration membrane, has the advantage that the solids fraction (i.e., cells and cell debris) can be retained, and that the membrane can be reused. In contrast, with dead-end filtration, the solids cannot be removed from the filter, which must be replaced after a single use. Also, a series of dead-end filters with decreasing pore size is normally required, with high-solids-capacity filters at the front end and sterilizing-grade membrane filters at the tail end. Optimization cross-flow filtration has been discussed by Maiorella et al.[99]

In recent years, research to eliminate the clarification step by directly adsorbing the product to the resin in an expanded bed has been ongoing.[100,101] Although clarification steps are omitted, adjustment of pH and conductivity may still be necessary to promote binding of the antibody to the matrix. Such adjustments may require dilution of the product stream and may lead to extensive cell lysis, increasing the DNA and protein load.

9.5.2 Chromatographies and Viral Clearance

Kenney[102] has discussed methods to purify MAbs. The purification of antibody by column chromatography relies on the partitioning of the antibody and impurities between two phases: a mobile phase, generally composed of an aqueous buffer solution, and a stationary phase or matrix, composed of a packed bed of a porous support material, such as agarose or silica with functional groups attached. Support materials vary with respect to properties such as rigidity, pore size, and bead size. For production scale chromatography, beads with diameters of 50–100 μm are generally used, giving rise to back pressures of only 1–3 bars.

9.5.2.1 Ion Exchange Chromatography

Ion exchange chromatography is commonly used for antibody purification.[103] The separation mechanism of this method relies on the binding of negatively charged molecules to a positively charged matrix or vice versa. Depending on the operating conditions and the antibody, either the antibody or the impurities will bind preferentially to the matrix. Anion exchange chromatography is useful for purifying therapeutic-grade MAbs as DNA and endotoxins bind to the anionic matrix, separating them from the product. The pH, ionic strength, and chemical composition of the buffers can be altered during chromatography and these changes can be made either stepwise or with a gradient to adjust binding of impurities and the product.

9.5.2.2 Affinity Chromatography

Affinity chromatography using immobilized protein A or protein G is popular for antibody purification. High purity levels (>95% by sodium dodecyl sulfate polyacrylamide gel electrophoresis; SDS-PAGE) can be achieved in a single step. Commercial matrices with ligands linked to cross-linked agarose, silica, or controlled pore glass beads are available. The dynamic capacity of these matrices is typically 10–20 mg of antibody per milliliter of packed matrix. As these matrices cannot be sanitized with caustic solutions, and since large-scale handling of concentrated alcohol solutions requires explosion-proof containment, other cleaning agents such as solutions of chaotropic salts must be used. An example of this method of purification is covered by Lee et al.[104]

Although this method of purification is very robust and not drastically affected by small changes in ionic strength and flow rates, it has two disadvantages; the cost of the matrix and ligand leakage. Protein A and G matrices are at least an order of magnitude more expensive than ion-exchange matrices. Since the robustness of this chromatography lends itself to easy automation and the high purity achieved saves on subsequent purity steps, the cost can be justified. Leakage of ligand from the support can be addressed by demonstrating that subsequent chromatography steps achieve the clearance of the ligand using very sensitive assay methods.[105]

9.5.2.3 Gel Permeation Chromatography

Gel permeation or size exclusion chromatography separates antibody from impurities on the basis of molecular size. This chromatography is useful if there is at least a twofold difference in molecular weight between the antibody and the impurities. It is quite useful in separating antibody aggregates and purifying large immunoglobulins like IgMs (900 kDa).[106]

Separation in gel permeation chromatography is achieved solely by a "sieving" mechanism that retards small molecules. Therefore, bed length is an important factor in the degree of purification obtained.

Also, the capacity of the column is determined by the volume of the sample applied and not by the amount of protein. In general, the sample volume may be 2–10% of the column volume and the bed length approximately 60–100 cm. This chromatography is therefore only suitable as a final polishing step where a concentrated and partially purified product stream can be applied.

9.5.2.4 Other Chromatographic Methods

Hydroxylapatite chromatography is a unique absorption chromatography used for antibody purification.[107,108] Hydroxylapatite is a crystalline form of calcium phosphate which adsorbs most MAbs at low concentrations of phosphate at neutral pH conditions, while serum proteins such as albumin and transferrin remain unadsorbed. MAbs can then be eluted by increasing the phosphate concentration. As sodium chloride and other ions do not interfere with antibody binding and elution, buffer exchange may not be necessary prior to hydroxylapatite chromatography. Hydrophobic interaction[109] and metal ion affinity[110] chromatography have also been used for antibody purification.

9.5.2.5 Optimization of Chromatographic Process and Scaleup

Purification schemes are designed to achieve as much purification as possible in the first chromatographic step, so that later steps can be optimized for the removal of small quantities of a few specific impurities. Affinity chromatography or ion-exchange chromatography are good candidates for the first step. It would be desirable to have the eluate from the first step be suitable for the next step. If pH and ionic strength conditions are not suitable, a buffer exchange step such as diafiltration is included between chromatographies. To achieve the desired degree of purification, two to four chromatographic steps are used. Where the final product specification calls for an extremely low level of antibody aggregates, gel filtration is frequently used as a final step. Gel filtration can serve as both an aggregate removal step and a buffer exchange step, transferring the antibody into the final formulation buffer.

Due to variability in size, charge, hydrophobicity, solubility, and stability of different MAbs, purification processes generally need to be specifically tailored to each individual antibody. Most human IgG MAbs bind to protein A or G and many murine IgG molecules can be made to bind by manipulation of the binding conditions such as the pH and salt concentration. For those IgGs that do not bind to protein A or G, ion exchange chromatography is typically used. Some IgG3 and IgM MAbs are particularly difficult to purify. They do not bind to protein A and have low solubility in the low conductivity buffers used in ion exchange. In such cases, ion exchange is attempted after the manipulation of pH or the addition of stabilizers.[111]

For large-scale operation, large beads are typically specified to enable high flow rates without high back pressure. These beads should be rigid or at least highly cross-linked chromatographic matrices that can withstand high operating pressures and flow rates. Column geometry also needs optimization for this type of chromatography. For most types of chromatography (except size exclusion), short and fat columns are preferred (diameter/height ratios of 3:5) in order to achieve higher throughput. However, the chromatographic bed must have a minimum bed height to achieve sufficient protein binding and resolution.

9.5.2.6 Viral Clearance

The presence of retroviruses in continuous mammalian cell lines has received a great deal of attention because of concern that these particles can potentially cause oncogenic events in man.[96] Reverse transcriptase assays, electron microscopy, and several other methods described in Section 9.2.2.2 are used to assess the presence of retroviruses in conditioned media.

In addition to endogenous retroviruses, there is always a concern about introducing unknown adventitious agents that are not easily detected by the test methods. Therefore, it becomes necessary to demonstrate virus removal during the product purification. It is advisable to include at least two specific virus removal steps such as low pH treatment, solvent-detergent treatment, affinity chromatography, or microfiltration[113] in the purification process.[114] These process steps should offer at least two different mechanisms of virus removal, e.g., chemical inactivation by solvent-detergent and physical removal by microfiltration. Once the purification process is finalized, validation studies should be carried out using a scaled-down version (typically 1/100-1/1000 of the actual scale) of the final process.[115] The validation study should include any endogenous retroviruses detected in the MCB/MWCB or a similar model virus and at least two to three additional model viruses with distinct characteristics such as resistance to chemical treatment, very small size, presence or absence of a lipid envelope, DNA or RNA, genome, etc. The CPMP guidelines on virus validation studies provide useful suggestions for selection of model viruses.[114] Process validation involves spiking a process step with a known large amount of the selected virus and monitoring its levels at the end of that process step. The actual virus reduction is determined by the viral loss during that step. The total reduction through the process is the sum of all the individual step reductions. Then the safety factor is calculated on the basis of total viral load (as determined by in process tests, see Section 9.2.2.3) minus the total reduction. It is advisable to achieve at least 4-6 log safety factor for the overall process.

9.5.2.7 Purification Process Validation

Process validation demonstrates that the production process performs as intended in a consistent manner. It must be demonstrated that the purification process will remove known impurities such as DNA and medium components, as well as potential contaminants such as viruses derived from the host cell lines.[116]

Validation data is normally gathered by analysis of full-scale manufacturing runs and also by "challenge" studies using model viruses, DNA, and process contaminants on scaled-down versions of the full-scale process. The detailed analysis of a small number of full-scale manufacturing runs can provide direct evidence that the purification process can consistently remove known impurities for which sensitive assays exist.

A similar approach using both small-scale challenge studies and analysis of full-scale production runs must be used to demonstrate the effect of reusing chromatography matrices. For the production of therapeutic MAbs where process hygiene is critical, both the process as well as the equipment have to be designed to achieve a very high degree of cleanliness. For example, threaded connections where bacterial deposits could accumulate should be avoided and highly polished stainless steels should be used for vessels and piping to minimize bacterial adhesion. Routine monitoring of raw materials, for example, water systems, and of both the manufacturing environment and the process stream is required to ensure that very high standards of hygiene are maintained.

9.5.3 Product Characterization Methods

The objective of product characterization is to monitor the integrity of structure and demonstrate elements particular to each individual antibody. In addition, product purity has to be confirmed. A simple set of assays is used for routine testing of a manufacturing process, while more complex testing is employed for structural characterization and for defining reference standards.

SDS-PAGE for purity, size exclusion high performance liquid chromatography (HPLC) for integrity and aggregation, activity or biological assays for potency, ultraviolet absorbance for concentration, and isotyping assays for identity are used for routine characterization of the product. Process contaminant assays for proteins (enzyme-linked immunosorbent assay; (ELISA), Western blotting, and DNA (hybridization or polymerase chain reaction; PCR) are also routinely used. Further characterization includes determining primary, secondary, and tertiary structure, carbohydrate content, charge isoforms, and hydrophobic interactions.

9.5.4 FORMULATION OF MAb PRODUCTS

MAbs are usually formulated in solution and less frequently as freeze-dried preparations. The development of a freeze-dried formulation can produce a product with an extended shelf life compared to solution and can facilitate storage at ambient temperature. However, freeze drying requires extensive process development.[117] Product integrity or stability during storage under different conditions can be followed by analytical methods such as SDS-PAGE, isoelectric focusing, reversed-phase HPLC, peptide mapping, and a specific activity assay such as ELISA. Additional non-routine stability tests may include techniques to follow secondary and tertiary structure such as circular dichroism, hydrophobic-interaction, or ion-exchange chromatography.

Formulation should provide a shelf-life in excess of 12 months stored under standard refrigeration conditions (2–8°C). In designing the formulation, the following points should be considered. Solubility and aggregation can normally be controlled by the same factors, e.g., pH, buffer, or detergent. However, they may not be directly related and therefore should be monitored independently. Oxidation of susceptible amino acid residues (e.g., methionine, cysteine, and tryptophan) is not a common problem with MAbs at pH <7. However, if there is a problem, it can be controlled by the addition of antioxidants. Deamidation is a commonly observed degradation process for MAbs and it can be controlled by maintaining pH at or below 7. Proteolysis can occur through either enzymatic or chemical mechanisms. It is minimized by optimizing pH or adding protease inhibitors, e.g., EDTA, to the buffer.

9.6 SCALEUP OF ANTIBODY PROCESSES

9.6.1 Issues Unique to Large-Scale Cultures and Processes

Use of a microporous frit sparger for efficient oxygen addition to the reactor is quite common. However, due to inefficient stripping of CO_2 by the slowly rising oxygen bubbles, the partial pressure of CO_2 has been shown to build up to three times the initial value levels, which are toxic to the cells.[118] This effect has been seen in 2500 l scale tanks,[40,119] where sparging with air as opposed to pure oxygen partially corrected the phenomenon. However, a foaming problem may arise with air sparging which can adversely affect cell growth. In airlift reactors, excessively sparging air or N_2 can strip CO_2 to extremely low levels[120] which may also be detrimental to culture performance.

Mixing in mammalian cell reactors is usually minimized to reduce any shear damage. However, this is a cause for concern as the reactor is scaled up. Typically, in a large bottom driven bioreactor, mixing at the top layer of liquid is rather poor. Therefore, care should be taken about any additions, such as caustic, from the top as there is a likelihood of poor bulk mixing. The poor mixing also hinders the breakup of foam which is formed at the top of the liquid by the air sparging. This can cause a number of problems such as poor ventilation of CO_2 and loss of any insoluble substrates in the foam layer. As the reactor scale increases, it is difficult to maintain the ratio of spin filter surface area to tank volume, complicating scaleup of perfusion reactors. Impeller tip speed shear and hydrostatic pressure also increase with scale. Current scaleup methodologies do not adequately address these problems. Processing times also increase with scale. Fortunately, most MAbs are relatively stable and not adversely affected by the increased residence times. Constructing a large-scale GMP facility for the production of therapeutics is a complex project and involves a number of considerations based on technology, regulations, and versatility of use. All these aspects are discussed by Srigley.[121]

9.6.2 Product Equivalence Upon Scaleup

Small-scale production processes are used to produce MAbs for initial phase I/II clinical trials and the process scaleup occurs as the clinical studies progress to the pivotal phase III stage. It is important that the product used for various stages of the clinical studies is structurally, biochemically, and functionally equivalent to the product to be offered on the market after the successful completion of clinical studies and licensing.[27] If significant process changes have occurred after or during the pivotal clinical trials, it may become necessary to perform bridging clinical studies to demonstrate *in vivo* product equivalence. Therefore, it is prudent to finalize the production process and facility prior to the initiation of pivotal clinical trials. However, since this may be economically unreasonable for a yet unproven product, the U.S. regulatory agency has recently suggested that the product for phase III clinical studies and the initial market launch may be produced in a pilot plant if produced under the appropriate GMP and GLP conditions. In this situation the product equivalence studies will have to be performed prior to introduction of the product from the full-scale production process in the market.[122]

The scale of production process may affect the product due to changes in shear, hydrostatic pressure, residence time, or mixing rates in a bioreactor or a chromatography column, number of cell doublings prior to and after the inoculation of the full-scale bioreactor hod steps in, etc. These process conditions may affect the product in various ways, e.g., glycoform distribution, deamidation, decarboxylation, oxidation, loss of terminal amino acids, or oligopeptides. Such modifications may change the binding affinity, biological activity, the *in vitro* and *in vivo* stability, or *in vivo* distribution of the product. Furthermore, the patterns of the related product and other contaminants may also change. Therefore, a variety of *in vitro* and *in vivo* tests should be developed to demonstrate product equivalence during and after process scaleup. For this purpose, product lots prepared at various stages of the development as well as multiple lots produced at the phase III clinical trial / post marketing stage should be compared using a variety of tests. The tests should include amino acid sequencing, electrophoretic and chromatographic methods, carbohydrate content and structure, circular dichroism, and mass spectroscopy. Immunological equivalence can be determined by ELISA, immunofluorescence, and antigenicity in primate models. Potency is the most important measurement. Binding affinity can be measured by ELISA or flow cytometry and activity by *in vitro* neutralization, antibody-dependent cellular cytotoxicity (ADCC), or complement-dependent cellular cytotoxicity (CDCC) assays. Pharmacokinetics and *in vivo* functional equivalence can be examined using rabbit or nonhuman primate animal models. *In vivo* functional equivalence can be examined if a suitable animal model for the disease or imaging is available. If significant changes in product characteristics are observed, then bridging clinical studies may be required to confirm equivalent clinical efficacy. It is most prudent, if not mandatory, to develop strategies for demonstration of product equivalence in close collaboration with the regulatory agencies.

9.7 CONCLUSIONS

Large-scale production of MAbs in mammalian cell culture foremost requires the development of cells lines that secrete antibody at high rates and can grow in a reactor environment. This environment most frequently requires that cells grow in suspended culture in airlift or stirred tank reactors. For higher volumetric (reactor-volume) productivity, medium is perfused through the reactor and the cells retained either physically or by gravity settling. Alternatively, cells are entrapped within fluidized bed or hollow fiber bioreactors, more commonly employed for intermediate scale production. Processes have been developed that result in crude antibody titers (concentration or yield) in fed-batch processes of over 1 g/l or volumetric productivities in perfusion processes of 0.6 g/l/day. To date, only relatively simple process monitoring and control are commonly applied for large-scale processing.

Recovery of antibody requires clarification of the cell broth, typically by centrifugation and/or filtration. Purification employs multiple column chromatography steps: generally, ion exchange or affinity chromatography coupled with additional ion exchange, gel permeation, or hydroxylapatite separation steps. The combination of multiple column chromatographic steps and one or more viral inactivation or removal steps typically affords sufficient assurance of viral clearance. Purified MAbs are characterized by standard biochemical and biophysical assays, coupled with some measure of potency or activity, typically antigen recognition or a biological assay. MAbs are commonly formulated in solution or, less frequently, as freeze-dried preparations.

Large-scale culture of MAbs poses unique issues of mixing and gas exchange, particularly with respect to removal of carbon dioxide from the culture. Validation of virus removal is of overriding concern for downstream processes. Both issues have been sufficiently addressed in the industry such that production of MAbs at scales reaching and exceeding hundreds of kilograms per year is fast becoming a reality.

9.8 ACKNOWLEDGMENTS

The authors thank R. W. Ellis and G. E. Mark for their support and encouragement and S. Pols for final preparation of this manuscript.

REFERENCES

1. Abraham, E., Wunderink, R., Silverman, H., Perl, T. M., Nasraway, S., Levy, H., Bone, R., Wenzel, R. P., Balk, R., and Allred, R., Efficacy and safety of monoclonal antibody to human tumor necrosis factor alpha in patients with sepsis syndrome. A randomized, controlled, double-blind, multicenter clinical trial. TNF-alpha-MAb sepsis study group, *JAMA*, 273, 934, 1995.
2. Osterhaus, A. and Uytdehaag, F., Lymphocyte hybridomas: production and use of monoclonal antibodies, in *Animal Cell Biotechnology, Vol. 2*, Spier R. E. and Griffiths, J. B., Eds., Academic Press, New York, 1985, 49.
3. Van Kroonenburgh, M. J. and Pauwels, E. K., Human immunological response to mouse monoclonal antibodies in treatment or diagnosis of malignant disease, *Nuclear Med. Commun.*, 9, 919, 1988.

4. Sawada, H. and Kitano, K., Antibody production in human hybridomas with growth associated production kinetics, in *ACS Symposium Series 604: Antibody Expression and Engineering*, Wang, H. Y. and Imanaka, T., Eds., American Chemical Society, Washington, D.C., 1995.
5. Bibila, T. A. and Robinson, D. K., In pursuit of the optimal fed-batch process for monoclonal antibody production, *Biotechnol. Prog.*, 11, 1, 1995.
6. Murakami, H., What should be focused in the study of cell culture technology for the production of bioactive proteins?, *Cytotechnology*, 3, 3, 1990.
7. Seaver, S. S., Enhancing monoclonal antibodies and hybridoma cell lines, *Cytotechnology*, 9, 131, 1992.
8. Huse, W., Sastry, L., Iverson, S. A., Kang, A. S., Alting-Nees, M., Burton, D. R., Benkovic, S. J., and Lerner, R. A., Generation of a large combinatorial library if immunoglobulin repertoire in phage lambda, *Science*, 246, 1275, 1989.
9. Ward, E. S., Gussow, D., Griffiths, A. D., Jones, P. T., and Winter, G., Binding activities of a repertoire of single immunoglobulin variable domain secreted from *Escherichia coli*, *Nature*, 341, 544, 1989.
10. Morrison, S. L., Johnson, M. J., Herzenberg, L. A., and Oi, V. T., Chimeric human antibody molecules: mouse antigen-binding domains with human constant region domains, *Proc. Natl. Acad. Sci. U.S.A.*, 81, 6851, 1984.
11. Larrick, J. W. and Fry, K. E., Recombinant antibodies, *Hum. Antibod. Hybridomas*, 2, 172, 1992.
12. Page, M. J. and Sydenham, M. A., High level expression of the humanized monoclonal antibody CAMPATH-1H in Chinese hamster ovary cells, *Bio/Technology*, 9, 64, 1991.
13. Fouser, L. A., Swanberg, S. L., Lin B.-Y., Benedict, M., Kellerher, K., Cumming, D. A., and Reidel, G. E., High level expression of a chimeric anti-ganglioside GD2 antibody: genomic kappa sequences improve expression in COS and CHO cells, *Bio/Technology*, 10, 1121, 1992.
14. Barnett, R. S., Limoli, K. L., Huynh, T. B., Ople, E. A., and Reff, M. E., Antibody production in Chinese hamster ovary cells using an impaired selectable marker, in *ACS Symposium Series 604: Antibody Expression and Engineering*, Wang, H. Y. and Imanaka, T., Eds., American Chemical Society, Washington, D.C., 1995, 27.
15. Robinson, D. K., DiStefano, D., Gould, S. L., Cuca, G., Seamans, T. C., Benincasa, D., Munshi, S., Chan, C. P., Strafford-Hollis, J., Hollis, G. F., Jain, D., Ramasubramanyan, K., Mark, G. E., and Silberklang, M., Production of engineered antibodies in myeloma and hybridoma cells: enhancements in gene expression and process design, in *ACS Symposium Series 604: Antibody Expression and Engineering*, Wang, H. Y. and Imanaka, T., Eds., American Chemical Society, Washington, D.C., 1995, 1.
16. Robinson, D. K., Seamans, T. C., Gould, S. L., DiStefano, D. J., Chan, C. P., Lee, D. K., Bibila, T., Glazomitsky, K., Munshi, S., Daugherty, B., O'Neill Palladino, L., Stafford-Hollis, J., Hollis, G. F., and Silberklang, M., Optimization of a fed-batch process for production of a recombinant antibody, *Ann. N. Y. Acad. Sci.*, 745, 285, 1994.
17. Bebbington, C. R., Renner, G., Thomson, S., King, Abrams, D., Yarranton, G. T., High-level expression of a recombinant antibody from myeloma cells using a glutamine synthetase gene as an amplifiable selectable marker, *Biotechnology*, 10, 169, 1992.
18. Kaufman R., Sharp P. A., and Latt, S. A., Evolution of chromosomal regions containing transfected and amplified dihydrofolate reductase sequences, *Mol. Cell. Biol.*, 3, 699, 1983.
19. Reff, M. E., High-level production of recombinant immunoglobulins in mammalian cells, *Curr. Opin. Biotechnol.*, 4, 573-576, 1993.

20. Mosser, D. D. and Massie, B., Genetically engineering mammalian cell lines for increased viability and productivity, *Biotech. Adv.*, 12, 253, 1994.
21. Bibila, T. A. and Flickinger, M. C., Use of a structured kinetic model of antibody synthesis and secretion for optimization of antibody production systems: II. Transient analysis, *Biotechnol. Bioeng.*, 39, 262, 1992.
22. Mercillle S. and Massie, B., Induction of apoptosis in nutrient-deprived cultures of hybridoma and myeloma cells, *Biotechnol. Bioeng.*, 44, 1140, 1994.
23. Mastrangelo, A. J. and Betenbaugh, M. J., Implications and applications of apoptosis in cell culture, *Curr. Opin. Biotechnol.*, 6, 198, 1995.
24. Itoh, Y., Ueda, H., and Suzuki, E., Overexpression of bcl-2, apoptosis suppressing gene: prolonged viable culture period of hybridoma and enhanced antibody production, *Biotechnol. Bioeng.*, 48, 118, 1995.
25. Kozack, R. W., Durfor, C. N., and Scribner, C. L., Regulatory consideration when developing biological products, *Cytotechnology*, 9, 203, 1992.
26. Center for Biologics Evaluation and Research, *Points to consider in the characterization of cell lines used to produce biologicals*, 1993.
27. Center for Biologics Evaluation and Research, *Points to consider in the manufacture and testing of monoclonal antibody products for human use*, 1994.
28. Commission of the European Communities Guidelines, *Production and quality control of human monoclonal antibodies*, 1990.
29. Lees, G. and Darling, A., *Biosafety Considerations in Monoclonal Antibodies — Princciples and Applications*, Wiley-Liss Inc., New York, 1995, 267.
30. Deo, Y. M., Ghebremariam, H., and Cloyd, M., Detection and characterization of murine ecotropic recombinant viruses in myeloma and hybridoma cells, *Hybridoma*, 13, 69, 1994.
31. Berthold, W., Gene stability in mammalian cells and protein consistency, *Biologicals*, 21, 95, 1993.
32. Wiebe, M. E. and Lin, N. S., Genetic stability of host cell and product, in *Regulatory Practice for Biopharmaceutical Production*, Lubiniecki, A. S., Ed., Wiley-Liss, New York, 1994.
33. Center for Biologics Evaluation and Research, *Supplement to the Points to Consider in the Production and Testing of New Drugs and Biologicals produced by Recombinant DNA Technology: Nucleic Acid Characterization and genetic Stability*, 1992.
34. Birch, J. R., Bonnerjea, J., Flatman, S., and Vranch, S., The production of monoclonal antibodies, in *Monoclonal Antibodies: Principles and Applications*, Birch J. R. and Lennox, E. S., Eds., Wiley-Liss, New York, 1995, 234.
35. Birch, J. R. and Arathoon, R., Suspension culture of mammalian cells, in *Large-Scale Mammalian Technology*, Lubiniecki, A. S., Ed., Marcel Dekker, New York, 1990, 251.
36. Radlett, P. J., Pay, T. W. F., and Graland, A. H. M., The use of BHK suspension cells for the commercial production of foot and mouth disease vaccines over a twenty year period, *Dev. Biol. Standard*, 60, 163, 1985.
37. Mizrahi, A., Production of human interferons: an overview, *Process Biochem.*, August, 9, 1983.
38. Phillips, A. W., Ball, G. D., Fantes, K. H., Finter, N. B., and Johnston, M. D., Experience in the cultivation of mammalian cells on the 8000 L scale, in *Large Scale Mammalian Cell Culture*, Feder, J. and Tolbert, W. R., Eds., Academic Press, Orlando, FL, 1985, 87.
39. Lebherz, W. B., Lee, S. M., Gustafson, M. E., Ricketts, R. T., Lufriu, I. F., Morgan, A. C., and Flickinger, M. C., Production of monoclonal antibodies by large-scale submerged hybridoma cultures, *In Vitro*, 21, 16A, 1985.
40. Aunins, J. G. and Henzler, H.-J., Aeration in Cell Culture Bioreactors, in *Biotechnology: A Multi-Volume Comprehensive Treatise, Vol. 3, 2nd edition*, Stephanopoulos, G. N., Pühler, A., and Stadler, P., Eds., VCH, Weinheim, Germany, 1993, 224.

41. Wagner, R. and Lehmann, J., The growth and productivity of recombinant animal cells in a bubble free aeration system, *Trends Biotechnol.*, 6:1011, 1988.
42. Rhodes, M. and Birch, J. R., Large-scale production of proteins from mammalian cells, *Bio/Technology*, 6, 518, 1988.
43. Onken, U. and Weiland, P., Airlift fermentors: construction, behavior and uses, *Adv. Biotechnol. Proc.*, 1, 67, 1983.
44. Merchuk, K. C. and Seigel, M. H., Airlift reactors in chemical and biological technology, *J. Chem. Tech. Biotechnol.*, 41, 105, 1988.
45. Smart, N. J., Gaslift fermentors: theory and practice, *Lab Pract.*, 9, 1984.
46. Katinger, H. and Scheirer, W., Mass cultivation and production of animal cells, in *Animal Cell Biotechnology, Vol. 1*, Spier, R. E. and Griffiths, J. B., Eds., Academic Press, Orlando, FL, 1985, 167.
47. Birch, J. R., Lambert, K., and Thompson, P. W., Antibody production with airlift fermentors, in *Large Scale Cell Culture Technology*, Lyderson, K., Ed., Hanser, New York, 1987, 1.
48. Himmelfarb, P., Thayer, P. S., and Martin, H. E., Spin filter culture: the propagation of mammalian cells in suspension, *Science*, 164, 555, 1969.
49. Griffiths, B., Perfusion system for cell cultivation, in *Large Scale Mammalian Technology*, Lubiniecki, A. S., Ed., Marcel Dekker, New York, 1990, 217.
50. Tolbert, W. R., Lewis, C., White, P. J., and Feder, J., Perfusion culture systems for production of mammalian cell biomolecules, in *Large Scale Mammalian Cell Culture*, Feder, J. and Tolbert, W., Eds., Academic Press Inc., New York, 1985, 97.
51. Avgerinos, G. C., Drapeau, D., Socolow, J. S., Mao, J., Hsiao, K., and Broeze, R. J., Spinfilter perfusion system for high density cell culture: production of recombinant urinary type plasminogen activator in CHO cells, *Bio/Technology*, 8, 54, 1990.
52. Deo, Y. M., Mahadevan, M. D., and Fuchs, R., Practical considerations in operation and scale up of spin filter based bioreactor for monoclonal antibody production, *Biotechnol. Prog.*, 12, 57, 1996.
53. Yabannavar, V. M., Singh, V., and Connelly, N. V., Mammalian cell retention in a spinfilter perfusion bioreactor, *Biotech. Bioeng.*, 40, 925, 1992.
54. Esclade, L. R. J., Carrel, S., and Peringer, P., Influence of the screen material on the fouling of spinfilters, *Biotechnol. Bioeng.*, 38, 159, 1991.
55. Yabannavar, V. M., Singh, V., and Connelly, N. V., Scaleup of spinfilter perfusion bioreactor for mammalian cell retention, *Biotech. Bioeng.*, 43, 159, 1994.
56. Kitano, K., Shintani, Y., Tsukamoto, K., Sasai, S., and Kida, M., Production of human monoclonal antibodies by heterohybridomas, *Appl. Microbiol. Biotechnol.*, 24, 282, 1986.
57. Takazawa, Y., Tokashiki, M., Hamamoto, K., and Murakami, H., High cell density perfusion culture of hybridoma cells recycling high molecular weight components, *Cytotechnology*, 1, 171, 1988.
58. Batt, B. C., Davis, R. H., and Kompala, D. S., Inclined sedimentation for selective retention of viable hybridoma in continuous suspension bioreactor, *Biotechnol. Prog.*, 6, 458, 1990.
59. Runstadler, P. W., Tung, A. S., Hayman, E. G., Ray, N. G., Sample, J. V. G., and DeLucia, D. E., Continuous culture with macroporous matrix, fluidized bed systems, in *Large Scale Mammalian Cell Culture Technology*, Lubiniecki, A. S., Ed., Marcel Dekker Inc., New York, 1990, 363.
60. Dean, R. C., Karkare, S. B., Phillips, P. G., Ray, N. G., and Runstadler, P. W., Continuous cell culture with fluidized sponge beads, in *Large Scale Cell Culture Technology*, Lydersen, B. K., Ed., Hanser Publishers, New York, 1987, 151.
61. Herschel, M. D. and Gruenberg, M. L., An automated hollow fiber system for the large-scale manufacture of mammalian cell secreted product, in *Large Scale Cell Culture Technology*, Lydersen, B. K., Ed., Hanser Publishers, New York, 1987, 113.

62. Griffiths, B., Perfusion systems for cell cultivation, in *Large Scale Mammalian Cell Culture Technology*, Lubiniecki, A. S., Ed., Marcel Dekker, New York, 1990, 217.
63. Yabannavar, V. M., Unpublished data.
64. Tolbert, W. R., Srigley, W. R., and Prior, C. P., Perfusion culture systems for large-scale pharmaceutical production, in *Animal Cell Biotechnology*, Vol. *3*, Spier, R. E. and Griffith, J. B., Eds., Academic Press, London, 1988, 373-393.
65. Shinmoto, H. and Dosako, S., Adaptation of mouse-human hybridomas to a protein-free medium, *Biotechnol. Lett.*, 15, 327, 1993.
66. Mather, J. P., Optimizing cell and culture environment for production of recombinant proteins, in *Gene Expression Technology, Methods in Enzymology, Vol. 185*, Goeddel, D. V., Ed., Academic Press, San Diego, 1990.
67. Aunins, J. Bibila, T., and Buckland, B. C., et al., Fluid mechanical considerations in industrial cell culture, Presented at Engineering Foundation Conference: Cell Culture Engineering IV, San Diego, CA, March 1994, 24.
68. Thomas, C. R., Al-Rubeai, M., and Zhang, Z., Prediction of mechanical damage to animal cells in turbulence, *Cytotechnology*, 15, 329, 1994.
69. Zhang, Z., Ferenczi, M. A., Lush, A. C., and Thomas, C. R., A novel micromanipulation technique for measuring the bursting strength of single mammalian cells, *Appl. Microbiol. Biotechnol.*, 36, 208, 1991.
70. Birch, J. R., Boraston, R. C., Metcalfe, H., Brown, M. E., Bebbington, C. R., and Field, R. P., Selecting and designing cell lines for improved physiological characteristics, *Cytotechnology*, 15, 11, 1994.
71. Bulter, M. and Christie, A., Adaptation of cells to non-ammoniagenic medium, *Cytotechnology*, 15, 87, 1994.
72. Maiorella, B., Inlow, D., and Howarth, W., Method of increasing product expression through solute stress, International Patent Application WO89/04867, 1989.
73. Schlumpp, B. and Schlaeger, E. J., Growth study of lactate and ammonia double-resistant clones of HL-60 cells, in *Animal Cell Technology: Developments, Processes, and Products*, Spier, R. E., Griffiths, J. B., and MacDonald, C., Eds., Butterworth-Heinemann, 1992, 183.
74. Oh, S. K. W., Vig, P., Chua, F., Teo, W. K., and Yap, M. G. S., Substantial overproduction of antibodies by applying osmotic pressure and sodium butyrate, *Biotechnol. Bioeng.*, 42, 601, 1993.
75. Blasey, H. D. and Benard, A. R., Repeated hybridoma batch culture with cell recycle, *Cytotechnology*, 13, 51, 1993.
76. Bushell, M. E., Bell, S. L., Scott, M. F., Spier, R. E., Wardell, J. N., and Sanders, P. G., Enhancement of monoclonal antibody yield by hybridoma fed-batch culture, resulting in extended maintenance of viable cell population, *Biotechnol. Bioeng.*, 44, 1099, 1994.
77. Maiorella, B., Hybridoma culture-optimization, characterization, cost, in *Harnessing Biotechnology for the 21st Century*. Proceedings of the Ninth International Biotechnology Symposium, Ladioch, M. and Bose, A., Eds., ACS, Salem, MA, 1992, 26.
78. Xie, L. and Wang, D. I. C., Applications of improved stoichiometric model in medium design and fed-batch cultivation of animal cells in bioreactor, *Cytotechnology*, 15, 17, 1994.
79. Robinson, D. K., Chan, C. P., Yu, Ip, C., Tsai, P. K., Tung, J.-S., Seamans, T. C., Lenny, A. B., Lee, D. K., Irwin, J., and Silberklang, M., Characterization of a recombinant antibody produced in the course of a high yield fed-batch process, *Biotechnol. Bioeng.*, 44, 727, 1994.
80. Bibila, T., Glazomitsky, K., Ranucci, C. S., Buckland, B. C., and Aunins, J. G., Monoclonal antibody process development using medium concentrates, *Biotechnol. Prog.*, 10, 87, 1994.

81. Kurokawa, H., Park, Y. S., Iijima, S., and Kobayashi, R., Growth characteristics in fed-batch culture of hybridoma cells with control of glucose and glutamine concentrations, *Biotechnol. Bioeng.*, 44, 95, 1994.
82. Bibila, T., Ranucci, C. S., Glazomitsky, K., Buckland, B. C., and Aunins, J. G., Investigation of NS0 cell metabolic behavior in MAb producing clones, *Ann. N. Y. Acad. Sci.*, 745, 277, 1994.
83. Banik, G. G. and Heath, C. A., Hybridoma growth and antibody production as a function of cell density and specific growth rate in perfusion culture, *Biotechnol. Bioeng.*, 48, 289, 1995.
84. Robinson, D. K., Widmer, J., and Memmert, K., Effect of specific growth rates on productivity in continuous open and partial cell retention animal cell bioreactors, *J. Biotechnology*, 22, 41, 1992.
85. Reddy, S. and Miller, W. M., Hybridoma antibody content and production rate in continuous culture: effect of dilution rate, *Biotech. Lett.*, 14, 1007, 1992.
86. Miller, W. M., Blanch, H. W., and Wilke, C. R., A kinetic analysis of hybridoma growth and metabolism in batch and continuous suspension culture: Effect of nutrient concentration, dilution rate, and pH, *Biotechnol. Bioeng.*, 32, 947, 1988.
87. Hu, W.-S. and Piret, J., Mammalian cell culture process, *Curr. Opin. Biotechnol.*, 3, 110, 1992.
88. Zhou, W. and Mulchandani, A., Recent advances in bioprocess monitoring and control, in *Recent Advances in Biosensors, Bioprocess Monitoring and Bioprocess Control*, ACS Symposium Series, Zhou, W. and Mulchandani, A., Eds., American Chemical Society, Washington D.C., 613, 89, 1995.
89. Zhou, W., Rehm, J., and Hu, W.-H., High viable cell concentration fed-batch cultures of hybridoma cells through on-line nutrient feeding, *Biotechnol. Bioeng.*, 46, 579, 1995.
90. Hansen, H. A., Madsen, N. M., and Emborg, C., An evaluation of fed-batch cultivation methods for mammalian cells based on model simulations, *Bioprocess Eng.*, 9, 205, 1993.
91. Noe, W., Schorn, P., Bux, R., and Bertholt, W., Fed-batch strategies for mammalian cell cultures, in *Animal Cell Technology: Products of Today, Prospects for Tomorrow*, Spier, R. E., Griffiths, J. B., and Berthold, W., Eds., Butterworth-Heinemann, Oxford, UK, 1994, 413.
92. Garg, V., Costello, M., and Czuba, B., Purification and production of therapeutic grade proteins, in *Purification and Analysis of Recombinant Proteins*, Seetharam, R. and Sharma, S., Eds., Marcel Dekker, New York, 1991, 29.
93. Brunner, K. H. and Henfert, H., Centrifugation, *Adv. Biotech. Proc.*, 8: 1, 1988.
94. Kempken, R., Preissmann, A., and Berthold, W., Clarification of animal cell cultures on a large scale by continuous centrifugation — downstream processing of a hybridoma cell culture using an industrial disc stack centrifuge; scale-up potential, *J. Ind. Microbiol.*, 14, 52, 1995.
95. Kempken, R., Pressman, A., and Berthold, W., Clarification of animal cell cultures on a large scale by continuous centrifugation, *J. Indust. Microbiol.*, 14, 52, 1995.
96. Ogez, J. R. and Builder, S. E., Downstream processing of proteins from mammalian cells, in *Large Scale Mammalian Cell Technology*, Lubiniecki, A. J., Ed., Marcel Dekker, New York, 1990, 396.
97. van Ries, R., Arathoon, W. E., Paoni, N. F., Sliwskowski, M. B., Lubiniecki, A. S., and Builder, S. E., A novel separation process for production of recombinant human tissue type plasminogen activator, unpublished data.
98. Arathoon, W. R., Builder, S. E., Lubiniecki, A. S., and van Ries, R. D., Process for producing biologically active plasminogen activator, European Patent Application 0248675.

99. Maiorella, B., Dorin, G., Carion, A., and Harano, D., Crossflow microfiltration of animal cells, *Biotechnol. Bioeng.*, 37: 121, 1991.
100. McCormick, D. K., Expanded bed adsorption, *Bio/Technology,* 11, 1059. 1993.
101. Batt, B. C., Yabannavar, V. M., and Singh, V., Expanded bed adsorption process for protein recovery from whole mammalian cell culture broth, *Bioseparation,* 5, 41, 1995.
102. Kenney, A. C., Large scale purification of monoclonal antibodies, in *Monoclonal Antibodies: Production and Application,* Mizrahi, A., Ed., New York: Alan R. Liss, 1989, 143.
103. Scott, R., Duffy, S., Moellering, B., and Prior, C., Purification of monoclonal antibodies from large scale mammalian cell culture perfusion systems, *Biotechnol. Prog.*, 3, 49, 1987.
104. Lee, S., Gustafson, M., Pickle, D., Flickinger, M., Muschik, G., and Moran, A., Large-scale purification of a murine antimelanoma monoclonal antibody, *J. Biotechnol.*, 4: 189, 1986.
105. Francis, R., Bonnerjea., J., and Hill, C., Validation of the re-use of protein A sepharose for the purification of monoclonal antibodies, in *Separations for Biotechnology 2,* Pyle, D. L., Ed., Elsevier Applied Science, New York, 1990, 491.
106. Jehanli, A. and Hough, D., A rapid procedure for the isolation of human IgM myeloma proteins, *J. Immunol. Methods,* 44, 199, 1981.
107. Bukovsky, J. and Kennett, R., Simple and rapid purification of monoclonal antibodies from cell culture supernatants and ascites fluids by hydroxylapatite chromatography on analytical and preparative scales, *Hybridoma,* 6, 219, 1987.
108. Stanker, L. H., Vanderlaan, M., and Juarex-Salinas, H., One step purification of mouse monoclonal antibodies from ascites fluid by hydroxylapatite chromatography, *J. Immunol. Methods,* 76: 157, 1985.
109. Guse, A. H., Milton, A. D., Schulzekoops, H., Muller, B., Roth, E., Simmer, B., Wachter, H., Weiss, E., and Emmrich, F., Purification and analytical characterization of an anti-CD4 monoclonal-antibody for human therapy, *Chromatography A,* 661, 13, 1994.
110. Casey, J. L., Keep, P. A., Chester, K. A., Robson, L., Hawkins, R. E., and Begent, R. H. J., Purification of bacterially expressed single-chain Fv antibodies for clinical-applications using metal chelate chromagraphy, *Methods,* 179, 105, 1995.
111. Jiskoot, W., Hoven, A., De Koning, A., Leering, M., Reubsaet, C., Crommelin, D., and Beuvery, E., Purification and stabilisation of a poorly soluble mouse IgG3 monoclonal antibody, *J. Immunol. Methods,* 138, 181, 1991.
112. Marcus-Sekura, C. J. and Kozak, R. W., Continuous cell lines and contaminant testing in regulatory practice for biopharmaceutical production, in *Regulatory Practice for Pharmaceutical Production,* Lubiniecki, A. S. and Vargo, S. A., Eds., Wiley-Liss, New York, 1994, 63.
113. Hirasaki, T., Ishikawa, G., Nakano, H., Manabe, S.-I., and Yamamota, N., Mechanism of virus removal by regenerated cellulose hollow fiber (BMM™), *Membrane,* 20, 135, 1995.
114. Revised CPMP Guidelines, *Virus validation studies: the design contribution, and interpretation of studies validating the inactivation and removal of viruses,* 1995.
115. Lubiniecki, A. S., Wiebe, M. E., and Builder, S. E., Process validation for cell culture-derived pharmaceutical proteins, in *Large Scale Mammalian Cell Technology,* Lubiniecki, A. J., Ed., Marcel Dekker, New York, 1990, 515.
116. Sofer, G. K. and Nystrom, L. E., *Process Chromatography, A Guide to Validation,* Academic Press, San Diego, 1989.
117. Franks, F., Freeze-drying: from empiricism to predictability, *Cryoletters,* 11, 93, 1990.

118. Aunins, J. G., Glazomitsky, K., and Buckland, B. C., Cell culture reactor design: known and unknown, in *BHRA Conference, 3rd International Conference, Bioreactor and Bioprocess Fluid Dynamics*, Nienow, A. W., Ed., BHRA Fluid Engineering, Cranfield, Bedford, England, 1993, 175.
119. Drapeau, D., Luan, Y.-T., Whiteford, J. C., Lavin, D. P., and Adamson, S. R., Cell culture scale-up in stirred tank bioreactors, paper presented at the Annual Meeting of the Society of Industrial Microbiology, Orlando, FL, August 1, 1990.
120. Birch, J. R., Lambert, K., Thompson, P. W., Kenney, A. C., and Wood, L. A., Antibody production with airlift fermentors, in *Large Scale Cell Culture Technology*, Lydrsen, B. K., Ed., Hanser, Munich, 1987, 1.
121. Srigley, W. R., Design and construction of manufacturing facilities for mammalian cell-derived pharmaceuticals, in *Large Scale Mammalian Cell Technology*, Lubiniecki, A. J., Ed., Marcel Dekker, New York, 1990, 567.
122. Schaffner, G., Haase, M., and Siegfried, G., Criteria for investigation of the product equivalence of monoclonal antibodies for therapeutic and *in vivo* diagnostic use in case of introduction of changes in the manufacturing process, *Biologicals*, 23, 253, 1995.

Chapter **10**

Production of Antibody Domains in Prokaryotes

Marc Better and Patrick Gavit

CONTENTS

0-8493-8547-4/97/$0.00+$.50

10.1 INTRODUCTION

In the recent past, scientists wishing to use prokaryotic hosts to produce antibody domains have been presented with a staggering number of options. Many expression systems have been described which utilize unique plasmid vectors, regulated promoters, and host strains, and an amazing array of antibody domains including Fab, $F(ab')_2$, single-chain antibody (SCA), and Fv. To the casual observer, this myriad of choices may seem daunting, but several important generalizations can be made. First, for most molecules of interest, a prokaryotic expression system can be identified that is useful for production. This statement may appear obvious, but until about 1985, mammalian lymphoid cells were the only source for antibody proteins. Second, antibody domains can be expressed both intracellularly in bacteria where they typically accumulate into insoluble inclusion bodies or they can be secreted from the bacterial cytoplasm where they often fold properly and can be recovered in an active form. Because each of these expression options presents some advantages (and disadvantages), planning is required to achieve optimal production goals.

The production of antibody domains in bacteria can be divided into two important steps; the first is protein expression while the second is product recovery and purification. For many uses where antibody domains are evaluated directly from bacterial cultures (for example, in screening applications), highly purified proteins may not initially be necessary. For other uses, especially where antibody domains are to be used as human pharmaceuticals, a highly purified and homogeneous product is essential. Clearly, the methods chosen for product expression will impact the methods available for subsequent processing. In this chapter, we will discuss the available options for both important aspects of antibody domain production.

10.2 ANTIBODY DOMAIN EXPRESSION: INTRACELLULAR VS. EXTRACELLULAR

Heterologous gene expression in *E. coli* often provides an opportunity to produce protein in large quantities. The exact form of a foreign protein produced in *E. coli*, however, will vary depending on many factors reflecting both the nature of the protein destined for expression and the type of expression system chosen. Proteins expressed in *E. coli* can remain soluble in the bacterial cytoplasm, become sequestered into inclusion bodies, be secreted across the cytoplasmic membrane, and accumulate in the periplasmic space, or in some cases accumulate in the bacterial growth medium. True secretion from *E. coli* is rare, however, most often it is the result of a specific mechanism for protein export.

Initial attempts to produce antibody molecules in bacteria relied on intracellular expression and formation of inclusion bodies, with subsequent *in vitro* refolding of individual antibody polypeptide chains to an active conformation. In these cases, the yield of individual antibody proteins produced intracellularly was high, but because the reassembly process was inefficient, only a small amount of an active antibody domain could be generated. As described in the first report of this type by Cabilly et al.,[1] the yield of correctly folded Fab protein was about 1.4% when the resolubilized peptides were refolded at 25 μg/ml, and hence this system was impractical for preparation of large quantities of recombinant material. Only recently has progress been made to increase the efficiency of this Fab refolding process (40% yield at 60 μg/ml).[2] In contrast to the refolding of a multisubunit protein such as Fab and Fv, *in vitro* refolding of SCA from insoluble inclusion bodies is somewhat more efficient, and this production strategy has been used widely.[3-5] In some instances, intracellular expression followed by *in vitro* folding remains a favored method of production, for example, with targeted fusions of antibody domains and cytotoxic proteins such as the *Pseudomonas* exotoxin.[6,7]

In 1988, two reports demonstrated for the first time that antibody domains could be secreted from *E. coli* and concurrently fold into an active configuration.[8,9] Addition of a bacterial leader peptide to the N-terminus of each of the antibody chains comprising either an Fab or Fv allowed for their transport across the bacterial cytoplasmic membrane where they associated into the proper configuration in the periplasmic space. Antibody domains could thereby be purified directly from bacterial cells or culture supernatant without subsequent protein refolding. Physical techniques such as electrospray mass spectrometry,[10] differential scanning calorimetry,[11] far UV circular dichroism,[12] and X-ray crystallography[13] have now demonstrated that antibody domains produced in this fashion from bacteria are correctly folded and of the expected molecular configuration. In recent years, many laboratories have utilized a similar secretion system to express antibody domains of various types, including Fab, $F(ab')_2$, SCA, Fv, and fusion proteins.

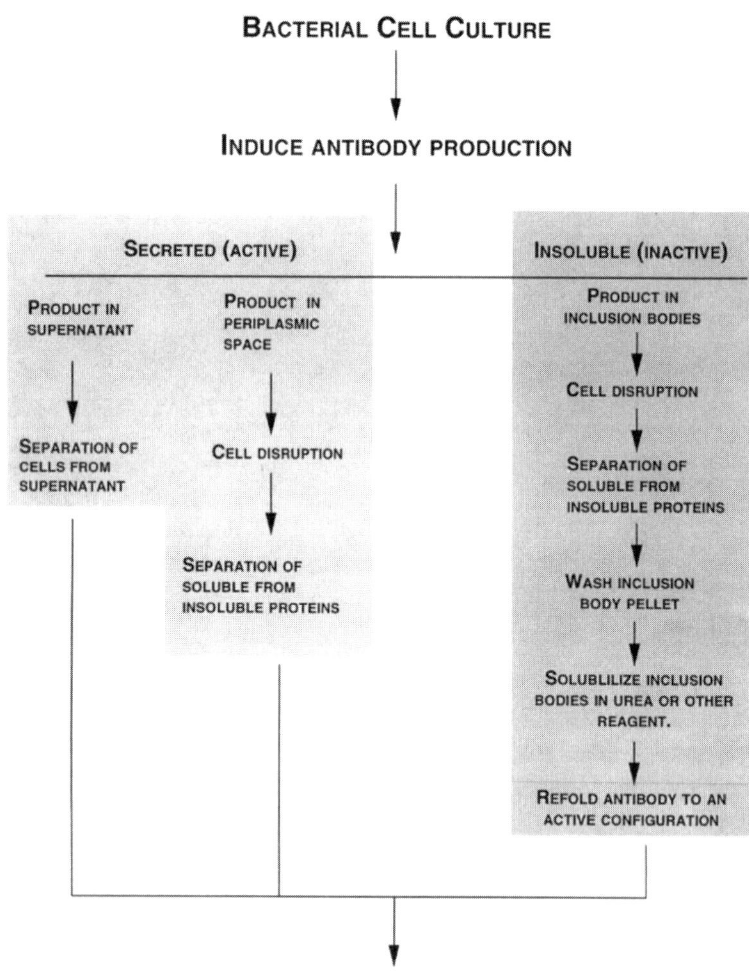

FIGURE 1
Process for recovery of secreted and insoluble antibody domains. A product recovered directly from a cell-free culture supernatant can be purified directly. To recover a product from the periplasmic space of *E. coli*, cells must be disrupted (either by osmotic shock or mechanical cell disruption) prior to product purification. An insoluble antibody domain must be separated from soluble proteins, solubilized, and refolded to an active form prior to purification.

In cases where a desired antibody domain can efficiently be recovered as a correctly folded, active protein from the periplasmic space or the culture supernatant, secretion provides the most convenient route for production. Figure 1 illustrates the general process flow for a model antibody domain being produced from a secreted vs. intracellular form. Particular advantages of a secretion process, especially if the product can be recovered directly from the culture medium, are that disruption of the cells is not necessary and the clarified, concentrated broth can be applied directly to a first step in protein purification (such as ion exchange chromatography). Not all attempts at protein secretion with antibody domains have met with equal success, however, as many details relating to expression can affect the efficiency and yield of a desired product.

10.3 EXPRESSION SYSTEMS FOR ANTIBODY DOMAINS

Although it is difficult to generalize about antibody domain production since many expression systems have been tried and many forms of antibody molecules have been expressed, certain features are required for successful expression. Perhaps most important is a strong regulated promoter which can efficiently initiate transcription at the desired time and minimize expression of recombinant product in the uninduced state. Certain promoters such as the *lac* promoter, which are transcribed at a relatively high rate even in the absence of an inducing agent, may be undesirable since constitutive expression of many antibody forms can inhibit cell growth[14] (perhaps in part a consequence of the accumulation of improperly folded intermediates), or allow selection of deletion mutants to appear. Tightly regulated bacterial promoters such as T7, *phoA*, and *araB* are ideal. Table 1 outlines many of the promoters that have been used most commonly to express antibody domains in *E. coli*. If an antibody domain is destined for intracellular accumulation, its expression from a strong regulated promoter is usually sufficient in conjunction with the standard set of *E. coli* transcriptional and translational regulatory sequences.[15] As with any protein expressed in *E. coli*, an effective ribosome binding site, initiation codon (ATG), and proper spacing between these regulatory sites is required.

For translocation of the antibody polypeptide across the cytoplasmic membrane of *E. coli*, a hydrophobic leader sequence must be linked to the N-terminus of the polypeptide chain. Most laboratories have utilized native bacterial leader sequences such as the *pelB*, *ompA*, *ompF*, and *stII* leader sequences. These secretion signal sequences all share structural features such as a charged N-terminus and a hydrophobic core. In general, the choice of leader sequence can affect the amount of a particular secreted product, although in some cases where antibody domains were linked to a number of leader sequences, equivalent product yield has resulted.[14]

TABLE 1

Expression Systems and Product Yield of Selected Antibody Domains

Promoter	Leader	Antibody Form	Shake Flask Soluble Yield[a] (mg/l)	Soluble or Insoluble[b]	Ref.
lambda	None	SCA	None	Insoluble	4
lambda	ompA	SCA	None	Insoluble	61
T7	None	Fab/SCA	None	Insoluble	62
T7	None	SCA	None	Insoluble	63
T7	None	SCA-fusion	None	Insoluble	7
tac	None	Fab	None	Insoluble	2
tac	ompF	Fab	None	Insoluble	64
trp	trp LE	SCA	None	Insoluble	5
lac	pelB	Fab, SCA	4–10	Soluble-periplasm	65
lac	ompA/phoA	Fv	0.2 (Purified yield)	Soluble-periplasm	9
lac	pelB	Fab	0.01–0.02	Soluble	66
lac	pelB	SCA	3.5	Soluble	14
T7	pelB	Fab	Very low	Soluble	67
T7	pelB	SCA	3.5	Soluble	24
tac	pelB	Fab	0.5–2	Soluble	68
tac	ompA	Fv	40	Soluble	28
tac	ompA	SCA	2.4	Soluble	23
tac	pelB	SCA	1–2	Soluble	69
araB	pelB	Fab	2	Soluble	8
lac	ompA	Fab	2	Soluble-periplasm	70
phoA	stII	Fab′	NA[c]	Soluble	12

[a] Shown is the amount of antibody domain recovered from culture supernatants or from the bacterial periplasm, either directly or after purification.

[b] Insoluble antibody domains were refolded to an active form. Soluble domains were evaluated directly or purified in an active form.

[c] NA, not applicable. In this case, only the Fab yield from a fermenter was described (1–2 g/l).

Note: This table illustrates the many promoters and leader sequences used to express antibody domains. This table is illustrative and does not present a comprehensive list of all described antibody expression systems. The yield of insoluble antibody domains from bacterial cultures is not shown.

10.4 PRODUCT YIELD FOR SECRETED ANTIBODY DOMAINS

The factors which affect the final product yield for secreted antibody domains, and secreted recombinant products from *E. coli* in general, are poorly understood. Notwithstanding, several reports describe expression of antibody domains in a secreted form with a yield approaching 1 g/l or higher.[12,16,17] To achieve such a prodigious yield, high cell density fermentation is required, although the fermentation process per se cannot guarantee a high yield. Perhaps the most important factor which affects product yield is the amino acid sequence of the particular molecule of interest, and how efficiently the nascent polypeptide chains can fold into the correct configuration in the environment of the bacterial periplasm.[14,18,19] In one of the first reports to detail a system for secretion of an antibody Fab, we noted that while 2 μg/ml of Fab could be recovered from the culture supernatant in a properly folded configuration, the majority of the expressed light chain remained cell associated in a non-native configuration.[20] Subsequent reports demonstrate that in many cases the majority of synthesized Fab, Fv, or SCA remains cell associated in an incorrectly folded state. In some cases, the vast majority or all of the antibody protein has folded incorrectly and remains cell associated. In several cases where an antibody domain was poorly expressed as a secreted protein, the cellular fate of antibody domains specifically designed for secretion through the periplasmic membrane was determined.[14,21] Unfortunately, antibody molecules can remain associated with the cell in an incorrectly folded form either in the periplasmic space, intracellularly, or in association with cell membranes. Subtle differences among antibody domains, even a single amino acid substitution, can greatly affect the overall folding rate and hence product yield.[22] In two reports, SCA molecules constructed from the same variable domains with the domain order reversed exhibited a profoundly different level of secreted product while the total amount of polypeptide product in the cell, primarily inclusion bodies, remained essentially constant.[21,23]

The product yield is a measure of both how efficiently the molecule folds in the environment of the bacterial cell and how efficiently it is expressed. Typically with strong, regulated bacterial promoters, transcription of the antibody gene is not limiting, but the efficiency of protein translation can limit product accumulation.[24] Most often, however, folding is the crucial aspect, and one that is difficult to address if product yield is low. Alteration in amino acid sequence which might increase expression level (by affecting the translation efficiency or folding rate) is possible either through direct selection for expression mutants or by increasing homology to proteins which are known to express well,[25] but may adversely influence the affinity of antibody for antigen.

A survey of published data reveals that most secreted antibody domains accumulate in the periplasmic space or culture supernatant in the range from barely detectable to about 40 μg/ml in a laboratory scale shake flask culture. Table 1 illustrates the reported yield of various secreted antibody products. When some of these molecules are expressed in a fermentor where cell densities of up to 5×10^{11} cells/ml can be achieved, an increase in total product of up to 500-fold or more may result.[24] Depending on the fermentation culture conditions, much of the correctly folded antibody domains may remain associated with the cells[12] (in the bacterial periplasm) or be released from the bacterial cells into the culture supernatant.[16,17] Typical fed-batch fermentation conditions provide sufficient nutrients to allow cell growth to an $OD_{550\ \sim100}$ prior to induction with an appropriate agent. Carter et al.[12] report 1–2 g/l of Fab′ after disruption of cells by sonication with approximately 100 mg/l in the culture medium. We reported Fab expression at up to 700 mg/l[16,17] directly from the cell-free culture supernatant. We have also expressed approximately fifteen additional antibody fragments to a titer of from 50 to 800 mg/l, and Pack et al.[26] and King et al.[27] have described the production of bivalent mini-antibodies at approximately 200 mg/l and Fv at 450 mg/l, respectively.

Bacterial growth temperature can also play an important role in determining product yield. Typically, growth temperatures in the range of 26 to 32°C are preferable to maximize the yield of recombinant antibody. Success is possible at 37°C,[12] however, and it is likely that unique folding properties of each antibody domain will influence the optimal growth temperature for bacterial cultures expressing antibody domains.

10.5 METHODS FOR ANTIBODY DOMAIN PURIFICATION

10.5.1 Product Recovery from Inclusion Bodies

To recover an antibody polypeptide from recombinant bacteria, cells are typically disrupted in lysis buffer and the insoluble inclusion bodies are separated by centrifugation.[3,6,7] The inclusion body pellet is then washed several times with buffer to separate soluble from insoluble *E. coli* proteins. In some cases, non-ionic detergent is included in the wash buffer.

Purification of antibody domains from inclusion bodies involves solubilization, followed by renaturation or refolding. Solubilization is normally done with a high concentration of urea or guanidine hydrochloride (typically 8 *M* or 6 *M*, respectively). Refolding can be accomplished by diluting the solubilized inclusion bodies into renaturation buffer and allowing the molecules to fold properly over a period of hours. Folding of immunofusion proteins which contain disulfide bonds can be facilitated in a redox buffer which allows disulfide interchange to occur. An example of a redox buffer that was successfully used to refold an immunofusion protein is 1 m*M* reduced glutathione and 0.1 m*M* oxidized glutathione.[6] Refolded antibody domain can then be purified by any of the methods described in the following section.

10.5.2 Recovery of Secreted Antibody Domains

While the purification of recombinant proteins from bacterial growth medium can avoid difficult issues associated with separation of inclusion bodies from whole cells such as cell disruption, resolubilization, and refolding, purification of secreted antibody domains presents other challenges. In cases where the proteins are translocated across the cytoplasmic membrane and accumulate in the periplasmic space, cells must still be disrupted prior to product purification. In those cases where the antibody domain accumulates directly in the culture supernatant, the secreted protein can represent only a small percentage of the total protein in the growth medium (due to partial cell lysis or selective permeabilization). In addition, soluble recombinant proteins can be somewhat more susceptible to proteolysis by endogenous bacterial proteases than are proteins in insoluble, inclusion bodies.

For preparation of antibody domains suitable as human pharmaceuticals, each purification process should include a number of selective steps designed to separate the antibody domain from other proteins, bacterial lipopolysaccharide, DNA, and other cellular components. An initial step that yields a high degree of purification is desirable, particularly to separate the antibody domain from the endogenous *E. coli* proteins in the growth medium or lysed cells. Affinity chromatography can often offer great specificity and the opportunity to obtain a high degree of purification in a single process step. An affinity step may be best suited to a position in the process stream where a clarified or partially purified feedstock can be applied. Since affinity chromatography media can have a relatively high cost compared with other types of media (i.e., ion exchange or hydrophobic interaction chromatography media), many users prefer to regenerate affinity resins for reuse. While leakage of affinity groups from most column support matrices is usually very low or undetectable, it may be neccesary to validate the removal of affinity ligands during the remaining downstream steps of the process. Described here are four affinity methods that are widely employed to purify secreted antibody domains and immunofusion proteins, or refolded antibody domains.

10.5.2.1 Protein G

Protein G is a cell wall protein from certain strains of groups G and C *streptococci* which binds to both IgG and Fab molecules.[28-30] The Fab binding site on protein G is distinct from the Fc binding site through which IgG binding is mediated.[31,32] Protein G is available in a variety of immobilized types, including recombinant forms,[33,34] which are produced in *E. coli*, and are modified to offer improvements over the native form. These improvements are sometimes helpful for purification of

IgG, for example, by removal of the albumin binding region of native protein G, incorporation of two IgG binding sites, and removal of the Fab binding portion.[34,35] Some altered forms of protein G resist proteolytic degradation and thereby provide a longer column life.

A number of approaches have been taken to produce an immobilized form of protein G which allows for high linear flow velocities, thus making it more amenable to large-scale purifications. Crosslinked agarose and glass bead supports are two examples of commonly available matrices which can be operated at high flow rates. Perfusion chromatographic media contain throughpores which allow convective transport to the interior of the particle to provide efficient access to short path length diffusive pores. This media configuration is amenable to high linear velocities since solute binding is less diffusion limited than conventional chromatographic media, and there is more efficient access to diffusive pores due to the convective throughpores. One other immobilized protein G format is a membrane affinity cartridge. Here the protein G is linked to the interior of hollow fibers through which the feedstream can be recirculated several times. High fluxes are possible because binding of solutes occurs during convective flow and is not diffusion limited.

Examples of antibody domain purification with protein G were recently described in which chimeric[11] and humanized[12] Fab were purified using protein G Sepharose Fast Flow (Pharmacia). Several factors can affect binding of Fab to protein G. First, the primary amino acid sequence is important since not all Fab molecules have affinity for protein G, and those that do exhibit widely varying binding affinity. Second, the protein G-Fab interaction is greatly affected by column loading conditions which need to be optimized for each particular antibody domain.

10.5.2.2 Protein A

Protein A is an IgG binding protein produced by *Staphylococcus aureus*. Specific domains of protein A bind tightly to the Fc portion of IgG, and protein A is used extensively to purify IgG. Protein A can also bind specifically to some Fab molecules.[36,37] The affinity of protein A for human Fab molecules is highly restricted to V_HIII molecules, although not all V_HIII chains bind to protein A,[38] and some nonhuman Fab molecules bind to protein A as well. Protein A was used to purify a humanized Fab domain recovered from the *E. coli* periplasm.[11] This Fab bound to a Prosep-A column (Bioprocessing) in phosphate buffered saline (PBS) with a capacity of about 6 mg/ml, and Fab eluted with 0.1 *M* glycine, pH 3.0. Affinity for protein A was antibody dependent, however, as the chimeric version of the same antibody did not bind to protein A. A potential drawback to the use of either protein A or protein

G is the harsh condition required for product elution, typically low pH. This condition could lead to denaturation and precipitation of the antibody domain.

10.5.2.3 Immobilized Metal Affinity Chromatography

One useful purification technique that has been applied widely to antibody domains involves the use of engineered affinity tails at the N or C terminus of a protein. For a review on the general use of affinity tails see Reference 39. One of the shortest affinity tails that can be incorporated onto a protein to aid in its purification is a metal chelate tail. This technique known as immobilized metal affinity chromatography (IMAC) or metal chelate affinity chromatography (MCAC) is based on the principle that certain amino acids form complexes with transition metal ions.[40,41] A commonly used chelating group is iminodiacetic acid (IDA) that is immobilized onto a rigid matrix; several IMAC resins are commercially available. In general, the resin is first charged with a metal ion and then sample is loaded. Product can be eluted in a variety of ways including pH reduction to protonate the histidine groups, addition of a chelating agent such as EDTA or EGTA to strip metal ions from the chelating groups, or addition of a competing ligand such as imidazole.

IMAC has been used to purify both Fv[42] and Fab[43] domains from *E. coli*. In these cases, a poly histidine tail was engineered onto the C-terminus of the protein. A Chelating Sepharose column (Pharmacia) was loaded with $ZnCl_2$ prior to sample addition, and the antibody was eluted with an imidazole gradient. Figure 2 shows the purification from *E. coli* growth medium of a SCA by this method. Here, the antibody domain included a His_6 C-terminal tail, and was purified using Chelating Sepharose Fast Flow (Pharmacia). The ability of this technique to yield a high degree of purification is apparent from Figure 2. In addition, poly histidine tails do not appear to disturb antigen binding.[42]

The strength of the interaction between metal chelate columns and proteins is largely dependent on the metal used and the configuration of histidine residues.[44]. In some cases a single accessible histidine is sufficient if Cu(II) is used, while two closely spaced histidine residues are sufficient if Zn(II) or Co(II) is used as a metal chelated to IDA.

10.5.2.4 Other Affinity Purification Techniques

Immobilized reactive dyes originally designed for the textile industry can sometimes be used for protein purification as they bind to specific classes of proteins.[45-47] They are thought to mimic biological substances like cofactors and effectors and can therefore be used for affinity purification of proteins which are normally substrates for these

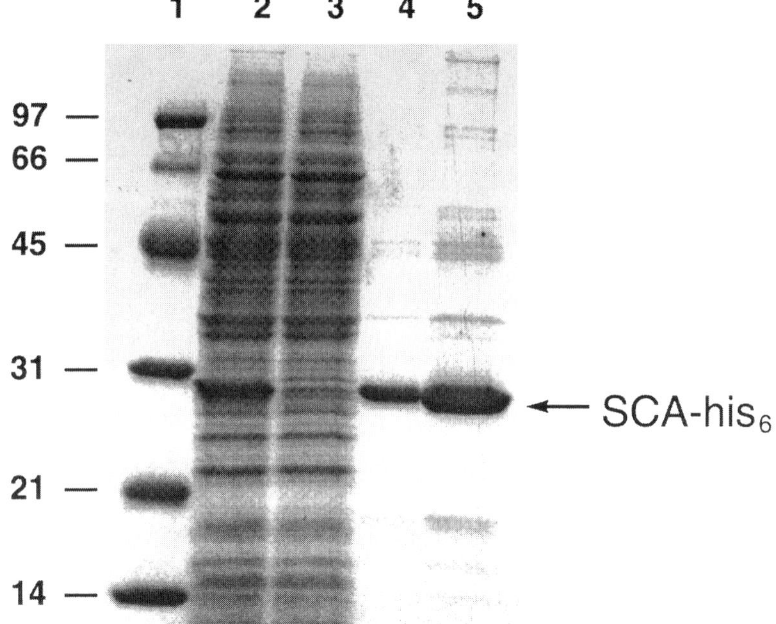

FIGURE 2
SDS-PAGE analysis of SCA-his$_6$ purification by IMAC. The SCA was expressed in *E. coli* as a secreted product and recovered directly from a cell-free fermentation broth that had been concentrated approximately fourfold.[48] A 50-ml column containing Chelating Sepharose (Pharmacia, 4.4 × 3.4 cm) was charged with 3 mg/ml $ZnCl_2$. The column was then equilibrated with 20 m*M* Tris-acetate, 0.5 *M* NaCl, pH 8.0, and the cell-free bacterial culture supernatant was loaded at 50 cm/h. The column was washed with 20 m*M* Tris-acetate, 0.5 *M* NaCl, pH 8.0, and the product was eluted with 10 m*M* sodium phosphate, 0.5 *M* NaCl, 40 m*M* EDTA, pH 7.0. Lane 1, size standards; lane 2, cell-free fermentation broth; lane 3, Chelating Sepharose flow through; lanes 4 and 5, Chelating Sepharose eluate (4 and 16 μg, respectively).

cofactors and effectors. While immobilized dyes are not typically being used to purify antibody domains alone, we have used this method to purify immunoconjugates and immunofusion proteins of antibody domains linked to plant ribosome inactivating proteins (RIP). Some of the RIP exhibit an affinity for Cibracon blue, and we have used columns containing this dye to purify Fab and $F(ab')_2$ conjugated to ricin toxin A chain and gelonin.[17,48]

Many types of antibody domains have been purified on antigen-based affinity columns or on anti-idiotype immunoaffinity columns. Antibody domains have also been fused to peptide tags that are recognized by monoclonal antibodies for purification. Similarly, antibody domains can be fused to whole proteins or protein domains to allow subsequent purification. For example, a strep tag affinity peptide can be bound to immobilized Streptavidin.[49] Another interesting and versatile approach is purification of antibody domains via a calmodulin fusion. Calmodulin allows purification via an anion-exchange resin or an immobilized organic calmodulin ligand.[50] In some cases, the peptide tag or fusion domain can be cleaved from the antibody domain after purification at an introduced protease-sensitive site.

Fusion of a peptide or protein to an antibody domain may also provide a helpful way of altering the molecular charge and thereby allow easier separation from contaminating (primarily acidic) *E. coli* proteins. A basic amino acid tail could be engineered onto an antibody domain for this purpose. For example, a polyarginine tail can be effective to assist purification of intracellular *E. coli* proteins.[51,52]

10.6 PURIFICATION OF SECRETED Fab AND IMMUNOFUSION PROTEINS

10.6.1 Purification Strategies

Previously, we described the purification of Fab and antibody domain immunofusion proteins from the culture supernatant of *E. coli* grown to a high cell density.[16,17,48] As an initial purification step, we loaded the concentrated culture supernatant onto a cation exchange resin since all of these proteins had relatively high isoelectric points, while the majority of the endogenous *E. coli* proteins are acidic, including those that appear in the growth medium with the recombinant antibody domains and immunotoxins.[16,51,53] This strategy achieved a high degree of purification early in the purification process. For antibody domains destined for use as pharmaceuticals, a cation exchange column early in the purification process can also remove DNA and endotoxin from the bacterial broth. The usefulness of this approach will be illustrated in the two purification examples which follow.

In the first example, we purified a humanized Fab from a concentrated fermentation broth. A flow diagram of the purification strategy is shown in Figure 3. Samples taken from each stage of the purification are shown in Figure 4. Analysis of these samples by SDS-PAGE demonstrates that significant purification was obtained with the initial cation exchange column (CM-Spherodex), since after this column, Fab is the predominant protein, see Figure 4, lane 3. The subsequent two steps, protein G and phenyl sepharose, remove the remaining protein impurities. Fab loss is minimal at each step, see Table 2. This purification strategy also effectively removes endotoxin and DNA. The CM-Spherodex column reduced the endotoxin and DNA by 3.4 and 2.7 logs, respectively, while the protein G step further reduced endotoxin by about 3.8 logs to <0.1 endotoxin units (EU)/mg Fab (undetectable).

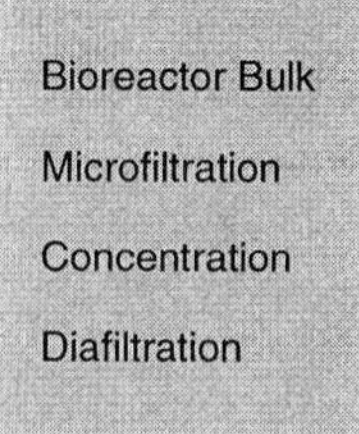

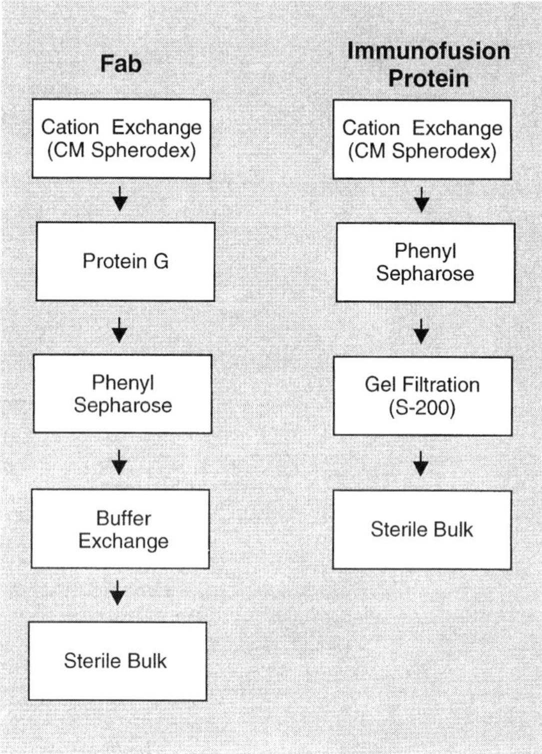

FIGURE 3
Flow diagram for recovery and purification of secreted antibody domains from bacterial fermentation broth. Details of the two processes are discussed in the text.

Hydroxyapatite (HAP), which is a relatively inexpensive alternative, could replace protein G with no loss of protein purity. Chromatography on HAP did not separate Fab and endotoxin as efficiently, however, as only about 1.5 log reduction in endotoxin occurred. Since

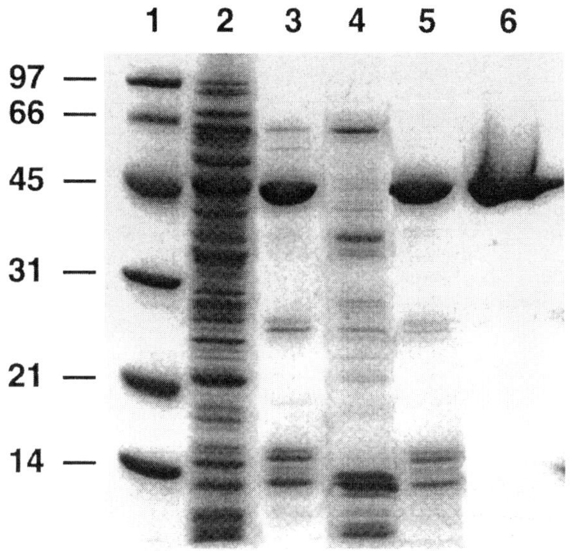

FIGURE 4
SDS-PAGE analysis of Fab purification. After removal of cells from a 10 liter *E. coli* fermentation batch, the growth medium was diafiltered into 20 m*M* HEPES, pH 6.8 (lane 2). This material was loaded onto a CM Spherodex column (Biosepra) and eluted with 20 m*M* HEPES, 75 m*M* NaCl, pH 6.8 (lane 3, CM Spherodex eluate). The eluate was loaded onto a protein G column (Prosep G from Bioprocessing) equilibrated in 20 m*M* HEPES, 75 m*M* NaCl, pH 6.8. Elution was accomplished with 100 m*M* glycine, 100 m*M* NaCl, pH 3.0. Lanes 4 and 5 are the protein G flow through and eluate, respectively. The protein G eluate was loaded onto a phenyl sepharose column (Pharmacia) equilibrated in 20 m*M* HEPES, 2 *M* $(NH_4)_2SO_4$, pH 6.8. Elution of the column was with 20 m*M* HEPES, 1 *M* $(NH_4)_2SO_4$, pH 6.8 (lane 6, phenyl sepharose eluate). Molecular weight size standard (Biorad) is shown in lane 1.

HAP is a charged amphoteric matrix, some endotoxin may bind and co-elute with Fab.

A different purification scheme was used to isolate an antibody immunofusion protein from *E. coli.* This fusion protein consists of the RIP gelonin coupled to Fab.[54] A flow diagram of the purification process is shown in Figure 3. The gelonin portion did not appreciably change the isoelectric point from that of Fab since gelonin itself has a relatively high isoelectric point. As for Fab, a cation exchange step led the purification process. A CM-Spherodex column removed the majority of the endogenous *E. coli* proteins, see Figure 5, lane 3. The main protein impurities after elution from this column, at around 30 kDa, were gelonin-related fragments as determined by Western analysis. The immunofusion protein was further purified by hydrophobic interaction chromatography on phenyl sepharose. The recovery at each step of the process is shown in Table 3.

TABLE 2

Fab Purification[a]

Sample	Total Fab (mg)	% Recovery	Endotoxin EU/mg Fab	Total Endotoxin	Log Reduction Endotoxin[b]	DNA conc. (pg/mg)	Total DNA (pg)	Log Reduction DNA[b]
Cell-free broth (diafiltered)	124.8	100	1.6E6	2.0E8		2.6E6	3.2E8	
CM-Spherodex FT	0.9	0.7						
CM-Spherodex eluate	127.3	102	5.7E2	7.3E4	3.4	4.5E3	5.7E5	2.7
Protein G FT	0	0						
Protein G eluate	108.1	86.7	<0.1	<10.8	>3.8	29	3.1E3	2.3
Phenyl sepharose FT	23.2	18.6						
Phenyl sepharose eluate	112.6	90.2				42	4.7E3	

[a] See the legend to Figure 4 for process details. Both DNA and endotoxin were efficiently removed from the sample by this procedure. FT refers to flow through.

[b] Shown is the log reduction from the previous step for DNA and endotoxin.

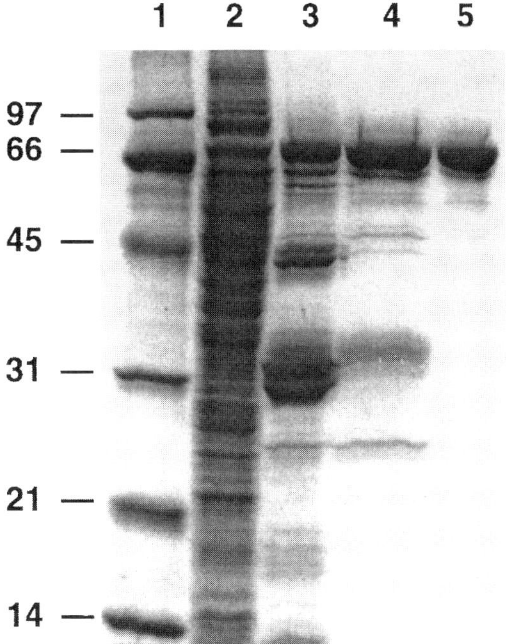

FIGURE 5
SDS-PAGE analysis of Fab-gelonin immunofusion[48] purification. After removal of cells from a 10 l *E. coli* fermentation run, the growth medium was diafiltered into 10 m*M* sodium phosphate, pH 7.0 (lane 2). This material was loaded onto a CM Spherodex column (Biosepra) equilibrated in 10 m*M* sodium phosphate, pH 7.0. The column was eluted with 10 m*M* sodium phosphate, 200 m*M* NaCl, pH 7.0 (lane 3, CM Spherodex eluate) and diluted twofold with 20 m*M* HEPES, 3 *M* $(NH_4)_2SO_4$, pH 7.0. The sample was then loaded onto a phenyl sepharose column (Pharmacia) equilibrated in 20 m*M* HEPES, 1.5 *M* $(NH_4)_2SO_4$, pH 7.0. This column was washed with 20 m*M* HEPES, 1.3 *M* $(NH_4)_2SO_4$, pH 7.0 and eluted with 20 m*M* HEPES, 0.9 *M* $(NH_4)_2SO_4$, pH 7.0 (lane 4, phenyl sepharose eluate). Finally, a Sephacryl S-200 gel filtration column was used to exchange the sample into 10 m*M* sodium phosphate, 150 m*M* NaCl, pH 7.0, as well as remove some protein impurities (lane 5, S-200 pool). Molecular weight size standard (Biorad) is shown in lane 1.

TABLE 3
Fab-gelonin Purification[a]

Sample	Volume (ml)	Concentration (mg/ml)	Total (mg)	% Recovery
Cell-free fermentation broth (diafiltered)	3200	0.17	557	100
CM-Spherodex eluate	304	1.79	544	97.7
Phenyl Sepharose eluate	215	2.21	475	85.3
S-200 pool	190	2.4	456	81.9

[a] See the legend to Figure 5 for process details.

Membrane adsorbers provide an alternative format for ion exchange chromatography of antibody domains. High flow rates can be achieved since solute binding to exchange groups occurs during convective flow and is not limited by the slower diffusion process. A strong cation exchange membrane adsorber was also used to purify a recombinant immunofusion of SCA and gelonin from *E. coli* growth media.[55] Capture of the immunofusion occurred at fluxes of 300 cm/h and at low pressures (<2 bar). The membrane exhibited a dynamic binding capacity of 1 mg/cm^2 (~50 mg/ml). Under these conditions, a 97% recovery and a tenfold increase in concentration of the immunofusion protein was achieved.

10.6.2 Separation of Similar Antibody Domain Forms

Recombinant proteins secreted from *E. coli* are sometimes susceptible to proteolysis either in the periplasmic space or in the culture supernatant, and proteolytic fragments of recombinant antibody domains such as Fab can complicate a purification process. During purification of one Fab′, we determined that most of the protein impurities present after the initial cation exchange chromatography step were indeed fragments of intact Fab′, (Figure 6). N terminal sequence analysis identified many of the bands as fragments of intact Fab′. The three proteins with a molecular mass of approximately 28 kDa could not be separated from intact Fab′ by chromatography on ion exchange, hydrophobic interaction chromatography, HAP, or protein G. They could, however, be separated by gel filtration in the presence of 8 *M* urea, (Figure 7). Separation did not occur in the absence of urea.

Denaturants may allow resolution of Fab fragments from the intact species for several reasons. First, perhaps the heavy (Fd) and light (kappa) chains, which can be resolved from intact Fab′ by SDS-PAGE, exist as a single associated, non-disulfide linked unit in solution held together by an interaction along the Fd-kappa hydrophobic interface. The peptide components which lack a proper interchain disulfide bond may therefore be the same molecular weight in solution as intact Fab′. Only addition of a denaturant or chaotropic salt, such as SDS, guanidine hydrochloride, or urea, will disrupt the noncovalent interaction of kappa and Fd chains and allow them to be separated from intact Fab′. Another possibility is that the resolving power of the gel filtration column is not sufficient to separate the kappa and Fd fragments from intact, native Fab′. Perhaps, fully denaturing the sample increases the effective radius of intact Fab′ and its fragments sufficiently to bring them into a more optimal resolving range of the gel filtration media. Proteolytic Fab fragments can be difficult to separate from intact Fab since they share many physical and chemical properties.

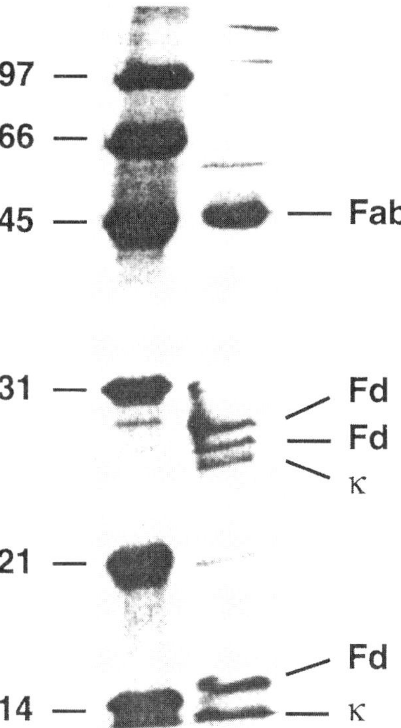

FIGURE 6
SDS-PAGE analysis of proteins in a preparation of Fab′ after chromatography on CM cellulose (Whatman). The identity of peptide contaminants was determined by N terminal sequencing. Molecular weight standards (Biorad) are shown in the left lane.

10.6.3 Separation of Bacterial Lipopolysaccharide

The amount of endotoxin in bacterial cultures can be quite high, as lipopolysaccharide (LPS) from the outer cell membrane of Gram-negative bacteria is continually shed into the growth medium. Endotoxin may be present in the *E. coli* culture supernatant at a concentration of 10^7 EU/ml in the Fab containing growth medium.[16] Since the lipid portion of LPS induces a pyrogenic or fever-causing reaction,[56] its removal from pharmaceutical products is essential.

A number of methods are known to remove endotoxins during the purification process. Affinity chromatography using immobilized polymyxin B, a cationic antibiotic, can be useful.[57,58] Immobilized histamine also has a high affinity for endotoxin.[59] As demonstrated above, however, endotoxin can be removed along with protein impurities during ion exchange, protein G, and HAP chromatography, and steps designed primarily for endotoxin removal may not be required. LPS is negatively charged and thus flows through cation exchange columns

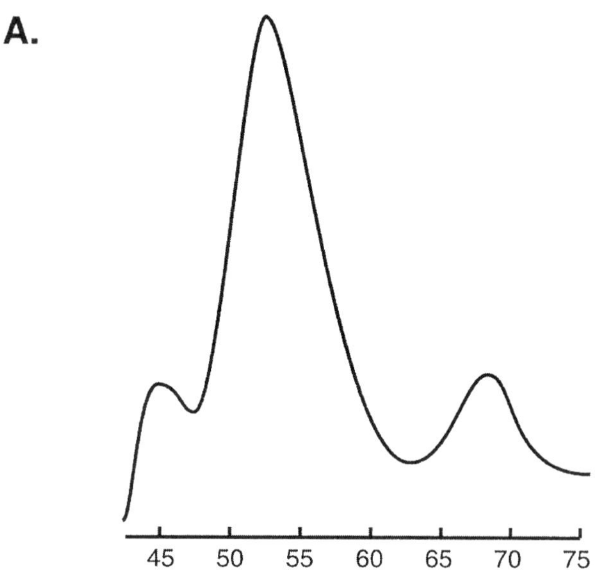

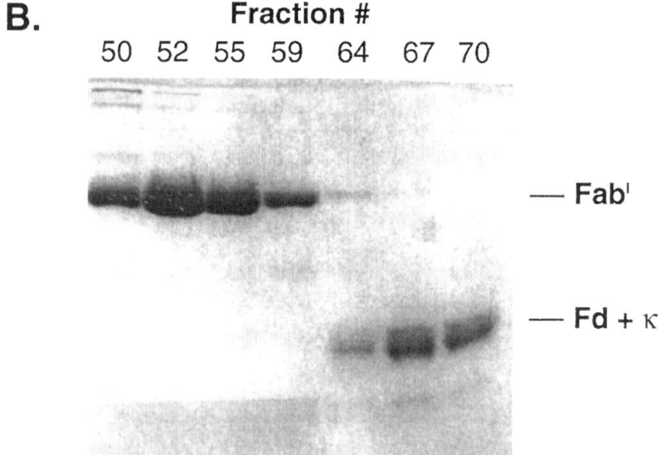

FIGURE 7
Removal of Fab′-related peptides by gel filtration on S-200 (Pharmacia). A CM cellulose (Whatman) eluate was loaded onto an S-200 column equilibrated in 8 M urea. Panel A shows the absorbance profile at 280 nm of material coming through the column. Panel B shows an SDS-PAGE analysis of various fractions that were collected from the column. The S-200 column was 2.5 × 70 cm and run at a flow rate of about 7.5 cm/h.

while bacterially expressed recombinant antibody domains typically bind due to their net positive charge. An anion exchange resin can likewise be incorporated into a purification protocol to bind endotoxin while the antibody product will flow through.[16,60] The usefulness of ion

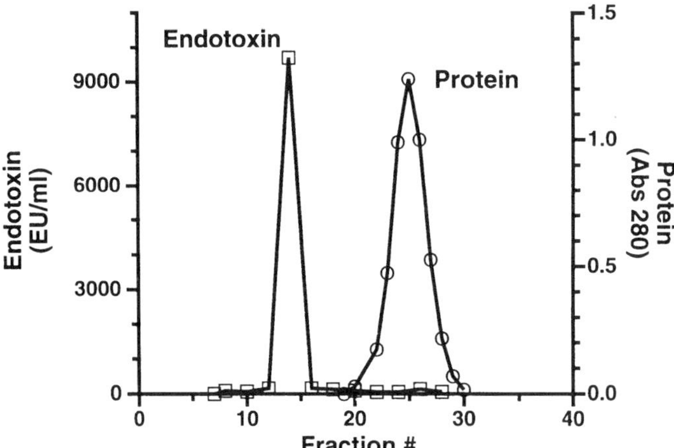

FIGURE 8
Separation of Fab and endotoxin by gel filtration on Sephacryl S-200 (Pharmacia). Samples containing Fab and endotoxin were loaded onto the column (2.2 × 42 cm) at 45 cm/h.

exchange chromatography to remove endotoxin is dependent upon the effective charge of the protein being purified. The greater the charge difference between the protein and endotoxin the more likely that separation will occur.

Gel filtration and ultrafiltration also can be very effective for endotoxin removal. These methods take advantage of the size difference between endotoxin in solution and the antibody domain. LPS from *E. coli* is generally of high molecular mass (>1000 kDa) and can be separated from Fab (molecular mass of ~45 kDa) using ultrafiltration membranes or gel filtration media. As an example, gel filtration was able to effectively separate LPS from Fab (Figure 8). Several factors can affect the resolving power of a gel filtration column, including column dimensions and buffer composition since the hydrodynamic radius of solutes can be affected by the aqueous environment. When designing processes, consideration should be given to achieving simultaneous removal of several classes of impurities, including protein, endotoxin, and DNA.

10.7 CONCLUSIONS

Antibody domains can efficiently be expressed in microorganisms and purified for use as either research reagents or pharmaceuticals. The selection of an appropriate expression system can be most useful to deliver the antibody domain into an appropriate bacterial compartment, either inside the cell, in the periplasmic space, or into the bacterial culture medium. When bacterial cultures are grown to a high cell density, the recombinant antibody proteins can often be recovered at a yield of 1 g/l or more. At this concentration, a purification strategy that separates the antibody domain from host bacterial proteins, DNA, and endotoxins is possible. Fortunately, antibody domains are stable in solution and can be purified with available technology. Many uses will undoubtedly be found for bacterially produced antibody domains.

REFERENCES

1. Cabilly, S., Riggs, A. D., Pande, H., Shively, J. E., Holmes, W. E., Rey, M., Perry, L. J., Wetzel, R., and Heyneker, H. L., Generation of antibody activity from immunoglobulin polypeptide chains produced in *E. coli*, *Proc. Natl. Acad. Sci. U.S.A.*, 81, 3273, 1984.
2. Buchner, J. and Rudolf, R., Renaturation, purification and characterization of recombinant Fab-fragments produced in *Escherichia coli*, *Bio/Technology*, 9, 157, 1991.
3. Whitlow, M., and Filpula, D., Single-chain Fv proteins and their fusion proteins. *Methods: A Companion to Methods in Enzymology*, 2, 97, 1991.
4. Bird, R. E., Hardman, K. D., Jacobson, J.W., Johnson, S., Kaufman, B. M., Lee, S.-M., Lee, T., Pope, S. H., Riordan, G. S., and Whitlow, M., Single chain antigen binding proteins, *Science*, 242, 423, 1988.
5. Huston, J. S., Levinson, D., Mudgett-Hunter, M., Tai, M.-S., Novotny, J., Margolies, M. N., Ridge, R. J., Bruccoleri, R. E., Haber, E., Crea, R., and Oppermann, H., Protein engineering of antibody binding sites: recovery of specific activity in an anti-digoxin single-chain Fv analogue produced in *Escherichia coli*, *Proc. Natl. Acad. Sci. U.SA.*, 85, 5879, 1988.
6. Spence, C., Nachman, M., Gately, M. K., Kreitman, R. J., Pastan, I., and Bailon, P., Affinity purification and characterization of anti-Tac (Fv)-C3-PE38KDEL: a highly potent cytotoxic agent specific to cells bearing IL-2 receptors, *Bioconj. Chem.*, 4, 63, 1993.
7. Batra, J. K., FitzGerald, D., Gately, M., Chaudhar, V. K., and Pastan, I., Anti-Tac (Fv)-PE40, a single chain antibody *Pseudomonas* fusion protein directed at interleukin-2 receptor bearing cells, *J. Biol. Chem.*, 265, 15198, 1990.
8. Better, M., Chang, C. P., Robinson, R. R., and Horwitz, A. H., *Escherichia coli* secretion of an active chimeric antibody fragment, *Science*, 240, 1041, 1988.
9. Skerra, A. and Plückthun, A., Assembly of a functional immunoglobulin Fv fragment in *Escherichia coli*, *Science*, 240, 1038, 1988.
10. Bourell, J. H., Clauser, K. P., Kelley, R., Carter, P., and Stults, J. T., Electrospray ionization mass spectrometry of recombinantly engineered antibody fragments, *Anal. Chem.*, 66, 2088, 1994.
11. Kelley, R. F., O'Connell, M. P., Carter, P., Presta, L., Eigenbrot, C., Covarrubias, M., Snedecor, B., Bourell, J. H., and Vetterlein, D., Antigen binding thermodynamics and anti-proliferative effects of chimeric and humanized anti-p185^{HER2} antibody Fab fragments, *Biochemistry*, 31, 5434, 1992.
12. Carter, P., Kelley, R. F., Rodrigues, M. L., Snedecor, B., Covarrubias, M., Velligan, M. D., Wong, W.-L. T., Rowland, A. M., Kotts, C. E., Carver, M. E., Yang, M., Bourell, J. H., Shepard, H. M., and Henner, D., High level *Escherichia coli* expression and production of a bivalent humanized antibody fragment, *Bio/Technology*, 10, 163, 1992.

13. Eigenbrot, C., Randeal, M., Presta, L., Carter, P., and Kossiakoff, A. A., X-ray structures of the antigen-binding domains from three variants of humanized anti p185HER2 antibody 4D5 and comparison with molecular modeling, *J. Mol. Biol.*, 229, 969, 1993.
14. Somerville, J. E., Goshorn, S. C., Fell, H. P., and Darveau, R. P., Bacterial aspects associated with the expression of a single-chain antibody fragment in *Escherichia coli*, *Appl. Microbiol. Biotechnol.*, 42, 595, 1994.
15. Gold, L. and Stormo, G. D., High-level translation initiation, in *Methods in Enzymology* 185, Goeddel, D. V., Ed., Academic Press, San Diego, 1990, chap. 7.
16. Gavit, P., Walker, M., Wheeler, T., Bui, P., Lei, S.-P., and Weickmann, J., Purification of a mouse-human chimeric Fab secreted from *E. coli.*, *Biopharm.*, 5, 28, 1992.
17. Better, M., Bernhard, S. L., Lei, S.-P., Fishwild, D. M., Lane, J., Carroll, S., and Horwitz, A. H., Potent anti-CD5 ricin A chain immunoconjugates from bacterially produced Fab′ and F(ab′)$_2$, *Proc. Natl. Acad. Sci. U.S.A.*, 90, 457, 1993.
18. Skerra, A. and Plückthun, A., Secretion and *in vivo* folding of the Fab fragment of the antibody MCPC603 in *Escherichia coli*: influence of disulfides and cis-proline, *Prot. Eng.*, 4, 971, 1991.
19. Knappik, A., Krebber, C., and Plückthun, A., The effect of folding catalysts on the *in vivo* folding process of different antibody fragments expressed in *Escherichia coli*, *Bio/Technology*, 11, 77, 1993.
20. Better, M. and Horwitz, A. H., Expression of engineered antibodies and antibody fragments in microorganisms, in *Methods in Enzymology — Immunochemical Techniques*, Vol. 178, 476–496, Langone, J. J., Ed., Academic Press, San Diego, 1989.
21. Anand, N. N., Mandal, S., MacKenzie, C. R., Sadowska, J., Sigurskjold, B., Young, N. M., Bundle, D. R., and Narang, S. A., Bacterial expression and secretion of various single-chain Fv genes encoding proteins specific for a *Salmonella* serotype B O-antigen, *J. Biol. Chem.*, 266, 21874, 1991.
22. Billiald, P., Motta, G., and Vauz, D. J., Production of a functional anti-scorpion hemocyanin scFv in *Escherichia coli*, *Arch. Biochem. Biophys.*, 317, 429, 1995.
23. Tsumoto, K., Nakaoki, Y., Ueda, Y., Ogasahara, K., Yutani, K., Watanabe, K., and Kumagai, I., Effect of the order of antibody variable regions on the expression of single-chain Hyhel 10 Fv fragment in *E. coli* and the thermodynamic analysis of its antigen-binding properties, *Biochem. Biophys. Res. Commun.*, 210, 546, 1994.
24. Better, M. and Horwitz, A. H., *In vivo* expression of antibody fragments, in *Protein Folding: In Vivo and In Vitro*, ACS Symposium Series 526, American Chemical Society, Washington, D.C., 1993.
25. Knappik, A., Bauer, K., and Plückthun, A., Improving the folding of antibodies by protein engineering, *J. Cell. Biochem., Suppl.*, 18D, 188, 1994.
26. Pack, P., Kujau, M., Schroeckh, V., Knüpfer, U., Wenderoth, R., Tiesenberg, D., and Plückthun, A., Improved bivalent miniantibodies with identical avidity as whole antibodies produced by high cell density fermentation of *Escherichia coli*, *Bio/Technology*, 11, 1271, 1993.
27. King, D. J., Byron, O. D., Mountain, A., Weir, N., Harvey, A., Lawson, A. D. G., Proudfoot, K. A., Baldock, D., Harding, S. E., Yarranton, G. T., and Owens, R. J., Expression, purification and characterization of B72.3 Fv fragments, *Biochem. J.*, 290, 723, 1993.
28. Bjork, L. and Kronvall, G., Purification and some properties of *Streptococcal* protein G, a novel IgG binding reagent, *J. Immunol.*, 133, 969, 1984.
29. Boyle, M. D. and Reis, K., Bacterial Fc receptors, *Bio/Technology*, 5, 697, 1987.
30. Reis, K. J., Hansen, H. F., and Bjorck, L., Extraction and characterization of IgG Fc receptors from group C and group G streptococci, *Mol. Immunol.*, 23, 425, 1986.
31. Erntell, M., Myhre, E. B., and Kronvall, G., Non-immune F(ab′)$_2$ binding to group C and G streptococci is mediated by structures on gamma chains, *Scand. J. Immunol.*, 21, 151, 1985.

32. Erntell, M., Myhre, E. B., Sjobring, U., and Bjorck, L., streptococcal protein G has affinity for both Fab and Fc-fragments of human IgG, *Mol. Immunol.*, 25, 121, 1988.
33. Fahnestock, S. R., Alexander, P., Nagle, J., and Filupa, D., Gene for an immunoglobulin-binding protein from a group G *Streptococcus*, *J. Bacteriol.*, 167, 870, 1986.
34. Fahnestock, S. R., Cloned streptococcal protein G genes, *Trends Biotechnol.*, 5, 79, 1987.
35. Goward, C. R., Murphy, J. P., Atkinson, T., and Barstow, D. A., Expression and purification of a truncated recombinant streptococcal protein G, *Biochem. J.*, 267, 171, 1990.
36. Erntell, M., Sjobring, U., Myhre, E. B., and Kronvall, G., Non-immune Fab- and Fc mediated interactions of avian Ig with *S. aureus* and group C and G streptococci, *Acta Pathol. Microbiol. Immunol. Scand.*, 96, 239, 1988.
37. Erntell, M., Myhre, E. B., and Kronvall, G., Non-immune $F(ab')_2$- and Fc-mediated interactions of mammalian immunoglobulins with *S. aureus* and group C and G streptococci, *Acta Pathol. Microbiol. Immunol. Scand.*, 94, 377, 1986.
38. Sasso, E. H., Silverman, G. J., and Mannik, M., Human IgA and IgG $F(ab')_2$ that bind to staphylococcal protein A belong to the V_HIII subgroup, *J. Immunol.*, 147, 1877, 1991.
39. Hammond, P. M., Atkinson, T., Sherwood, R. F., and Scawen, M. D., Manufacturing new-generation proteins, part 1: The technology, *Biopharm*, 4, 16, 1991.
40. Fatiadi, A., Affinity chromatography and metal chelate affinity chromatography, *CRC Crit. Rev. Anal. Chem.*, 18, 1, 1987.
41. Porath, J., High performance immobilized-metal-ion affinity chromatography of peptides and proteins, *J. Chromatog.*, 443, 3, 1988.
42. Skerra, A., Pfitzinger, I., and Plückthun, A., The functional expression of antibody Fv fragments in *Escherichia coli*: improved vectors and a generally applicable purification technique, Bio/*Technology*, 9, 273, 1991.
43. Skerra, A., A general vector, pASK84, for cloning, bacterial production, and single-step purification of antibody Fab fragments, *Gene*, 141, 79, 1994.
44. Sulkowski, E., Purification of proteins by IMAC, *Trends Biotechnol.*, 3, 1, 1985.
45. Stellwagen, E., Chromatography on immobilized reactive dyes, *Methods Enzymol.*, 182, 343, 1990.
46. Knight, E. and Fahey, D., Human fibroblast interferon, an improved purification, *J. Biol. Chem.*, 256, 3609, 1989.
47. Kawano, T., Kozutsumi, Y., Kawasaki, T., and Suzuki, A., Biosynthesis of *N*-glycolylneuraminic acid-containing glycoconjugates. Purification and characterization of the key enzyme of the cytidine monophospho-*N*-acetylneuraminic acid hydroxylation system, *J. Biol. Chem.*, 269, 9024, 1994.
48. Better, M., Bernhard, S. L., Fishwild, D. M., Nolan, P. A., Bauer, R. J., Kung, A. H. C., and Carroll, S. F., Gelonin analogs with engineered cysteine residues form antibody immunoconjugates with unique properties, *J. Biol. Chem.*, 269, 9644, 1994.
49. Skerra, A., Use of the tetracycline promoter for the tightly regulated production of a murine antibody fragment in *Escherichia coli*, *Gene*, 151, 131, 1994.
50. Neri, D., de Lalla, C., Petrul, H., Neri, P., and Winter, G., Calmodulin as a versatile tag for antibody fragments, *Bio/Technology*, 13, 373, 1995.
51. Brewer, S. J. and Sassenfeld, H. M., The purification of recombinant proteins using C-terminal polyarginine fusions, *Trends Biotechnol.*, 3, 119, 1985.
52. Sassenfeld, H. M. and Brewer, S. J., A polypeptide fusion designed for the purification of recombinant proteins, *Bio/Technology*, 2, 76, 1984.
53. Atkinson, A., The purification of microbial enzymes, *Process Biochem.*, 8, 9, 1973.
54. Better, M., Bernhard, S. L., Williams, R. E., Leigh, S., Bauer, R. J., Kung, A. H. C., Carroll, S. F., and Fishwild, D. M., T cell-targeted immunofusion proteins from *E. coli.*, *J. Biol. Chem.*, 270, 14951, 1995.

55. Wang, W. K., Lei, S.-P., Monbouquette, H. G., and McGregor, W. C., Membrane adsorber process development for the isolation of a recombinant immunofusion protein, *Biopharm*, 8, 52, 1995.
56. Brade, H., Brade, L., Schade, Zahringer, V. U., Holst, O., Kuh, H., Rozalski, A., Rohrscheidt, E., and Rietschel, E. T., Structure, endotoxicity, immunogenicity, and antigenicity of bacterial lipopolysaccharides, in *Bacterial Endotoxins: Pathophysiological Effects, Clinical Significance and Pharmocological Control*, Levin, J., Cate, J., Buller, H., Van Deventer, S., and Sturk, A., Eds., Alan R. Liss, Inc., New York, 17, 1988.
57. Duff, G. W., Waisman, D. M., and Atrins, E., Removal of endotoxin by a polymyxin B affinity column, *Clin. Res.*, 30, 565A, 1982.
58. Issekutz, A. C., Removal of gram-negative endotoxin from solutions by affinity chromatography, *J. Immunol. Methods*, 61, 275, 1983.
59. Minobe, S., Tadashi, S., Tosa, T., and Chibata, I., Characteristics of immobilized histamine for pyrogen adsorption, *J. Chromatogr.*, 262, 193, 1983.
60. Shibatani, T., Kakimoto, T., and Chibata, I., Purification of high molecular weight urokinase from human urine and comparative study of two active forms of urokinase, *Thromb. Haemostasis*, 49, 91, 1983.
61. Gibbs, R. A., Posner, B. A., Filpula, D. R., Dodd, S. W., Finkelman, M. A. J., Lee, T. K., Wroble, M., Whitlow, M., and Benkovic, S. J., Construction and characterization of a single-chain catalytic antibody, *Proc. Natl. Acad. Sci. U.S.A.*, 88, 4001, 1991.
62. Condra, J. H., Sardana, V. V., Tomassini, J. E., Schlabach, A. J., Davies, M.-E., Lineberger, D. W., Graham, D. J., Gotlib, L., and Colonno, R. J., Bacterial expression of antibody fragments that block human rhinovirus infection of cultured cells, *J. Biol. Chem.*, 265, 2292, 1990.
63. Lake, D. F., Lam, K. S., Peng, L., and Hersh, E. M., Molecular cloning, expression and mutagenesis of an anti-insulin single chain Fv (scFv), *Mol. Immunol.*, 31, 845, 1994.
64. Shibui, T., Munakata, K., Matsumoto, R., Ohta, K., Matsushima, R., Morimoto, Y., and Nagahari, K., High-level production and secretion of a mouse-human chimeric Fab fragment with specificity to human carcinoembryonic antigen in *Escherichia coli*, *Appl. Microbiol. Biotechnol.*, 38, 770, 1993.
65. McGregor, D. P., Molloy, P. E., Cunningham, C., and Harris, W. J., Spontaneous assembly of bivalent single chain antibody fragments in *Escherichia coli*, *Mol. Immunol.*, 31, 219, 1994.
66. Cheung, S. C., Dietzschold, B., Koprowski, H., Notkins, A. L., and Rando, R. F., A recombinant human Fab expressed in *Escherichia coli* neutralizes rabies virus, *J. Virol.*, 66, 6714, 1992.
67. Ward, V. K., Schneider, P. G., Kreissig, S. B., Hammock, B. D., and Choudhary, P. V., Cloning, sequencing and expression of the Fab fragment of a monoclonal antibody to the herbicide atrazine, *Prot. Eng.*, 6, 981, 1993.
68. Alfthan, K., Takkinen, K., Sizmann, D., Seppälä, I., Immonen, T., Vanne, L., Keränen, S., Kaartinen, M., Knowles, J. K. C., and Teeri, T. T., Efficient secretion of murine Fab fragments by *Escherichia coli* is determined by the first constant domain of the heavy chain, *Gene*, 128, 203, 1993.
69. Takkinen, K., Laukkanen, M.-L., Sizmann, D., Alfthan, K., Immonen, T., Vanne, L., Kaartinen, M., Knowles, J. K. C., and Teeri, T., An active single-chain antibody containing a cellulase linker domain is secreted by *Escherichia coli*, *Prot. Eng.*, 4, 837, 1991.
70. Anand, N. N., Dubuc, G., Phipps, J., MacKenzie, C. R., Sadowska, J., Young, N. M., Bundle, D. R., and Narang, S. A., Synthesis and expression in *Escherichia coli* of cistronic DNA encoding an antibody fragment specific for a *Salmonella* serotype B-antigen, *Gene*, 100, 39, 1991.

Chapter 11

Emerging Production Systems for Antibody Therapeutics

Andy J. R. Porter, Kate J. Bentley, Pauline M. Cupit, and T. Paul Wallace

CONTENTS

0-8493-8547-4/97/$0.00+$.50

11.1 INTRODUCTION

The number of antibodies undergoing development as therapeutics has increased dramatically over recent years. This has required the large-scale, commercial manufacture of clinical grade material. The antibody production process chosen must meet several criteria depending on the ultimate use of the antibody. In particular, for clinical applications, the process must be safe, efficient, and cost effective; these criteria are relaxed if the antibody is for small-scale research use.

Relatively new, mammalian cell culture expression systems have been developed that can provide high expressing cell lines, but other single cell processes are now being developed that use other cell types. These may be of particular use for the rapid and inexpensive expression of antibody fragments, and may provide alternative expression systems for some applications where other considerations (such as glycosylation pattern) are not important. Other exciting and developing technologies include the expression of antibodies in plants and transgenic animals. Each of these systems (discussed below) has its merits, and it is probable that each system will find a niche in the growing field of commercial antibody production.

11.2 TRANSGENIC PLANTS

Higher plants provide the major supply of food and foodstuffs for man's life on earth and in addition a source of fuels, fibers, oils, detergents, and dyes. Until recently most medical compounds had their origins in plant tissues, for example, the heart stimulant digitalis from foxglove, and opium from the poppy plant. Today, most new drugs are synthesized by chemists and biochemists in pharmaceutical companies. However, as the production of transgenic plants is now routine in many laboratories, engineered plants are regarded by many as having enormous commercial potential for the large-scale production of recombinant therapeutic biomolecules.[1,2] Exploiting plants as solar powered bioreactors is often referred to as "molecular-" or "biofarming."

11.2.1 Biofarming

The more traditional fermentation-based systems for the production of recombinant proteins require substantial capital investment and, for animal cell cultures, expensive growth media. In contrast, the upstream production costs for plants are probably lower than for any other system. Modern plant agriculture has already established many of the techniques required for the manufacture of huge quantities of biomass, and scale up simply requires the planting of additional acreage. Using 1990 figures for soybean, production costs prior to extraction of a recombinant protein accumulating at 10 g/kg of total protein would be as little as $0.1/g.[3] In addition, being eukaryotes, the post-translational processing of large multimeric proteins presents few problems to plant expression systems. In microbial systems, such proteins are often toxic or are expressed as insoluble aggregates that require expensive and lengthy resolubilization and refolding to recover function.

The cloning of a transgenic plant still remains a relatively slow process and therefore plants will never replace the conventional microbial systems for the initial characterization and engineering of recombinant proteins. However, plant transformation techniques usually result in the stable integration of foreign DNA into the plant genome and therefore, by simple cross-breeding techniques, new genes and multiple transgenes can be introduced into plants. Furthermore, this genetic information can be easily stored at low cost for many years as plant seeds.

Concern about the economics of purifying biomolecules from plant tissues is the single most important issue limiting the exploitation of plants as a novel expression system. Downstream processing methodologies must be developed if a plant-derived biomolecule of sufficiently high purity for therapeutic use is ever to be produced. Techniques are required which allow the purification and concentration of a recombinant protein present at low levels compared to the total plant biomass. A novel procedure for the partitioning of recombinant proteins from the bulk of seed proteins has already been described[4] and much research effort is continuing in this area.

11.2.2 Antibody Production by Plants

Foreign DNA can be stably introduced into plant cells using *Agrobacterium tumifaciens*-mediated gene transfer, particle bombardment (Biolistics), electroporation, and even microinjection. These genes can be driven by a range of constitutive, inducible, and tissue specific promoters, can contain affinity tags for detection and purification, and can be designed to include signal sequences to enable proteins to enter the secretory pathway or be targeted to different plant cell compartments.[5,6] As the cloning of transgenic plants has become increasingly routine, a growing number of groups have reported the expression of full length antibodies and antibody fragments (Table 1).

TABLE 1

Expression of Antibodies in Plants

Antibody Molecule	Antigen	Plant Species
Single domain (dAb)	Substance P (neuropeptide)	Tobacco[7]
scFv	Phytochrome A	Tobacco[8,9]
scFv	Artichoke mottle crinkle virus coat protein	Tobacco[10]
scFv	2-phenyl-oxazol-5-one	Tobacco[11]
Single chain antibody (scAb)[12]	Herbicides paraquat and atrazine	Tobacco[13]
Fab and IgG	Human creatine kinase	Tobacco and *Arabidopsis*[14]
IgG	Transition state analog	Tobacco[15,16]
IgG	Fungal cutinase	Tobacco[17]
Secretory IgG/A	*Streptococcus mutans* adhesin	Tobacco[18]
IgM	NP (4-hydroxy-3-nitro-phenyl) acetyl hapten	Tobacco and *Acetabularia mediterranea*[19,20]

11.2.2.1 Whole Antibodies

The first intact immunoglobulin expressed in plants was the mouse IgG1 monoclonal antibody (MAb) 6D4, which recognizes a synthetic transition state analog phosphonate ester.[15] Production of this MAb in transgenic tobacco plants proceeded in two stages: (1) the *Agrobacterium*-mediated transformation of cDNAs encoding either the antibody heavy or light chains; transgene expression was driven by a constitutive promoter and separate, heavy and light chain specific, stable lines selected and (2) sexual crossing of individual plants expressing either the heavy or light chains to produce F1 progeny expressing both chains.

Intact antibody was extractable from F1 plants and was shown to have a similar binding specificity as the parent 6D4 MAb. Plants accumulated significant amounts of functional protein (1% total plant protein) only if the mouse signal sequence coding region was retained in the original vector.[15,21] This suggests that plants recognize the mouse signal sequences and that targeting of the separate chains to the plant endoplasmic reticulum (ER), which contains protein disulfide isomerases and protein chaperonins, may be necessary for correct assembly and stability. Following assembly, the antibodies are then secreted and localized in the apoplast, a large stable aqueous environment external to the cell.

Since those original experiments, double transformation techniques and single expression vectors have been used to produce transgenic plants expressing different functional IgG1 and IgM antibodies as well as IgG/IgA hybrids (Table 1). As observed with microbial systems, expression yields in plants vary considerably, from 0.05 to 1.5% total soluble protein.[14,15] In *E. coli* the primary sequence of the antibody often determines yield and stability.[22] However, in plants, as in stable mammalian cell expression systems, the observed variation in expression yield is more likely the result of position effects resulting from the random integration of the foreign DNA into the plant genome.

Recently, the assembly of a functional multimeric secretory IgA (SIgA) recognizing *Streptococcus mutans* has been described in plants.[18] SIgA is the predominant form of immunoglobulin found in secretions from mucosal surfaces and is a dimeric molecule made up of two IgA molecules linked by a small polypeptide J chain. A fourth polypeptide, secretory component (SC), is also associated with the antibody complex and confers a degree of resistance to proteolysis at mucosal surfaces such as the gastrointestinal tract.

Attempts to produce a monoclonal SIgA in mammalian cells have met with limited success because of the complex nature of the protein. To express SIgA in plants a four-step cloning procedure was used.[18] The first two steps were as described above for MAb 6D4 and resulted in the selection of plant lines expressing monomeric IgA. These plants were crossed with a plant expressing the J chain protein and resulted in the selection of plants expressing dimeric IgA. Finally, these were crossed with a plant expressing the SC polypeptide and progeny producing a fully functional dimeric SIgA were identified. This example illustrates the remarkable ability of plant cells to synthesize, assemble, and secrete complex, multimeric recombinant proteins.

11.2.2.2 Antibody Fragments

Most of the various antibody fragment structures which have been expressed in *E. coli* have also now been expressed in plants. These include Fab, scFv, scAb, and single domain antibodies (Table 1). In general, the assembly requirements of antibody fragments are less stringent than for whole antibodies and processing through the ER is not always essential. The inclusion of plant signal sequences allows antibody fragments to be targeted to intracellular compartments or to the extracellular space. A number of scFv and scAb constructs[13] have been used to produce functional antigen-binding protein in both the plant cytoplasm[8,10] and apoplast.[9,13] When an scFv recognizing phytochrome A was targeted to the cytoplasm the extractable expression yield was only 0.06% total plant protein.[8] However, when the same scFv was expressed via the plant secretory pathway, using a PR1 tobacco signal sequence, expression yields increased tenfold.[9] The protein:mRNA ratio was significantly higher for plants expressing the secretory construct suggesting increased stability of the secreted scFv protein and/or an increased rate of translation of the scFv mRNA.

Different antibody fragments have been expressed in plants for a number of possible applications including:

1. Immunomodulation — an scFv recognizing a conserved epitope on the plant regulatory receptor, phytochrome A has been expressed in tobacco resulting in plants which produced seed with poor phytochrome-dependent light-mediated promotion of germination.[8,9]
2. Crop protection — an scFv recognizing the coat protein of an artichoke mottled crinkle virus has been expressed in the cytoplasm of transgenic tobacco resulting in plants less susceptible to infection by the target virus.[10]
3. Bioremediation — functional scAbs which separately recognize the herbicides paraquat and atrazine have been expressed in tobacco.[13] The ability of these plants to sequester low levels of these herbicides from aqueous environments is currently being evaluated.

11.2.3 Immunotherapy Using Plant-Derived Antibodies

11.2.3.1 Whole Antibodies

Despite the enormous therapeutic and commercial potential of recombinant antibodies only three have been approved for therapeutic use by the U.S. Food and Drug Administration (FDA), although over seventy are currently in clinical trials. Passive immunization studies require relatively large quantities of MAbs for *in vivo* clinical evaluation. Producing this antibody in mammalian cell lines is very expensive and therefore plants may provide an alternative bulk supply of antibody at low cost. A key issue in the development of plant-based antibody products is that the presence of complex plant-specific glycans, rather than mammalian-derived glycans, on the Fc portion of the heavy chain may increase their immunogenicity, affect biodistribution, and alter certain of the biological properties of the antibody.

Plant glycans have been shown to be immunogenic. Immunization of animals with plant glycoproteins can often result in non-specific polyclonal sera containing a mixture of both anti-polypeptide and anti-glycan antibodies.[23] However, a detailed study of the immunogenicity of plant antibodies has not yet been carried out. MAb 6D4 made in plants bound to the lectin concanavalin A in a similar manner to the parental murine MAb, confirming the presence of core high mannose glycans on the plant heavy chain. The plant antibody, however, would not react with *Ricinis communis* agglutinin or wheat germ agglutinin suggesting that the terminal plant glycan residues differ from those of the murine MAb.[16] Strategies to remove the plant glycans by simple chemical cleavage or by engineering out the N linked glycosylation site or even using mutant plants lacking key enzymes involved in the glycosylation pathway,[24] may reduce the immunogenicity of antibodies synthesized by plants but will also alter the biological activity of the recombinant product (see Chapter 1).

The generation of a multimeric secretory IgA form of MAb Guy's 13 was noted earlier. This MAb recognizes the cell-surface adhesin of the bacteria *S. mutans* which is the causative agent of dental caries. Topical application of MAb Guy's 13 in a primate model reduced both the severity and establishment of the disease.[25] IgA is the predominant form of immunoglobulin found in the oral cavity and at other mucosal surfaces, therefore the IgA form is proposed as a topical treatment for dental caries. Quantities of this antibody are currently being purified from plants for clinical trials to establish whether regular oral application will result in control of dental caries without inducing mucosal or systemic immune responses. Targeting expression of the SIgA to edible organs of plants, allowing antibody delivery to the oral cavity in foodstuffs, is an exciting future possibility.

11.2.3.2 Antibody Fragments

Antibody fragment expressed in plants should display similar properties to the same products derived from other systems. In most cases antibody fragments lack glycosylation sites so this potential problem is avoided for systemic administration. Plant-derived antibody fragments may in the future provide a cheap supply of antigen-binding proteins for the targeted delivery of chemotherapeutic drugs, toxins, and diagnostic agents. Agracetus Inc. (Middleton, WI) is currently expressing an antibody BR96 in transgenic soybean. In preclinical trials the MAb expressed in mammalian cell lines has shown some promise as a vehicle for the delivery of the chemotherapeutic drug doxorubicin to breast, colon, ovarian, and lung tumors.[26]

A number of toxins (ricin, abrin, saporin), which have already been used as partners with antibody fragments, are themselves derived from plants. Production of immunoconjugates directly in plants may result in increased efficiency of conjugate synthesis at reduced costs.

The ability of antibody fragments to penetrate tissues and the absence of the Fc portion of the molecule, avoiding events associated with activation of effector functions, make them ideal candidate molecules for topical applications. The cost-effective production of plant-derived, immunogenically "safe" antibody fragment formulations, for inclusion in prophylactic topical preparations, may be a promising new application.

11.2.4 Potential of Plant Antibodies as Pharmaceuticals

Plants clearly have the potential to become a cost-effective system for the bulk production of antibodies and antibody fragments. If this potential is to be realized then downstream processing methodologies must be developed for the production of quantities of high purity product. The recent successful targeting of a functional scFv to plant seeds, and their long term storage in seeds, is a positive development toward this aim.[11] Plant production will eliminate fears about contamination of products with animal viruses, a major concern of antibody produced in mammalian cell lines. The need to consider the consequences of difference in glycosylation means careful choice of antibody form is essential.

Expression of antibodies in plants would permit access to immunotherapeutic technology by the developing world, where the costs of establishing fermentation systems for the production of recombinant proteins are often prohibitive. The exciting possibility of administering antibody by oral or topical application of plant tissues, eliminating costly downstream purification expenditure, may also benefit developing countries.

If immunotherapeutic targets and applications are chosen carefully, then plant expression systems may have a promising future.

11.3 METHYLOTROPHIC YEASTS AND FILAMENTOUS FUNGI

The yeast *Saccharomyces cerevisiae* has been widely used for the production of recombinant proteins. As an expression host it is subject to some limitations, in particular, a tendency to hyperglycosylate glycoproteins resulting in a product with significantly altered properties. Alternative expression hosts capable of authentic post-translational modification have recently been developed and include the methylotrophic yeasts (*Pichia pastoris, Hansenula polymorpha*) and filamentous fungi (*Trichoderma reesei, Aspergillus niger*). Two of these microorganisms, *P. pastoris* and *T. reesei,* are considered here.

11.3.1 *P. pastoris* Expression Systems

Like all methylotrophs, *P. pastoris* is able to grow on methanol as its sole source of carbon as it possesses a highly regulated methanol utilization pathway. The initial reaction of this pathway is catalyzed by the enzyme alcohol oxidase which is absent on cells grown on glucose, glycerol, and ethanol but can form up to 30% of the total cell protein in methanol-induced cells.[27] *P. pastoris* has two genes which code for alcohol oxidase, namely *AOX1* and *AOX2*.[28,29] However, most of the alcohol oxidase activity in the cell is encoded by *AOX1*. Hence, this promoter has been incorporated into most *P. pastoris* vectors. The *AOX1* gene is regulated by a catabolite repression/derepression and induction mechanism.[30] When methanol is the sole carbon source, the *AOX1* gene is efficiently transcribed, under other growth conditions it is repressed.

Many of the *P. pastoris* expression vectors are so-called shuttle vectors containing components which allow propagation and selection both in *P. pastoris* and *E. coli,* thus allowing routine vector manipulations in *E. coli.* The most widely used selection marker is the histidinol dehydrogenase gene (*HIS4*) for complementation of the auxotrophic host.[31] In addition to *HIS4,* some vectors contain the *Tn903* G418 resistance gene which affords the advantage of identifying high copy transformants.[32] Heterologous expression in *P. pastoris* may be internal or secreted. For naturally secreted proteins such as antibodies, the reducing environment of the cytoplasm is not conducive to disulfide bond formation. Secretion can be achieved with a signal peptide and *Pichia* expression vectors often use either a native acid phosphatase (*PHO1*) signal sequence or more commonly the *S. cerevisiae* α-factor pre-pro leader peptide.

For the generation of stable production strains, the expression plasmids are normally integrated into the host genome. Integration may occur by either gene replacement or insertion as a result of homologous recombination between shared sequences of the vector and host.[31,33] Although this generally results in recombinants with a single copy of the gene, spontaneous gene insertion events can also occur.[34] However, to obtain increased levels of the expressed protein multiple tandem integrations are necessary.[34]

11.3.2 *T. reesei* Expression Systems

The filamentous fungi *T. reesei* produces a complex of cellulase degrading enzymes. The major cellulase, cellobiohydrolase I (CHBI) constitutes approximately 50% of the total protein secreted.[35] Thus, the promoter from CHBI is used for the expression of proteins in *T. reesei*. This promoter is induced with cellulase or small oligosaccharides such as cellobiose or sophorose. Like yeasts, targeted integration of the expression cassette into the genome ensures stability of the production strains. The signal sequence from CHBI is used to direct the secretion of the protein into the culture media. Transformants can be selected on the basis of resistance to phleomycin or their ability to utilize acetamide as the sole nitrogen source.

11.3.3 Recombinant Protein Production by *P. pastoris and T. reesei*

Contrary to *S. cerevisiae*, hyperglycosylation is generally not a problem for *P. pastoris*. In a comparative study, invertase secreted from *P. pastoris* displayed a lower number of mannose units at the site of N linked glycosylation, typically 8-14, compared to greater than 40 in the *S. cerevisiae* secreted invertase.[36] Furthermore, *P. pastoris* did not contain any terminal α1,3-mannose linkages which are responsible for the immunogenicity of *S. cerevisiae* glycoproteins; however, in a different study, a significant proportion of the HIV gp120 secreted in *P. pastoris* was found to be hyperglycosylated.[37]

11.3.3.1 Expression Yield

The use of efficient inducible promoters, combined with high cell densities in simple defined media, make both *P. pastoris* and *T. reesei* powerful and cost-effective expression systems. *P. pastoris* has been used successfully for high level expression of various secreted proteins with potential therapeutic applications including a recombinant pertactin

(P69) from *Bordetella pertussis*,[38] produced at 3 g/l, a tetanus toxin fragment C,[33] produced at a level of 12 g/l, and human tumor necrosis factor[39] produced at 10 g/l.

11.3.3.2 Antibody Fragments

To date, no complete antibodies have been expressed in either *P. pastoris* or *T. reesei*. However, a soluble functional scFv fragment, specific for a recombinant human leukemic inhibitory factor, has successfully been expressed in *P. pastoris* using the *S. cerevisiae* α-factor prepro signal sequence.[40] Yields of 100 mg/l were recovered from the culture media directly. A single chain antibody (scAb)[12] fragment directed against the isoenzyme human type V acid phosphatase has been expressed in *P. pastoris*. The yield of the fragment was increased by up to 100-fold over *E. coli* cultures, however, these fragments did not bind the target antigen as well as the scAb expressed from *E. coli* (P. M. C. C, unpublished data).

An active Fab fragment derived from a murine anti-2-phenyloxazolone has been produced in *T. reesei*[41] at a level of 1 mg/l. When the Fab fragment was fused to the cellulase CBHI the yield was increased to 40 mg/l. Fermentation of the CHBI-Fab improved the level still further to 150 mg/l, however, there was no improvement in the yield of extractable Fab fragment.

11.3.4 Potential of Yeast and Fungal Proteins as Pharmaceuticals

While *E. coli* and *S. cerevisiae* have proved useful hosts for the expression of recombinant proteins, extensive clinical use has been limited by poor biological activity, the co-purification of bacterial toxins, or immunogenicity of the final product. In contrast, *P. pastoris* and *T. reesei* are non-pathogenic, and recombinant proteins are expressed free of toxins, allergens, and pyrogens and with reduced hyperglycosylation, limiting immunogenicity.[36,42] Both have been granted GRAS (generally regarded as safe) status by the FDA and may be considered as novel commercial candidates for the large-scale production of safe, therapeutic antibodies and antibody fragments and like plants may be ideal for the cost-effective production of bulk antibody for topical applications.

11.4 BACULOVIRUS/INSECT CELLS

A wide variety of eukaryotic and prokaryotic proteins have been expressed in a correctly processed and biologically active form using the baculovirus/insect cell expression system[43-46] and it presents a potentially attractive alternative to the use of mammalian cells or bacteria for the production of recombinant antibodies. Insect cells are capable of carrying out the post-translational modifications necessary for the secretion of correctly assembled and processed antibody, i.e., signal peptide cleavage, disulfide bond formation, and N- and O-linked glycosylation. In addition, recombinant protein expression levels using this system can be very high, with some heterologous proteins comprising up to 50% of total cell protein, although expression levels for different proteins vary considerably, from 1 to >500 mg/l.

11.4.1 Baculovirus Infection

The baculovirus/insect cell expression system generally consists of an expression vector based on the *Autographa californica* nuclear polyhedrosis virus (AcNPV), which is used to infect *Spodoptera frugiperda* (fall armyworm) cells, although other NPV viruses and cell types or insect larvae may be used, for example, *Bombyx mori* nuclear polyhedrosis virus (BmNPV) and *B. mori* (silkworm) cells or larvae. Baculoviruses possess a double-stranded, circular genome of 128 kilobases (kb) surrounded by an enveloped, rod-shaped capsid. During wild-type NPV infection at least three phases of viral gene expression can be distinguished, early (0–6 h post-infection; p.i.), late (6–20 h p.i.), and very late (20–72 h p.i.), and two distinct forms of virus are produced. First, at about 12–18 h p.i., enveloped viruses (EV) bud out from the infected cell and proceed to infect neighboring cells in an insect host, these EV also being important in spreading infection in cultured insect cells. At the very late stage of infection, i.e., at 20–72 h p.i., occluded virus (OV) embedded in polyhedra, referred to as occlusion bodies (OBs), form in the cell nucleus. Such OBs consist essentially of the polyhedrin protein, an abundantly expressed, virally encoded protein. A second viral protein, p10, is also expressed at a high level in the very late stage of infection and causes insect cells to lyse, releasing the OBs. These OV, while being important for the horizontal transfer of virus to new insect hosts, are not important for the propagation of virus in insect cell culture. Hence, the polyhedrin and p10 proteins, which comprise up to 50% of the total protein synthesized in infected insect cells, are not essential for virus replication *in vitro*.

11.4.1.1 Baculovirus Expression Systems

Recombinant baculovirus expression vectors are constructed by the replacement of one of the above, non-essential genes, usually polyhedrin, with the coding region of the desired protein so that high levels of expression are driven by the strong, late polyhedrin promoter following infection. The AcNPV genome is too large for the efficient introduction of the foreign gene by conventional DNA cloning techniques. Instead a two-step procedure is followed in which the gene to be expressed is first inserted into a vector containing a viral expression cassette flanked by viral DNA sequences. This transfer vector is co-transfected with viral genomic DNA into insect cells, in which homologous recombination leads to the targeted integration of the foreign gene into the polyhedrin locus. Originally, recombinants were identified by their inability to form OBs in the insect cell nucleus (since the polyhedrin protein is no longer expressed), with plaques appearing clear rather than opaque. However, screening was made difficult as the recombination event is relatively inefficient, recombinants making up only 0.1–1% of progeny virus. An improved system has since been described[47-49] which reduces the background of non-recombinant, parental-type viruses to approaching 0%.

11.4.2 Antibody Production by Baculovirus/Insect Cells

Expression of antibody in the baculovirus/insect cell system has been achieved both by co-infection with separate heavy chain- and light chain-encoding viruses[50-52] and by infection with a double recombinant virus encoding both chains.[51-54] In addition, co-infection with three recombinant virus-types encoding heavy chain, light chain, and J chain resulted in the secretion of dimeric IgA.[50] Several strategies have been followed in the construction of a double recombinant virus. Heavy and light chain co-expression from a single, dicistronic message under the control of one copy of the polyhedrin promoter was found to be unsuccessful.[51] A complete dicistronic mRNA was produced but the second gene in the message was not translated at a detectable level, despite attempts to optimize the context between the stop codon of the first gene and the initiation codon of the second. In contrast, infection with a recombinant virus containing the heavy and light chain coding regions under the transcriptional control of separate copies of the polyhedrin promoter, with the transcription units arranged in an opposite orientation, resulted in the expression of both chains and the secretion of intact antibody.[51] A different study[52] concluded that expression cassettes arranged in tandem were unstable, being deleted by a homologous recombination event. Use of a double recombinant virus ensures that every infected cell receives heavy and light chain transcription units in a 1:1 ratio. There is, however, some evidence to suggest that a 1:1 co-infection ratio is not necessarily optimal for antibody yield. In one study,[55] co-infection with the light chain-encoding virus in a fourfold excess over the heavy chain-encoding virus resulted in a twofold higher yield of secreted CAMPATH-1H antibody, demonstrating a potential advantage to the use of separate heavy and light chain-encoding viruses. In addition, co-expression using separate viruses can be convenient, for example, to investigate different antibody forms (IgG, Fab, etc.) using a common light chain.

The successful production of antibody in the baculovirus/insect cell expression system has been reported by several groups, using vectors based on AcNPV to infect *Spodoptera frugiperda* cells[50-53] and BmNPV-derived vectors to infect *B. mori* cells and larvae.[54] Whole antibody molecules (IgG[51-54] and monomeric and dimeric IgA[50]) and an scFv molecule[56] have been expressed at a low to moderate level (from 1 to ~30 mg/l in cell culture, 800 mg/l in the hemolymph of infected larvae), and in each case the heavy and light chains were correctly processed, with cleavage of the signal peptide sequence and glycosylation of the heavy chain (N linked in the case of IgG, N, and O linked in the case of IgA).

11.4.3 Potential of Baculovirus Antibodies as Pharmaceuticals

11.4.3.1 Biological Activity

Insect cell-derived antibody has been found to bind antigen with the same specificity as native hybridoma- or ascites-derived MAbs,[51,52] or recombinant MAb expressed in a transfected mammalian cell culture.[15] The ability of the recombinant antibody to drive effector functions may be important, for example, if it is to be used therapeutically, and the limited studies reported present encouraging results. A murine IgG2a MAb, CO17-1A, expressed in the baculovirus/insect cell system showed comparable antibody-dependent cellular cytotoxicity (ADCC) activity to that of the native, ascites-derived material.[52] Similarly, other preliminary studies[55] suggest that the humanized IgG1 antibody, CAMPATH-1H, derived from insect cells shows comparable ADCC activity to material expressed in a transfected Chinese hamster ovary (CHO) cell line. The ability of insect-derived material to drive complement-dependent cellular cytotoxicity (CDCC) is less clear. An insect cell-derived murine IgG2a MAb was capable of binding C1q but at a lower level than ascites-derived material.[54] The ascites-derived material had, however, been protein A-purified unlike that from the insect system and hence the reduced C1q binding of the latter may simply have been due to competition from contaminating protein. Other preliminary studies,[55] however, also suggest that insect cell-derived MAb is less efficient than mammalian cell-derived material at mediating the CDCC effector function activity. The efficiency with which insect cell-derived antibody recruits human host cell effector molecules, and hence their suitability for particular therapeutic uses, requires further, more rigorous investigation.

11.4.3.2 Glycosylation

Glycosylation has been demonstrated in the baculovirus/insect cell system by observing differences in heavy chain mobility when infected insect cells are cultured in the presence of tunicamycin[51] and heavy chain sensitivity to endoglycosidase F/glycopeptidase F.[53] However, the nature of the carbohydrate addition has not been analyzed. It was originally assumed that recombinant glycoproteins expressed in insect cells would have a simple, high-mannose carbohydrate addition. Indeed, endogenous insect cell-specific proteins show a low level of processing of the carbohydrate addition to a complex form,[57] instead having an oligomannosidic structure with only two or three mannose units, and often being fucosylated. More recently, however, it has been shown that some heterologous proteins expressed in baculovirus-infected insect cells have a complex-type oligosaccharide addition[58,59] showing that at least some insect cell types do contain the enzymatic machinery needed for carbohydrate residue addition and trimming. Not all recombinant glycoproteins expressed in insect cells have a complex glycosylation pattern, and so it seems that such processing is directed by the protein itself, rather than being a general feature of baculovirus infection. In addition, it appears that the nature of the carbohydrate side chain of at least some glycoproteins is dependent on the time post-infection. Human plasminogen harvested within 20 h p.i. contained high-mannose side chains while material harvested from 60–96 h p.i. contained predominantly complex bi-, tri-, and tetra-antennary structures.[60] In another study,[61] however, HIV-1 envelope proteins harvested 24 h p.i. were glycosylated while proteins harvested between 24–72 h p.i. were predominantly nonglycosylated. Even if the immunoglobulin heavy chain synthesized in insect cells does have a complex-type glycosylation pattern, it is highly likely that the actual carbohydrate residues present will be different to those added in any other cell type, since glycosylation is species-, tissue-, and cell-type specific.[62,63]

It is known that the glycosylation pattern can affect the antibody's ADCC and CDCC activity[64,65] and hence any differences in the activity of insect cell-derived MAb and mammalian cell-derived MAb may be due to glycosylation. In addition, the insect-type glycosylation pattern on recombinant antibody synthesized in the baculovirus/insect cell system may affect its immunogenicity and *in vivo* half-life if administered for therapeutic purposes.

11.4.3.3 Expression Yield

Antibody expression levels in the baculovirus/insect cell system, like the majority of other secretory proteins, are generally poor (IgG up to 30 mg/l)[53] compared to intracellular proteins (e.g., β-galactosidase at 200 mg/l).[66] The expression of some secretory proteins is improved by the use of insect-[67] or baculovirus-specific[61] signal peptides, however, a similar increase may not necessarily be achieved for antibody production since the improvement appears to be protein dependent.[68] One study[69] attempted to increase the yield of secreted antibody by co-expression of murine heavy chain binding protein (BiP), important in immunoglobulin assembly in mammalian cells, in the infected insect cells. Intracellular levels of functional antibody and soluble immunoglobulin were higher, but secreted levels were not, indicating that some step after chain assembly, for example, disulfide bond formation, glycosylation, or oligosaccharide trimming, was limiting. Late in infection, when the polyhedrin promoter which drives heterologous protein expression is highly active, the host cell's post-translational processing and secretory apparatus may be compromised due to a virtual shutdown in the synthesis of host cell-specific proteins from 18–24 h p. i.[70] Higher levels of active material have been reported for some recombinant proteins, e.g., protein kinase -Cδ and the β subunit of human gonadotrophin, using a transcriptionally weaker but earlier acting viral promoter, e.g., the basic protein promoter which shows peak activity in the late phase of infection, at ~12 h p. i.[71,72] Use of the early phase promoter, immediate early 1 (IE1), which is most active from 0–6 h p.i. did not lead to a higher yield of functional CAMPATH-1H compared to the polyhedrin promoter.[55] It is possible, however, that use of a late phase promoter, e.g., the basic protein promoter or a non-viral constitutively active promoter, with higher transcriptional activity than the IE1 promoter, may give higher yields of functional material than the very late polyhedrin promoter.

Thus far, the antibody expression levels achieved in the baculovirus/insect cell system are lower than those achieved with an amplified, mammalian cell line, the more usual choice for recombinant antibody production (e.g., yields of ~200 mg/l are routinely achieved using the CHO/dihydrofolate reductase[73] or NS0/glutamine synthetase[74] amplification systems and yields as high as 800 mg/l have been reported for the latter system[75]). In addition, the mammalian cell lines have the added advantage of being a continuous production system, rather than the transient infection system and avoid the potential problems associated with recombinant protein expression in insect cells whose post-translational modification and secretory apparatus may be compromised. The use of the constitutively active IE1 promoter in stably transfected insect cells has been described for human tissue plasminogen activator (tPA) production,[76] however, expression levels were considerably lower than had previously been achieved for tPA in amplified CHO cells[76] (~0.5 mg/l compared to ~200 mg/l). Hence, until expression levels in the system are improved, it seems that antibody expression in recombinant baculovirus-infected cells or in stably transfected insect cells may not be a viable alternative to the more usual eukaryotic protein expression host, i.e., mammalian cells.

11.5 GRAM-POSITIVE BACTERIA

Bacillus subtilis is the gram-positive bacterium most commonly used for the expression of foreign proteins. It is easily grown, can be genetically manipulated, and has been granted GRAS status by the FDA. Furthermore, it has the ability to secrete proteins into the extracellular medium, unlike *E. coli* which generally secretes proteins only as far as the periplasmic space. This property can potentially simplify the downstream purification of proteins secreted from *B. subtilis* which makes it an attractive organism for the cost-effective, large-scale expression of recombinant proteins for therapeutic applications.

11.5.1 *Bacillus subtilis* Expression Systems

B. subtilis naturally secretes several proteases into the growth medium which can degrade foreign proteins, dramatically reducing their yield.[77] This problem can largely be overcome by the generation of mutant strains (e.g., GP263 and WB600) which exhibit reduced extracellular protease production.[77-79] A second disadvantage that has limited the general application of *B. subtilis* as an expression system, is the need for regulated, inducible vectors. Such vectors have now been developed and, in the main, use one of: the *B. subtilis* sucrose-inducible *sacB* gene system, temperature-sensitive repressor systems, or the *E. coli lac* system.[80-87]

B. subtilis has a complex transcriptional arrangement with several RNA polymerases differing in the nature of their subunits. Each polymerase recognizes different conserved promoter -35 and -10 regions, and in this way families of genes are transcribed by different polymerases at different stages of the growth, stationary, and sporulation phases. The organism's translational machinery is similarly specific and requires the presence of a complementary sequence to the 16S rRNA Shine-Dalgarno sequences 5′ of the initiation codon.[88] Foreign gene expression therefore requires suitable promoter regions that will be recognized by *B. subtilis*. Several promoters are available from *B. subtilis* genes, *Bacillus* phage and *E. coli*.[89] Enhanced expression can be achieved if the promoter contains certain regulatory sequences. P_{Lev} is such a promoter; it contains the regulatory region of *sacB* (the sucrose-inducible gene for *B. subtilis* levansucrase). When this is combined in a plasmid with the gene for a *sacB*-regulatory protein (*sacY*, under the control of a strong promoter, P43) expression of a foreign protein is enhanced 18-fold.[77] Although codon usage in *B. subtilis* is quite variable, it is not thought to limit the expression yield.[90]

Secretion of a protein into the extracellular medium requires the presence of a suitable signal sequence and signal sequence processing site. Secretory protein signal sequences in gram-positive bacteria have a similar structure to those from *E. coli*, with a positively charged N-terminus followed by a stretch of hydrophobic amino acids and a signal sequence processing site immediately N terminal to the mature protein. However, differences from *E. coli* include additional positively charged residues at the N terminus, and a slightly longer hydrophobic stretch.[91]

11.5.2 Expression of Antibody Fragments in *B. subtilis*

If the above criteria are met, antibody fragments can be expressed in *B. subtilis*, and secreted into the extracellular medium. Of particular note is the expression of an anti-digoxin scFv (VL-linker-VH format) in the protease deficient WB600 strain.[92] The *sacB* signal sequence was used and the whole gene was under the control of the strong *B. subtilis* promoter P43. This gene construct was contained within the scFv expression vector pATD2, which is a derivative of pUB18. ScFv was expressed and, importantly, could be purified directly from the medium using an ouabain-sepharose affinity column. N terminal amino acid sequence analysis of the purified scFv showed the signal sequence was correctly removed. VH and VL genes could also be expressed independently, but this did not lead to the recovery of functional Fvs in the medium, probably because of the slow rate of association of VH and VLs in the dilute environment.

11.5.2.1 Biological Activity and Expression Yield

Anti-digoxin scFv, purified from the *B. subtilis* growth medium, had a similar affinity constant to the original whole antibody, and retained original specificity.[92] This is in contrast with some antibody fragments expressed in *E. coli*, where there is often a need for the antibodies to be purified and renatured from intracellular inclusion bodies; such procedures can lead to a significant reduction in biological activity.

In a separate study an anti-fluorescein scFv was expressed in *B. subtilis*. The expression construct also included a poly histidine tail to facilitate one-step purification from the cell culture medium using immobilized metal affinity chromatography.[93]

Despite the merits of the *B. subtilis* expression system, yields of the anti-digoxin scFv were only up to 5 mg/l. Interestingly this is greater than the levels obtained when the scFv was expressed in *E. coli*

(0.38 mg/l).[92] In *E. coli*, functional expression levels have been shown to be greatly influenced by the primary sequence of the antibody fragment.[22]

11.5.3 Potential of *B. subtilis* Expression Systems

As with other prokaryotes, *B. subtilis* can only be realistically considered as a host for the expression of antibody fragments, rather than whole antibodies, as it is not able to glycosylate proteins, and so typical mammalian post-translation modifications will not be made. The utilization of *B. subtilis* as an expression system is lagging behind that of *E. coli*. However, it is probable that the attraction of the extracellular secretion pathway, and the recognition of the bacterium's GRAS status, will ensure the system is further developed. In particular, a fuller understanding of the protein secretion pathway, which exhibits both similarities and differences with that of *E. coli*, should enable the development of *B. subtilis* strains with enhanced secretory properties for the low cost, large-scale production of antibody fragments.

11.6 TRANSGENIC ANIMALS

The expression of foreign proteins in the milk of transgenic animals represents a very attractive production method. Advantages over other expression systems include the genetically stable and renewable source, potentially high yields, mammalian post-translation processing system, and the ease of protein purification. Cattle, sheep, and goats are being used to produce pharmaceutical products in milk. The current major disadvantage is the time and cost for development of sufficient numbers of the transgenic animals.

11.6.1 Antibody Production Methods

11.6.1.1 Large-Scale Expression

The strategy most commonly used involves cloning of the foreign gene under the control of a promoter and regulatory elements that direct expression of a gene for a host milk protein. The gene is then introduced, by microinjection, into the pronuclei of fertilized oocytes, where it becomes integrated into the host's DNA. The fertilized, transgenic oocytes are then introduced into a surrogate mother. The recombinant protein should be expressed in mammary gland epithelial cells of progeny only during lactation.[94-98] This technology is being applied and actively developed by a number of biotechnology companies.[99]

The yield of proteins expressed in the milk of transgenic animals depends upon the animal used, the host promoter and regulatory sequences, the site of integration of the gene into the host DNA, and the gene copy number. The foreign gene itself can also significantly affect the expression levels; the use of genomic DNA (with all the elements that can affect gene transcription, mRNA stability and translation) instead of cDNA, may improve yields.[97,100,101]

Purification of the foreign protein from milk is simplified because relatively few types of proteins are present in milk. Furthermore, milk production in most animals is a sterile process and, depending on the regularity of milking, the proteins may be present in the milk for only a short period of time prior to purification, thereby reducing possible degradation often associated with alternative, cell culture expression systems. For proteins with a nutritional application, or biomedical proteins that can be taken orally, purification may simply require concentration of the whey fraction and other procedures commonly used in the dairy industry.[96]

The expression of functional antibodies in transgenic animals is complicated by the need for co-expression of the two genes for the heavy and light chains, and then the proper association of these protein chains. This was first achieved for the expression of an anti-cancer antibody in the milk of transgenic mice. These mice had been generated by the co-injection of the antibody heavy and light chain genes, under the control of a casein promoter, into one-cell mouse embryos. The antibody produced was functional, and the yield was 4 g/l. Subsequently, the expression of antibodies in transgenic goats was reported.[102]

11.6.2 Potential of Transgenic Animals for Pharmaceutical Production

Several foreign proteins, expressed in the milk of transgenic animals, are being developed for clinical trials due to begin in early 1996.[99] The particular advantages of the use of transgenic animals include: typical mammalian glycosylation pattern, relatively low cost and simple downstream purification of the protein, stable production source, and high yields. Disadvantages include the complexity and expense of the process to develop the transgenic animals. Careful consideration should also be given to the type of animal used; for instance, it has been calculated that 300 transgenic cows will be required to provide the estimated annual need of human serum albumin, but this number rises to 8300 if goats are used.[99]

Future developments are likely to include the exploitation of ES cells, and in particular, the use of homologous recombination to specifically introduce a foreign antibody gene into a mouse milk protein gene. In this way, the transgenic mouse is instructed to produce high levels of only one recombinant antibody. At the moment, the use of ES cells is restricted to mice; further research is required to extend these ES technologies to the more productive ruminants.

In general, the use of transgenic animals for the production of antibodies is lagging behind their use for the production of other proteins, primarily because of the complexity of the antibody molecule. However, recent signs are that these problems are being overcome and transgenic animals are likely to become an increasingly popular source of therapeutic proteins, including antibodies.

11.7 CONCLUSIONS

It is probable that each of the methods described above will be developed further for the production of antibody therapeutics. In due course the advantages and disadvantages of the different processes will be better understood, which will lead to different methods being chosen for specific applications, for example, where post-transcriptional modification is an issue. However, it is likely that in the not too distant future one or more of the processes described here will compete with "traditional" mammalian and *E. coli* expression systems for the production of antibody therapeutics.

The major factors governing the selection of a particular expression system will be economic and regulatory; commercial commitment to a particular novel production method will depend on that method's ability to provide a cost-effective and safe product. The regulatory approval of products produced by one of these emerging methods will encourage others to follow the same strategy.

REFERENCES

1. Whitelam, G. C., The production of recombinant proteins in plants, *J. Sci. Food Agric.*, 68, 1, 1995.
2. Goddijn, O. J. M., and Pen, J., Plants as bioreactors, *Trends Biotechnol.*, 13, 379, 1995.
3. Hiatt, A., Antibodies produced in plants, *Nature*, 344, 469, 1990.
4. van Rooijen, G. J. H. and Moloney, M. M., Plant seed oil-bodies as carriers for foreign proteins, *Bio/Technology*, 13, 72, 1995.
5. Weising, K., Schell, J., and Kahl, G., Foreign genes in plants: transfer, structure, expression and applications, *Annu. Rev. Gen.*, 22, 421, 1988.
6. Gasser, C. S. and Fraley, R. T., Transgenic crops, *Sci. Am.*, 266, 34, June 1992.

7. Benvenuto, E., Ordas, R. J., Tavazza, R., Ancora, G., Biocca, S., Catteneo, A., and Galeffi, P., Phytoantibodies: a general vector for the expression of immunoglobulin domains in transgenic plants, *Plant Mol. Biol.*, 17, 865, 1991.
8. Owen, M. R. L., Gandecha, A., Cockburn, W., and Whitelam, G. C., Synthesis of a functional anti-phytochrome single-chain Fv protein in transgenic tobacco, *Bio/Technology*, 10, 790, 1992.
9. Firek, S., Draper, J., Owen, M. R. L., Gandecha, A., Cockburn, W., and Whitelam, G. C., Secretion of a functional single-chain Fv protein in transgenic tobacco plants and cell suspension cultures, *Plant Mol. Biol.*, 23, 861, 1993.
10. Tavladoraki, P., Benvenuto, E., Trinca, S., de Martinis, D., Cattaneo, A., and Galeffi, P., Transgenic plants expressing a functional single-chain Fv antibody are specifically protected from virus attack, *Nature*, 366, 469, 1993.
11. Fiedler, U. and Conrad, U., High level production and long term storage of engineered antibodies in transgenic tobacco seeds, *Bio/Technology*, 13, 1090, 1995.
12. McGregor, D. P., Molloy, P. E., Cunningham, C., and Harris, W. J., Spontaneous assembly of bivalent single chain antibody fragments in *Escherichia coli, Mol. Immunol.*, 31, 219, 1994.
13. Longstaff, M., Axis Genetics Ltd, Babraham, Cambridge, U.K. personal communication, 1996.
14 De Neve, M., De Loose, M., Jacobs, A., van Houdt, H., Kaluza, B., Weidle, U., van Montague, M., and Depicker, A., Assembly of an antibody and its derived antibody fragment in *Nicotiana* and *Arabidopsis, Transgenic Res.*, 2, 227, 1993.
15. Hiatt, A. C., Cafferkey, R., and Bowdish, K., Production of antibodies in transgenic plants, *Nature*, 342, 76, 1989.
16. Hein, M. B., Tang, Y., McCleod, D. A., Janda, K. D., and Hiatt, A. C., Evaluation of immunoglobulins from plant cells, *Biotechnol. Prog.*, 7, 455, 1991.
17. van Engelen, F. A., Schouten, A., Molthoff, J. W., Roosien, J., Salinas, J., Dirkse, W. G., Schots, A., Gommers, F. J., Jongsma, M. A., Bosch, D., and Stiekema, W. J., Coordinate expression of antibody subunit genes yields high levels of functional antibodies in roots of transgenic tobacco, *Plant Mol. Biol.*, 26, 1701, 1994.
18. Ma, J. K.-C., Hiatt, A., Hein, M., Vine, N. D., Wang, F., Stabila, P., van Dolleweerd, C., Mostov, K., and Lehner, T., Generation and assembly of secretory antibodies in plants, *Science*, 268, 716, 1995.
19. During, K., Hippe, S., Kreuzaler, F., and Schell, J., Synthesis and self-assembly of a functional monoclonal antibody in transgenic *Nicotiana tabacum, Plant Mol. Biol.*, 15, 281, 1990.
20. Stieger, M., Neuhaus, G., Momma, T., Schell, J., and Krezaler, F., Self assembly of immunoglobulins in the cytoplasm of the alga *Acetabularia mediterranea, Plant Sci.*, 73, 181, 1991.
21. Hiatt, A. and Mostov, K., Assembly of multimeric proteins in plant cells: characteristics and uses of plant derived antibodies, in *Transgenic plants: Fundamentals and Applications*, Hiatt, A., Ed., Marcel Dekker Inc., New York, 1993, 221.
22. Knappick, K. and Pluckthun, A., Engineered turns of a recombinant antibody improve its *in vivo* folding, *Prot. Eng.*, 8, 81, 1995.
23. Faye, L., Gomrod, V., Fitchette-Laine, A.-C., and Chrispeels, M. J., Affinity purification of antibodies specific for Asn-linked glycans $\beta 1 \rightarrow 2$ xylose, *Anal. Biochem.*, 209, 104, 1993.
24. von Schwaewen, A., Sturm, A., O'Neil, J., and Chrispeels, M. J., Isolation of a mutant Arabidopsis plant that lacks *N*-acetyl glucosaminyl transferase I and is unable to synthesise golgi-modified complex N-linked glycans, *Plant Physiol.*, 102, 1109, 1993.
25. Lehner, T., Caldwell, J., and Smith, R., Local passive immunization by monoclonal antibodies against antigen I/II in prevention of dental caries, *Infect. Immun.*, 50, 796, 1985.

26. Moffit, A. S., Exploring plants as a new vaccine source, *Science*, 268, 658, 1995.
27. Couderc, R. and Baratti, J., Oxidation of methanol by the yeast, *Pichia pastoris*. Purification and properties of the alcohol oxidase, *Agric. Biol. Chem.*, 44, 2279, 1980.
28. Ellis, S. B., Brust, P. F., Koutz, P. J., Waters, A. F., Harpold, M. M., and Gingeras, T. R., Isolation of alcohol oxidase and two other methanol regulatable genes from the yeast *Pichia pastoris, Mol. Cell. Biol.*, 5, 1111, 1985.
29. Cregg, J. M., Madden, K. R., Barringer, K. J., Thill, G. P., and Stillman, C. A., Functional characterization of the two alcohol oxidase genes from the yeast *Pichia pastoris, Mol. Cell. Biol.*, 9, 1316, 1989.
30. Tschopp, J. F., Brust, P. F., Cregg, J. M., Stillman, C. A., and Gingeras, T. R., Expression of the *lacZ* gene from two methanol-regulated promoters in *Pichia pastoris, Nucl. Acids Res.*, 15, 3859, 1987.
31. Cregg, J. M., Barringer, K. J., Hessler, A. Y., and Madden, K. R., *Pichia pastoris* a host system for transformations, *Mol. Cell. Biol.*, 5, 3376, 1985.
32. Scorer, C. A., Clare, J. J., McCombie, W. R., Romanos, M. A., and Sreekrishna, K., Rapid selection using G418 of high copy number transformants of *Pichia pastoris* for high-level foreign gene expression, *Bio/Technology*, 12, 181, 1994.
33. Cregg, J. M., Tschopp, J. F., Stillman, C., Siegel, R., Akong, M., Craig, W. S., Buckholz, R. G., Madden, K. R., Kellaris, P. A., Davis, G. R., Smiley, B. L., Cruze, J., Torregrossa, R., Veliçelebi, G., and Thill, G. P., High-level expression and efficient assembly of hepatitis B surface antigen in the methylotrophic yeast, *Pichia pastoris, Bio/Technology*, 5, 479, 1987.
34. Clare, J. J., Rayment, F. B., Ballantine, S. P., Sreekrishna, K., and Romanos, M. A., High-level expression of tetanus toxin fragment C in *Pichia pastoris* strains containing multiple tandem integrations of the gene, *Bio/Technology*, 9, 455, 1991.
35. Durand, H., Clanet, M., and Tiraby, G., Genetic improvement of *Trichoderma reesei* for large scale cellulase production, *Enzyme Microb. Technol.*, 10, 341, 1988.
36. Tschopp, J. F., Sverlow, G., Kosson, R., Craig, W., and Grinna, L., High-level secretion of glycosylated invertase in the methylotrophic yeast, *Pichia pastoris, Bio/Technology*, 5, 1305, 1987.
37. Scorer, C. A., Buckholz, R. G., Clare, J. J., and Romanos, M. A., The intracellular production and secretion of HIV-1 envelope protein in the methylotrophic yeast *Pichia pastoris, Gene*, 136, 111, 1993.
38. Romanos, M. A., Clare, J. J., Beesley, K. M., Rayment, F. B., Ballantine, S. P., Makoff, A. J., Dougan, G., Fairweather, N. F., and Charles, I. G., Recombinant *Bordetella pertussis* pertactin (P69) from the yeast *Pichia pastoris*: high-level production and immunological properties, *Vaccine*, 9, 901, 1991.
39. Sreekrishna, K., Nelles, L., Potenz, R. H. B., Cruze, J. A., Mazzaferro, P. K., Fish, W., Fuke, M., Holden, K. A., Phelps, D. A., Wood, P. J., and Parker, K. A., High level expression, purification, and characterization of recombinant human tumor necrosis factor synthesized in the methylotrophic yeast *Pichia pastoris, Biochemistry*, 28, 4117, 1989.
40. Ridder, R., Schmitz, R., Legay, F., and Gram, H., Generation of rabbit monoclonal antibody fragments from a combinatorial phage display library and their production in the yeast *Pichia pastoris, Bio/Technology*, 13, 255, 1995.
41. Nyyssönen, E., Penttilä, M., Harkki, A., Saloheimo, A., Knowles, J. K. C., and Keränen, S., Efficient production of antibody fragments by the filamentous fungus *Trichoderma reesei, Bio/Technology*, 11, 591, 1993.
42. Harkki, A., Uusitalo, J., Bailey, M., Pentillä, M., and Knowles, J. K. C., A novel fungal expression system: secretion of active calf chymosin from filamentous fungus *Trichoderma reesei, Bio/Technology*, 7, 169, 1989.
43. Miller, L. K., Baculoviruses as gene expression vectors, *Annu. Rev. Microbiol.*, 42, 177, 1988.

44. Griffiths, C. M., Baculovirus expression vectors: advances and applications, *Exp. Opin. Ther. Patents*, 4, 1065, 1994.
45. Luckow, V. A. and Summers, M. D., Trends in the development of baculovirus expression vectors, *Bio/Technology*, 6, 47, 1988.
46. O'Reilly, D. R., Miller, L. K., and Luckow, V. A., *Baculovirus Expression Vectors: A Laboratory Manual*, WH Freeman and Company, New York, 1992.
47. Davies, A. H., Current methods for manipulating baculoviruses, *Bio/Technology*, 12, 47, 1994.
48. Kitts, P. A., Ayres, M. D., and Possee, R. D., Linearization of baculovirus DNA enhances the recovery of recombinant virus expression vectors, *Nucleic Acids Res.*, 18, 5667, 1990.
49. Kitts, P. A. and Possee, R. D., A method for producing recombinant baculovirus expression vectors at high frequency, *BioTechniques*, 14, 810, 1993.
50. Carayannopoulos, L., Max, E. E., and Capra, J. D., Recombinant human IgA expressed in insect cells, *Proc. Natl. Acad. Sci. U.S.A.*, 91, 8348, 1994.
51. Hasemann, C. A. and Capra, J. D., High-level production of functional immunoglobulin heterodimer in a baculovirus expression system, *Proc. Natl. Acad. Sci. U.S.A.*, 87, 3942, 1990.
52. Nesbit, M., Fang Fu, Z., McDonald-Smith, J., Steplewski, Z., and Curtis, P. J., Production of a functional monoclonal antibody recognizing human colorectal carcinoma cells from a baculovirus expression system, *J. Immunol. Methods*, 151, 201, 1992.
53. zu Putlitz, J., Kubasek, W. L., Duchene, M., Marget, M., von Specht, B. U., and Domdey, H., Antibody production in baculovirus-infected insect cells, *Bio/Technology*, 8, 651, 1990.
54. Reis, U., Blum, B., von Specht, B. U., Domdey, H., and Collins, J., Antibody production in silkworm cells and silkworm larvae infected with a dual recombinant *Bombyx mori* nuclear polyhedrosis virus, *Bio/Technology*, 10, 910, 1992.
55. Bentley, K. J., unpublished data, 1995.
56. Laroche, Y., Demaeyer, M., Stassen, J. M., Gansemans, Y., Demarsin, E., Matthyssens, G., Collens, D., and Holvoet, P., Characterization of a recombinant single-chain molecule comprising the variable domains of a monoclonal antibody specific for human fibrin fragment D-dimer, *J. Biol. Chem.*, 266, 16343, 1991.
57. Kretzschmar, E., Geyer, R., and Klenk, H. D., Baculovirus infection does not alter *N*-glycosylation in *Spodoptera frugiperda* cells, *Biol. Chem.*, 375, 323, 1994.
58. Jarvis, D. L. and Summers, M. D., Glycosylation and secretion of human tissue plasminogen activator in recombinant baculovirus-infected insect cells, *Mol. Cell. Biol.*, 9, 214, 1989.
59. Davidson, D. J., Fraser, M. J., and Castellino, F. J., Oligosaccharide processing in the expression of human plasminogen cDNA by lepidopteran insect (*Spodoptera frugiperda*) cells, *Biochemistry*, 29, 5584, 1990.
60. Davidson, D. J. and Castellino, F. J., Asparagine-linked oligosaccharide processing in lepidopteran insect cells. Temporal dependence of the nature of the oligosaccharides assembled on asparagine-289 of recombinant plasminogen produced in baculovirus vector infected *Spodoptera frugiperda* (IPLC-SF-21AE) cells, *Biochemistry*, 30, 6167, 1991.
61. Murphy, C. I., McIntire, J. R., Davis, D. R., Hodgdon, H., Seals, J., and Young, E., Enhanced expression, secretion, and large-scale purification of recombinant HIV-1 gp120 in insect cells using the baculovirus egt and p67 signal peptides, *Prot. Expr. Purif.*, 4, 349, 1993.
62. Rademacher, T. W., Parekh, R. B., and Dwek, R. A., Glycobiology, *Annu. Rev. Biochem.*, 57, 785, 1988.

63. James, D. C., Freedman, R. B., Hoare, M., Ogonah, O. W., Rooney, B. C.,Larionov, O. A., Dobrovolsky, O. V., and Jenkins, N., *N*-glycosylation of recombinant human interferon-γ produced in different animal expression systems, *Bio/Technology*, 13, 592, 1995.
64. Tsuchiya, N., Endo, T., Matsuta, K., Yoshinoya, S., Aikawa, T., Kosuge, E., Takeuchi, F., Miyamoto, T., and Kobata, A., Effects of galactose depletion from oligosaccharide chains on immunological activities of human IgG, *J. Rheumatol.*, 16, 285, 1989.
65. Wright, A. and Morrison, S. L., Effect of altered C_H2-associated carbohydrate structure on the functional properties and *in vivo* fate of chimeric mouse-human immunoglobulin G1, *J. Exp. Med.*, 180, 1087, 1994.
66. Jarvis, D. L., Fleming, J. G. W., Kovacs, G. R., Summers, M. D., and Guarino, L. A., Use of early baculovirus promoters for continuous expression and efficient processing of foreign gene products in stably transformed Lepidopteran cells, *Bio/Technology*, 8, 950, 1990.
67. Tessier, D. C., Thomas, D. Y., Khouri, H. E., Laliberte, F., and Vernet, T., Enhanced secretion from insect cells of a foreign protein fused to the honeybee melittin signal peptide, *Gene*, 98, 177, 1991.
68. Jarvis, D. L., Summers, M. D., Garcia, A., and Bohlmeyer, D. A., Influence of different signal peptides and prosequences on expression and secretion of human tissue plasminogen activator in the baculovirus system, *J. Biol. Chem.*, 268, 16754, 1993.
69. Hsu, T. A., Eiden, J. J., Bourgarel, P., Meo, T., and Betenbaugh, M. J., Effects of co-expressing chaperone BiP on functional antibody production in the baculovirus system, *Prot. Expr. Purif.*, 5, 595, 1994.
70. Miller, R. K., Trimarchi, R. E., Browne, D., and Pennock, G. D., A temperature-sensitive mutant of the baculovirus *Autographa californica* nuclear polyhedrosis virus defective in an early function required for further gene expression, *Virology*, 126, 376, 1983.
71. Rankl, N. B., Rice, J. W., Gurganus, T. M., Barbee, J. L., and Burns, D. J., The production of an active protein kinase C-δ in insect cells is greatly enhanced by the use of the basic protein promoter, *Prot. Expr. Eng.*, 5, 346, 1994.
72. Sridhar, P. and Hasnain, S. E., Differential secretion and glycosylation of recombinant human chorionic gonadotrophin (βhCG) synthesized using different promoters in the baculovirus expression vector system, *Gene*, 131, 261, 1993.
73. Page, M. J. and Sydenham, M. A., High level expression of the humanized monoclonal antibody CAMPATH-1H in Chinese hamster ovary cells, *Bio/Technology*, 9, 64, 1991.
74. Bebbington, C. R., Renner, G., Thomson, S., King, D., Abrams, D., and Yarranton, G. T., High-level expression of a recombinant antibody from myeloma cells using a glutamine synthetase gene as an amplifiable selectable marker, *Bio/Technology*, 10, 169, 1992.
75. Birch, J. R. and Froud, S. J., Mammalian cell culture systems for recombinant protein production, *Biologicals*, 22, 127, 1994.
76. Weidle, U. H., Buckel, P., and Wienberg, J., Amplified expression constructs for human tissue-type plasminogen activator in Chinese hamster ovary cells: instability in the absence of selective pressure, *Gene*, 66, 193, 1988.
77. Wu, X.-C., Lee, W., Tran, L., and Wong, S.-L., Engineering a *Bacillus subtilis* expression-secretion system with a strain deficient in six extracellular proteases, *J. Bacteriol.*, 173, 4952, 1991.
78. Sloma, A., Rudolph, C. F., Rufo, G. A., Sullivan, B. J., Theriault, K. A., Ally, D., and Pero, J., Gene encoding a novel extracellular metalloprotease in *Bacillus subtilis*, *J. Bacteriol.*, 172, 1024, 1990.

79. Sloma, A., Rufo, G. A., Rudolph, C. F., Sullivan, B. J., Theriault, K. A., and Pero, J., Bacillopeptidase F of *Bacillus subtilis*: purification of the protein and cloning of the gene, *J. Bacteriol.*, 172, 1470, 1990.
80. Zukowski, M. M. and Miller, L., Hyperproduction of an intracellular heterologous protein in a *sacU*^{h} mutant of *Bacillus subtilis, Gene,* 46, 247, 1986.
81. Edelman, A., Joliff, G., Klier, A., and Rapoport, G., A system for the inducible secretion of proteins from *Bacillus subtilis* during logarithmic growth, *FEMS Microbiol. Lett.*, 52, 117, 1988.
82. Zukowski, M. M., Miller, L., Cogswell, P., and Chen, K., Inducible expression system based on sucrose metabolism genes of *Bacillus subtilis,* in *Genetics and Biotechnology of Bacilli,* Vol. 2, Ganesan, A. T. and Hoch, J. A., Eds., Academic Press, San Diego, 1988, 17.
83. Wong, S.-L., Development of an inducible and enhancible expression and secretion system in *Bacillus subtilis, Gene,* 83, 215, 1989.
84. Osburne, M. S., Craig, R. J., and Rothstein, D. M., Thermoinducible transcription system for *Bacillus subtilis* that utilizes control elements from temperate phage Φ105, *J. Bacteriol.*, 163, 1101, 1984.
85. Breitling, R., Sorokin, A. V., Ellinger, T., and Behke, D., Controlled gene expression in *Bacillus subtilis* based on the temperature-sensitive λ*cI* repressor, in *Genetics and Biotechnology of Bacilli,* Vol. 3, Ganesan, A. T. and Hoch, J. A., Eds., Academic Press, San Diego, 1990, 3.
86. Yansura, D. G. and Henner, D., Use of the *Escherichia coli lac* repressor and operator to control gene expression in *Bacillus subtilis, Proc. Natl. Acad. Sci. U.S.A.,* 81, 439, 1984.
87. Le Grice, S. F. J., Regulated promoter for high-level expression of heterologous genes in *Bacillus subtilis, Methods Enzymol.*, 185, 201, 1990.
88. Doi, R. H., Wong, S.-L., and Kawamura, F., Potential use of *Bacillus subtilis* for secretion and production of foreign protein, *Trends Biotechnol.*, 4, 232, 1986.
89. Harwood, C. R., *Bacillus subtilis* and its relatives: molecular biological and industrial workhorses, *Trends Biotechnol.*, 10, 247, 1992.
90. Ogasawar, A. N., Markedly unbiased codon usage in *Bacillus subtilis, Gene,* 40, 145, 1985.
91. Perlman, D. and Halvorson, H. O., A putative signal peptidase recognition site and sequence in eukaryotic and prokaryotic signal peptides, *J. Mol. Biol.*, 176, 391, 1983.
92. Wu, X.-C., Ng, S.-C., Near, R. I., and Wong, S.-L., Efficient production of a functional single-chain antidigoxin antibody via an engineered *Bacillus subtilis* expression-secretion system, *Bio/Technology,* 11, 71, 1993.
93. de Ferra, F., Tortora, C., Tosi, E., and Grandi, G., Expression system for scFv in *B. subtilis,* EMBO and IRBM workshop on: molecular repertoires and methods of selection, Gubio, Italy, 1993.
94. Wright, G., Carver, A., Cottom, D., Reeves, D., Scott, A., Simons, P., Wilmut, I., Garner, I., and Colman, A., High level expression of active human alpha-1-antitrypsin in the milk of transgenic sheep, *Bio/Technology,* 9, 830, 1991.
95. Carver, A. S., Dalyrymple, M. A., Wright, G., Cottom, D. S., Reeves, D. B., Gibson, Y. H., Keenan, J. L., Barrass, J. D., Scott, A. R., Colman, A., and Garner, I., Transgenic livestock as bioreactors: stable expression of human alpha-1-antitrypsin by a flock of sheep, *Bio/Technology,* 11, 1263, 1993.
96. Lee, S. H. and de Boer, H. A., Production of biomedical proteins in the milk of transgenic dairy cows: the state of the art, *J. Controlled Release,* 29, 213, 1994.
97. Houdebaine, L.-M., Production of pharmaceutical proteins from transgenic animals, *J. Biotechnol.*, 34, 269, 1994.
98. Maga, E. A. and Murray, J. D., Mammary gland expression of transgenes and the potential for altering the properties of milk, *Bio/Technology,* 13, 1452, 1995.

99. Rudolph, N. S., Advances continue in production of proteins in transgenic animal milk, *Gen. Eng. News*, 15(18), 8, 1995.
100. Whitelaw, C. B. A., Archibald, A. L., Harris, S., McClenaghan, M., Simons, J. P., and Clark, A. J., Targeting expression to the mammary gland: intronic sequences can enhance the efficiency of gene expression in transgenic mice, *Transgen. Res.*, 1, 3, 1991.
101. Hurwitz, D. R., Nathan, M., Barash, I., Ilan, N., and Shani, M., Specific combinations of human serum albumin introns direct high level expression of albumin in transfected COS cells and in the milk of transgenic mice, *Transgen. Res.*, 3, 365, 1994.
102. Meade, H., Ditullio P., and Pollock, D., Transgenic production of antibodies in milk, International patent publication WO95/17085, 1995.

Part IV

Recombinant Antibodies in the Clinic

Chapter **12**

DEVELOPMENT OF ZENAPAX®: A HUMANIZED ANTI-TAC ANTIBODY

John Hakimi, Diane Mould, Thomas A. Waldmann, Cary Queen, Claudio Anasetti, and Susan Light

CONTENTS

0-8493-8547-4/97/$0.00+$.50

12.1 INTERLEUKIN-2 AND ITS ACTIONS AT THE INTERLEUKIN-2 RECEPTOR

Interleukin-2 (IL-2) and the IL-2 receptor (IL-2R) comprise a well-characterized ligand-receptor system that plays a key role in the induction of immune responses. T-cell-mediated immune responses require that T cells undergo a transformation from a resting to an activated state. Activation of these cells requires two signals.[1] The first is initiated when appropriately processed and presented antigen interacts with the 90-kDa polymorphic heterodimeric T-cell surface receptor for the specific antigen. The second is characterized by the expression of IL-2 and high-affinity IL-2R by the T cell. Although the interaction between appropriately presented antigen and its target receptor determines specificity for a given immune response, the interaction of IL-2 and high-affinity IL-2R determines the magnitude and duration of that response.[1]

12.1.1 Interleukin 2 (IL-2)

Interleukin-2, a glycoprotein made up of 133 amino acids, has an apparent molecular mass of 15.5 kDa.[2] Because it regulates the clonal expansion of T cells, IL-2 plays a central role in the cellular immune response.[3] IL-2 mediates its biologic effects by binding to specific receptors on the surfaces of activated T lymphocytes. It facilitates both antibody formation and cell-mediated immune responses. IL-2 serves not only as the essential growth factor for T lymphocytes, but also acts on other cells in the immune system including macrophages, B lymphocytes, natural killer (NK) cells, lymphokine-activated killer (LAK) cells, and immature thymocytes. Oligodendrocytes of the central nervous system proliferate in response to IL-2.[3] IL-2 is thus a pleiotropic mediator exerting multiple effects via specific receptors on a wide variety of cells.[4]

12.1.2 The Interleukin-2 Receptor (IL-2R)

IL-2 exerts its effects on T lymphocytes by binding to the IL-2R. The IL-2R is composed of three distinct membrane components: the α chain (T-cell activation antigen (Tac), IL-2Rα), the β chain (IL-2Rβ), and the α chain (IL-2Rγ); (Figure 1).[5,6] The genes encoding these receptor subunits have been cloned and characterized. IL-2Rβ and IL-2Rγ are members of a recently defined superfamily of cytokine receptors characterized by four conserved cysteines and the sequence, WSXWS (Trp-Ser-X-Trp-Ser motif).[6,7] The IL-2Rβ/IL-2Rγ complex, which is normally expressed on select resting T and B cells and NK cells, as well as LAK cells, mediates signaling and receptor internalization.

Most resting T, B, and NK cells express IL-2Rβ and IL-2Rγ, but not IL-2Rα (or Tac). Tac is expressed only after these cells are activated as a result of interaction with a foreign antigen or with IL-2. The IL-2Rα subunit associates with the IL-2Rβ/IL-2Rγ subunits, forming the high-affinity IL-2R complex. Tac found unassociated with the intermediate IL-2R complex or expressed alone by genetic engineering has a low affinity for IL-2 and does not mediate any known biological signal. An antibody or pharmacological agent that selectively destroys or inactivates Tac-bearing cells would be expected to inhibit nascent or ongoing immune responses and, depending on its binding properties, may not suppress natural (nonspecific) immunity or a specific immune response to a new antigen once immunosuppressive therapy has been terminated. Moreover, the constitutive expression of Tac on the surface of certain types of tumor cells suggests that an anti-Tac antibody may also be useful in the treatment of such tumors.[8]

It should also be noted that Tac is the only subunit of IL-2R that is specific for IL-2. The β subunit is also a component of the IL-15 receptor

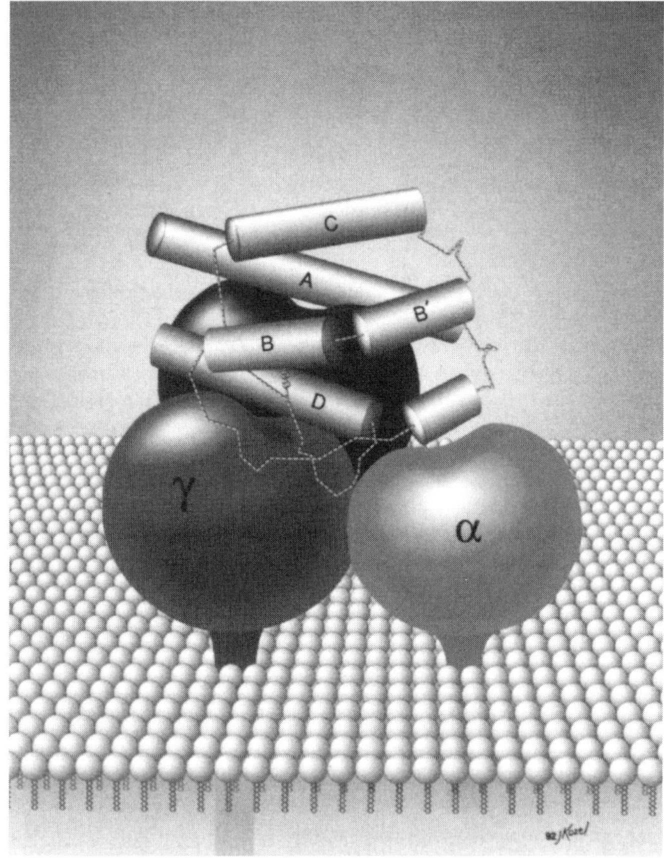

FIGURE 1
Model of IL-2 interactions with α, β, and γ receptor subunits. Predicted sites of interaction between IL-2 and receptor subunits are based on mutational and epitope-mapping studies. The helical model of IL-2 structure is based on recent modifications of the original crystallographic predictions. The indicated interaction of γ chain with the carboxy terminal D helix is supported by studies showing that alteration of specific amino acids in the carboxyl terminal yields mutant forms of IL-2 that bind to α chains and β complexes, but not to intermediate-affinity receptors. (From Voss, S. D. et al., *Proc. Natl. Acad. Sci. U.S.A.*, 90, 2428, 1993. With permission.)

and the γ subunit is shared with the IL-4, IL-7, IL-9, and IL-15 receptors. This unique feature supports the theory that an anti-Tac antibody would be a highly specific inhibitor of immune responses.[9,10]

A murine monoclonal IgG2a (murine anti-Tac, MAT) that was demonstrated to bind to IL-2Rα,[11,12] was originally identified by Waldmann and collaborators[13] on the basis of its ability to bind to activated human T cells or to select Epstein-Barr virus (EBV) transformed human B cells, but not to resting T cells. *In vitro,* MAT was found to inhibit antigen- and mitogen-induced human T-cell proliferation; allogeneic human cytolytic T-cell responses; T-cell-dependent, pokeweed mitogen-activated human B-cell immunoglobulin production; IL-2-dependent proliferation of mitogen-activated human B-cell immunoglobulin production;[14] IL-2-dependent proliferation of mitogen-activated human B cells;[15] and IL-2-dependent proliferation of IL-2-activated human NK/LAK cells.[16] Anti-Tac had no effects on cells that do not express IL-2Rα, demonstrating the biologic specificity of this antibody and thus its high potential for efficacy in the clinical setting.

12.1.3 Roles of Interleukin-2 in Allograft Rejection, Graft-vs.-Host Disease, Autoimmune Disease, and Malignancy

A large body of literature has implicated IL-2 and IL-2R in the pathogenesis of graft rejection, autoimmune disease, and malignancy. These findings, and the robust and specific *in vitro* properties of MAT as well, have prompted its evaluation — as well as other monoclonal antibodies (MAbs) directed against IL-2R — in animal models of a number of different clinical conditions.

12.1.3.1 Allograft Rejection

A central feature of the complex series of events leading to allograft rejection is the activation of T cells.[17,18] This process, which is initiated when T cells recognize intracellularly processed fragments of foreign proteins, is amplified by autocrine T-cell proliferation that occurs as a consequence of the expression of IL-2 that is dependent on T-cell activation and the expression of high-affinity (i.e., α, β, and γ subunit-containing) IL-2R.[18] Cytokine production and the expression of activation-induced cell-surface receptors results in the emergence of antigen-specific T cells that infiltrate the graft and contribute to its destruction.[19]

While a variety of immunosuppressive regimens have been employed for the prevention of allograft rejection, all are associated with characteristic side effects.[18,19] Several studies have demonstrated the efficacy of murine MAbs directed against IL-2R in animal models of transplantation. Kirkman et al.[20,21] have shown that treatment of mice with murine anti-IL-2R antibodies (either M7/20 or AMT-13) prolongs cardiac allograft survival. Kupiec-Weglinski et al.[22] reported similar results for another anti-IL-2R antibody (ART18). Reed et al.[23] demonstrated that administration of MAT significantly prolonged the survival of renal allografts in cynomolgus monkeys. All of these results suggested strongly that anti-IL-2R antibodies, including MAT, might be useful in the prevention of graft rejection in human solid organ transplant recipients. Studies which directly evaluated this possibility are reviewed below.

12.1.3.2 Acute Graft-vs.-Host Disease

Acute graft-versus-host disease (GVHD) is a major clinical complication of allogeneic bone marrow transplantation (ABMT), especially when the donor is unrelated to the recipient.[24-26] Despite extensive efforts at prophylaxis with conventional agents such as cyclosporin, methotrexate, and methylprednisolone, most patients who receive ABMT from unrelated donors still develop GVHD.[26]

Acute GVHD is now thought to be the result of a "cytokine storm" in which IL-2 and the IL-2R may play a role.[24,25] Reactive donor T cells proliferate as a function of interaction with host antigens and secrete several cytokines, including IL-2. IL-2 production appears to be an important marker for GVHD, since it has been demonstrated that the precursor frequency of anti-host-specific IL-2-producing cells is predictive for GVHD in HLA-identical sibling transplants.[27] Because the binding of IL-2 to IL-2R mediates T-cell proliferation, the use of MAbs directed against this receptor offers a rational approach to both prophylaxis against, and treatment of, GVHD in patients undergoing ABMT. Another attractive aspect of this approach is the possibility of targeting and selectively destroying activated T cells. In theory, anti-IL-2R antibodies should be relatively selective compared with other conventional immunosuppressive agents or pan–T-cell antibodies because they should have no effect on resting T cells that do not express IL-2Rα.[28] The potential therapeutic efficacy of blocking the interaction of IL-2 and IL-2R in ameliorating GVHD has been demonstrated in an animal model,[29,30] prompting the evaluation of several such preparations in patients who have undergone ABMT. These studies are reviewed below.

12.1.3.3 Autoimmune Disease

The central role of T cells in the pathology of autoimmune disease is well established.[31,32] Evidence for T-cell activation and abnormal Tac expression has been noted in numerous autoimmune diseases including rheumatoid arthritis, systemic lupus erythematosus, scleroderma, pulmonary sarcoidosis, and human T-cell lymphotropic virus type I (HTLV-I)-associated tropical spastic paraparesis.[31] Furthermore, animal studies have demonstrated that antibodies directed against IL-2R provide significant protection against induced autoimmune diseases that can be passively transferred by T cells to naive recipients.[32] Thus, antibodies directed against IL-2R may also prove to be effective for the treatment of human patients with autoimmune diseases.

12.1.3.4 Malignancy

Tac is expressed by T cells from patients with a variety of lymphoproliferative disorders including Hodgkin's disease, well-differentiated lymphocytic lymphomas, intermediate lymphocytic lymphomas, follicular or follicular and diffuse poorly differentiated lymphomas, mixed B- and T-cell lymphomas, large-cell lymphomas, and hairy cell leukemias.[33]

Expression of Tac is of particular interest in adult T-cell leukemia (ATL) associated with the retrovirus HTLV-I. In this leukemia, malignant cells tend to infiltrate the skin; patients also experience hypercalcemia and a profound immunodeficient state.[34] All malignant T cells in patients with this disease express Tac.[35,36] The HTLV-I virus produces a protein called *tax* which increases the transcription of both IL-2 and Tac.[34] In the early phase of ATL, this abnormal expression is thought to be responsible for the uncontrolled proliferation of these cells,[35] which may be stimulated in an autocrine manner by IL-2.[37] Thus, an antibody directed against Tac may provide a rational approach to therapy in patients with this malignancy.

12.1.3.5 Summary

Results of animal experiments demonstrated the efficacy of murine anti-Tac antibodies for a number of disease states. These findings led to clinical trials of several of these preparations and ultimately to the humanization of MAT and clinical evaluation of HAT.

12.2 DEVELOPMENT OF THE HUMANIZED ANTI-Tac ANTIBODY (Zenapax®, HAT)

12.2.1 Limitations of Murine Anti-IL-2R Antibodies in Human Patients

While animal experimental studies demonstrated the efficacy of a number of anti-IL-2R antibodies, results obtained with these preparations in human patients have been quite variable and in many cases, disappointing. In general, the results of these trials have pointed out the important limitations of murine preparations for the treatment of clinical patients.

12.2.1.1 Allograft Rejection

Soulillou and colleagues[38-40] carried out a series of studies that compared the efficacy and tolerability of rat MAb (33B3.1) with rabbit anti-thymocyte globulin (ATG) for the prevention of rejection in patients who received cadaveric renal allografts. While their initial report indicated that the MAb was as effective and better tolerated than ATG,[38] subsequent studies demonstrated a significant superiority of ATG over the rat anti-Tac antibody.[39,40]

Kirkman et al.[41] compared the efficacy of standard triple immunosuppressive therapy (cyclosporin, azathioprine, and prednisone) vs. MAT delivered with the same treatment (with reduced cyclosporin) for the prevention of rejection in 80 patients who received renal allografts. While the addition of MAT significantly delayed the time to first rejection from 7.6 ± 6.3 days to 12.5 ± 6.3 days, there were no differences in actual or actuarial graft or patient survival between the two groups. Therapy with MAT appeared to be limited by the development of anti-idiotypic antibodies.

12.2.1.2 GVHD

Hervé et al.[42] assessed the efficacy of a murine MAb directed against IL-2R (B-B10) in 32 patients early in the course of GVHD, after 48 h of treatment with glucocorticoids. Twenty-one of these patients had complete responses to treatment and six had partial responses. Surprisingly, only 1 of 14 patients tested developed anti-idiotypic antibodies against the murine MAb. Anasetti et al.[28] reported less encouraging results with a murine MAb (2A3) directed against IL-2Rα. They tested this preparation in 11 patients who developed glucocorticoid-refractory GVHD following ABMT. One patient, in whom the skin was the only involved organ, had a complete response to treatment and two patients had partial responses. Of the total antibody infusions, 14% were complicated by adverse events which included fever, respiratory distress, hypertension, hypotension, and chills. Of the eight patients evaluated, four had IgM antibody responses and one had an IgG response to the murine MAb.

Blaise et al.[43] and Belanger et al.[44] have reported results for a large number of patients who received prophylactic treatment against GVHD following ABMT with a rat monoclonal antibody (33B3.1) directed against IL-2Rα. In the initial trial,[43] administration of this antibody along with methotrexate and cyclosporin appeared to reduce the incidence of GVHD in a sample of 15 patients. However, a larger prospective study that included 64 consecutively treated patients provided no evidence of reduced GVHD relative to a group of 89 historical control patients.[44] Most of the patients treated in the larger study developed IgM or IgG antibodies to the rat MAb and pharmacokinetic analysis demonstrated that 50% of the patients in this trial may have had serum MAb levels that were subtherapeutic. However, there was no significant correlation between serum levels of the MAb and the development of antibodies to it.[44] Blaise et al.[45] compared the efficacy of standard methotrexate plus cyclosporin therapy with the standard therapy plus 33B3.1 in 101 randomly assigned leukemia patients. In this prospective study, the anti-IL-2R antibody did not significantly affect the frequency or severity of GVHD, but did delay its onset. At median followup of 58 months, the 33B3.1-treated group had lower leukemia-free survival due to an increase in the rate of late relapses.

Cuthbert et al.[46] and Herbelin et al.[47] evaluated B-B10 (BT563) in a total of 29 patients with acute corticosteroid-resistant GVHD. In the first trial, complete responses were observed in 4 of 14 patients and partial responses were noted in an additional 4 patients.[46] In the second, complete responses were observed in 10 of 15 patients and one additional patient had a partial response. Ten of the 15 patients are long-term survivors and free of chronic GVHD.[47]

In summary, results obtained with murine MAbs directed against IL-2R in the prevention or treatment of GVHD have been quite mixed. The reason for the marked differences among the results obtained in different trials is not clear, but the variability does suggest that a murine preparation that lacks the ability to mediate antibody-dependent cell-mediated toxicity (ADCC) and has poor pharmacokinetics may not provide the most effective approach to modulating IL-2R and thus T-cell function in humans with GVHD.

12.2.1.3 Malignancy

Waldmann et al.[48] evaluated the efficacy of MAT in patients with ATL. Conventional chemotherapy is ineffective in patients with this disease, but given the fact that ATL cells constitutively express IL-2Rα and binding of IL-2 to this receptor may be necessary for the uncontrolled proliferation of these lymphocytes (see above), blockade of IL-2Rα offers a rational approach to the treatment of these patients. These investigators treated 19 patients with ATL using MAT: two patients developed complete remissions; four patients developed a partial remission; and one patient had a mixed remission. Remission was associated with a return to normal serum calcium levels, improvement in liver function tests, and, in some cases, amelioration of the profound immunodeficiency characteristic of ATL.

12.2.2 Humanization of a Murine Anti-Tac Antibody

While the results of Waldmann et al.[48] in patients with ATL and several of the trials of murine anti-IL-2R antibodies in patients with GVHD appear encouraging, the clinical efficacy of mouse and rat MAbs directed against IL-2R is likely to be limited for two important reasons. First, they are recognized as foreign and neutralized when patients develop antibodies to them, usually within the first month of treatment.[49] This immune response speeds the clearance of murine preparations and reduces their circulating half-life ($t_{1/2}$). Murine antibodies generally have half-life values of less than 50 h when infused into human patients, while values for human antibodies generally exceed 100 h.[50,51] When a long-circulating half-life is necessary for the clinically relevant biologic activity of the antibody, the limitations of murine preparations are obvious.[52] Second, therapeutic antibodies of murine origin are often less effective than human antibodies in recruiting human immune-effector functions such as ADCC and complement fixation. These limitations have prompted the development and testing of humanized versions of one of the murine anti-IL-2Rα antibodies, MAT.

Queen and associates[53] produced humanized chimeric and hyperchimeric forms of the murine anti-IL-2Rα antibody by genetic engineering. A hyperchimeric humanized antibody (HAT, humanized anti-Tac, Zenapax®) was constructed in two stages. First, the six complementarity-determining regions (CDRs) of the MAT light- and heavy-chain variable domains were combined with the variable framework regions of human Eu antibody. Several additional amino acids were retained from the MAT framework to maintain the conformation of the CDRs within the binding domain. The next step in the preparation of HAT was the combination of the light- and heavy-chain variable regions with human κ and γ1 constant regions, respectively. These combined genes were expressed in SP2/0 mouse myeloma cells. Thus, in HAT, the major portions of the original murine MAb that were retained were the hypervariable segments critical to the specificity of epitope binding. The total retained mouse segments account for less than 10% of the protein mass, making HAT more than 90% human.[49]

12.3 PROPERTIES OF HAT: PRECLINICAL DATA

Junghans and associates[49] carried out extensive *in vitro* analyses of the characteristics of HAT and compared them with those of both MAT and a chimeric form of MAT.

12.3.1 *In Vitro* Studies

In vitro experiments demonstrated that HAT maintains high affinities for antigen and effectively blocks T-cell activation and proliferation. This new preparation did not demonstrate complement-mediated cytotoxicity, but it did show the capability of inducing ADCC on human cells, a property not possessed by MAT.[49]

12.3.1.1 *Binding to Antigen*

The active fractions of the chimeric antibodies and HAT were evaluated for their ability to bind to the IL-2Rα-expressing human T-cell line — HUT-102. All of these antibodies and MAT showed binding in the range of 60 to 80%. Scatchard analysis demonstrated a K_a of 9×10^9 M^{-1} for both the murine and chimeric antibodies and 3×10^9 M^{-1} for the hyperchimeric antibody.

12.3.1.2 *Inhibition of IL-2-Dependent, Antigen-Induced, T-Cell Proliferation*

One critical property of MAT is its ability to block antigen-induced T-cell proliferation in assays that measure the response of sensitized T cells to antigen. This property was fully retained by both chimeric and hyperchimeric antibodies. All of the antibodies blocked thymidine incorporation in a dose-dependent manner for both tetanus-toxoid and influenza-virus stimulants. The mean antibody concentrations required for 50% inhibition of T-cell proliferation were in the range of 0.5 to 1.0 μg/ml (3–7 nM). Similar results were obtained in mixed lymphocyte reaction cultures and phytohemagglutinin (PHA)–activated T-cell blast-proliferation assays.

12.3.1.3 *ADCC*

Murine antibodies are frequently unable to promote ADCC in assays with human effectors and nucleated target cells displaying natural antigens.[54] However, this ability to recruit cellular effector mechanisms is presumed to be an important determinant of the therapeutic efficacy of any antibody whether its target is tumor or normal activated T cells.[49] Mouse anti-Tac antibody is unable to promote ADCC even when administered in combination with 7G7/B6, another monoclonal antibody specific for IL-2 receptor.[49,55] In contrast, both the chimeric and hyperchimeric forms of MAT demonstrate significant ADCC (Figure 2). This activity was modestly augmented with higher effector cell/target cell (E/T) ratios and was stimulated when effector cells were activated with IL-2.[49] ADCC is an *in vitro* activity which cannot be demonstrated in the presence of human serum. Thus, the real biological significance of this activity remains to be demonstrated.

12.3.1.4 *Synergism with a Humanized Antibody Directed at the β-Chain of IL-2R*

In vitro studies using murine antibodies directed against the α and β chains of the IL-2R complex have demonstrated synergism between

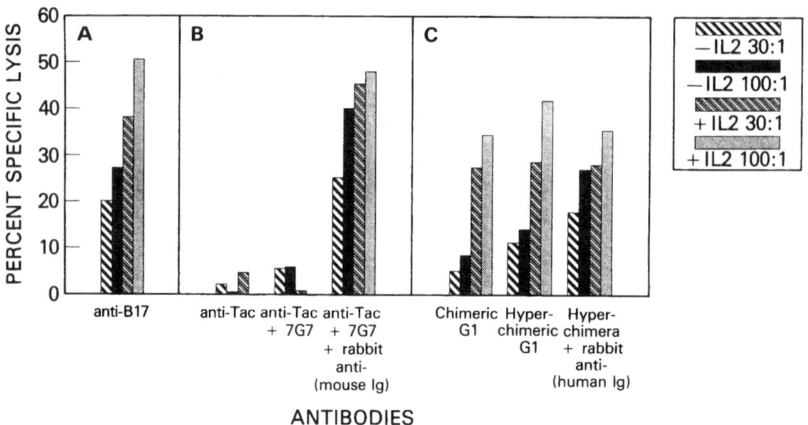

FIGURE 2
Antibody-dependent cell-mediated cytotoxicity with a chimeric anti-IL-2Rα antibody and HAT. The first two bars in each set represent results with E/T ratios of 30:1 and 100:1, respectively, without IL-2 activation. The second pair shows the same ratios with IL-2 activation. (From Junghans, R. P. et al., *Cancer Res.*, 50, 1495, 1990. With permission.)

these preparations in inhibiting IL-2-mediated responses.[56] Experiments reported by Hakimi et al.[57] have demonstrated that such synergism is also demonstrated by humanized preparations. They showed that HAT exhibits synergism with a humanized Mikβ1 antibody directed at the β chain of the IL-2R. Their results demonstrated that this antibody acted synergistically with HAT to prevent proliferation of PHA-T-cell blasts. However, synergy with these two humanized anti-IL-2R antibodies was not observed *in vivo* in the cynomolgus cardiac allograft model.[58]

12.3.2 *In Vivo* Experiments

The binding of HAT exhibits strict species specificity toward its antigen-binding site. HAT, like other anti-human IL-2Rα antibodies, binds only to primate IL-2Rα and does not bind to the analogous protein in rodents. Therefore, HAT was evaluated exclusively in various primate models to assess its pharmacokinetics, immunogenicity, efficacy, and potential toxicities.

12.3.2.1 Pharmacokinetics

Hakimi et al.[59] evaluated the pharmacokinetics of HAT in cynomolgus monkeys. The pharmacokinetic properties, that is the half-life and area under the serum concentration vs. time curve (AUC) values, of

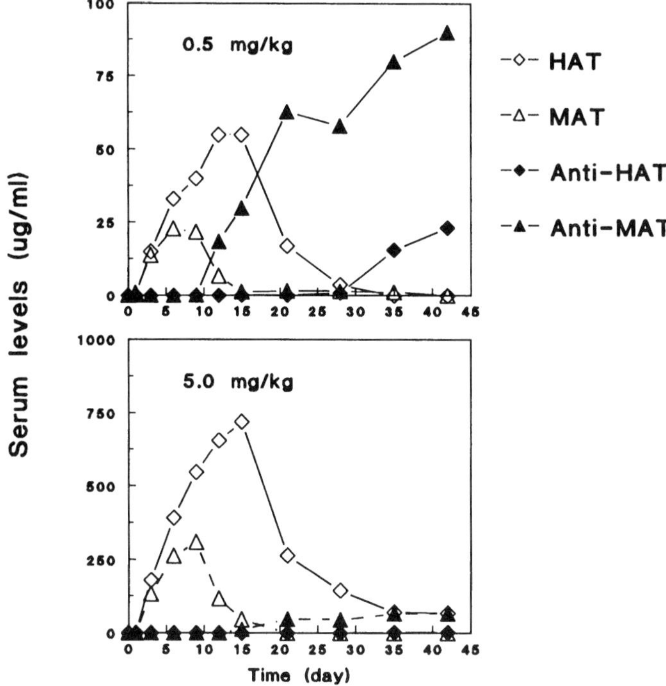

FIGURE 3
Serum concentrations of anti-Tac and anti-anti-Tac antibodies after 14 days of once-daily dosing with 0.5 or 5.0 mg/kg of HAT or MAT.

HAT were also significantly different from those of MAT. The mean half-life of a single dose of HAT was 214 h which was four- to fivefold greater than the half-life value determined for MAT (48 h). The AUC value for HAT following a single 5.0-mg/kg intravenous dose was twofold greater than that for MAT (26,657 vs. 11,442 μg.h/ml). The AUC, a measure of systemic exposure, was reduced in monkeys that were previously treated with HAT or MAT and developed anti-anti-Tac antibodies.

The multiple-dose pharmacokinetic profiles for HAT and MAT were also substantially different.[59] The mean maximum serum concentrations following once-daily dosing for 14 days with 0.5 or 5.0 mg/kg of HAT were 57 ± 20 μg/ml and 726 ± 115 μg/ml, respectively (Figure 3). These same values for the 0.5 and 5.0 mg/kg doses of MAT were 26 ± 9 μg/ml and 311 ± 47 μg/ml, respectively.

Brown et al.[50] also compared the pharmacokinetic profiles of iodinated HAT and MAT in monkeys. They reported a harmonic mean half-life of 103 h for HAT and 38 h for MAT.

12.3.2.2 Immunogenicity

The immunogenicity of HAT was evaluated in a cynomolgus monkey study.[59] In this study, monkeys were treated with daily doses of 0.0, 0.05, 0.5, or 5.0 mg/kg of HAT or MAT for 14 days, rested for 28 days, and rechallenged with a single intravenous dose of 5 mg/kg of HAT or MAT. Analyses of monkey sera for anti-HAT and anti-MAT antibodies demonstrated that HAT was less immunogenic than MAT. MAT-treated monkeys developed anti-MAT antibodies during the 14-day treatment period at all doses tested, which was preceded by a rapid reduction in serum MAT concentrations. At a comparable dose of anti-Tac antigen, anti-HAT antibody titers were five- to tenfold lower than anti-MAT antibody titers, and the antibodies were not detected until several days after the 14-day dosing regimen was completed. The lack of anti-HAT antibodies resulted in higher maximum and trough serum concentrations. Furthermore, a single high (5.0 mg/kg) intravenous bolus dose of MAT administered to naive monkeys on day 42 was sufficient to evoke a primary antibody response within 13 days, while a similar (5.0 mg/kg) intravenous bolus of HAT on day 42 did not induce a measurable antibody response. Similar trends in immunogenicity patterns and correlation with observed pharmacokinetic properties were noted in monkeys with cardiac allografts receiving HAT as discussed in Section 12.3.2.3.[50]

The binding specificity of the monkey anti-HAT and anti-MAT responses was determined.[57] The results demonstrated that the monkey anti-MAT response was a mixture of anti-isotypic and anti-idiotypic antibodies, while the anti-HAT response was predominantly anti-idiotypic (i.e., the antibodies were directed against the CDRs of anti-Tac). In a second study[60] using 12 humanized anti-Tac variants differing in CDR sequences, most of the anti-idiotypic response to HAT in monkeys was found to be directed against conformations composed wholly or in part of CDR regions H1, H2, and L3.

All of these results indicate that HAT is less immunogenic than MAT in nonhuman primates. This results in the potential for a longer drug exposure, thus improving the pharmacokinetic behavior of the humanized form of the anti-Tac antibody. The reduced immunogenicity and substantially longer elimination half-life of HAT suggests that it can be administered in a more acceptable dosing regimen and that the humanized antibody can be significantly more effective than the murine antibody in humans.

12.3.2.3 Pharmacologic Effects

Brown et al.[50] compared the efficacy and immunogenicity of HAT and MAT in a primate model of cardiac allograft survival. In this trial, monkeys that received cardiac allografts were either untreated or received 1.0 mg/kg of HAT or MAT every other day until graft rejection occurred. The grafts in the untreated monkeys were rejected in an average of 9.20 ± 0.48 days. In the MAT-treated animals, rejection occurred at an average of 14.0 ± 1.98 days and in the HAT-treated monkeys, the average time to rejection was 20.0 ± 0.55 days (p <0.001 vs. untreated and p <0.02 vs. MAT-treated animals).

Rejection in the MAT-treated monkeys was preceded by the development of anti-MAT antibodies and a concomitant decline in the trough serum concentration of MAT from 10 μg/ml to below the limits of assay detection (Figure 4A). In contrast, rejection in monkeys receiving HAT occurred when serum HAT levels were still high and anti-HAT antibodies were not yet detectable (Figure 4B). This suggests that the development of anti-MAT antibodies may have contributed to the allograft rejection in the monkeys that received the murine preparation, but that rejection in the HAT-treated animals was probably not associated with the development of antibodies to the humanized preparation.[50] These results, like those from the studies evaluating the immunogenicity and pharmacokinetics of HAT and MAT in cynomolgus monkeys, support the conclusion that the humanized antibody is much more likely to be effective in humans than the murine preparation.

12.3.2.4 Toxicity

The potential toxicity of HAT has been evaluated in a variety of species. Single-dose studies of HAT in mice, rats, and rabbits with doses up to 125 mg/kg resulted in no deaths or clinical symptoms of toxicity.[61] The toxicity of HAT was also evaluated in a 28-day study in which monkeys received daily intravenous boluses of up to 15 mg/kg for 28 days. There were no clinical signs of toxicity and no treatment-related changes in complement components (C3a, C4a, and C5a) or in lymphocyte phenotype markers (CD4 and CD8). HAT was well tolerated at all doses tested. Brown et al.[50] also noted no evidence of toxicity in HAT-treated monkeys that received cardiac allografts. All of these data suggest that HAT should be safe for administration to humans.

12.4 CLINICAL EXPERIENCE

12.4.1 Pharmacokinetics

Model-independent pharmacokinetic analyses for HAT in clinical trials have been reported.[62] Data from 20 patients with GVHD who

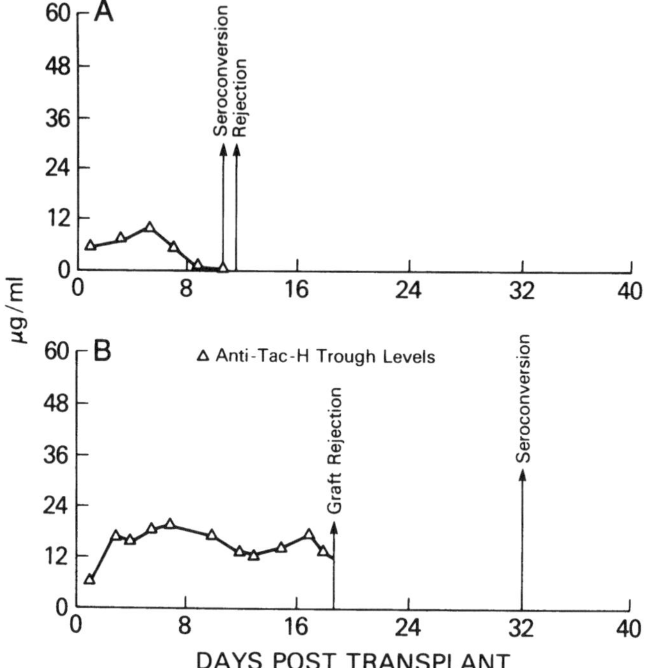

FIGURE 4
MAT and HAT serum concentration-time profiles in cynomolgus monkeys treated with MAT (A) or HAT (B) (given daily as i.v. bolus injections until time of rejection). Note that cardiac graft rejection in the MAT-treated animal occurs shortly after the appearance of anti-MAT antibodies and a decrease of serum MAT to undetectable levels. Graft rejection in the HAT-treated monkey occurred well before the appearance of anti-HAT antibodies and while trough serum concentrations of HAT were still >10 µg/ml. (From Brown, P. S. et al., *Proc. Natl. Acad. Sci. U.S.A.*, 88, 2663, 1991. With permission.)

received either 0.5, 1.0, or 1.5 mg/kg of HAT were evaluated, and the results of Anasetti et al.[62] indicated that the pharmacokinetics were characterized by a long terminal elimination half-life, a low systemic clearance, and a small volume of distribution (Figure 5). These kinetics are typical of other humanized IgG antibodies.[53]

Mould et al.[63] carried out a more extensive model-dependent analysis of HAT concentrations in the sera of the patients in the study by Anasetti et al.[62] and reported that the pharmacokinetics for this humanized MAb were well described by the two-compartment model with an overall harmonic mean half-life of 138 h (range, 115.5–173.3 h). The half-life for HAT in man was shorter than that in monkeys. This may be attributed to differences in clearances of human IgG molecules between monkey and man or to disease-induced changes that are reflected in decreased protein clearance in monkeys.[64]

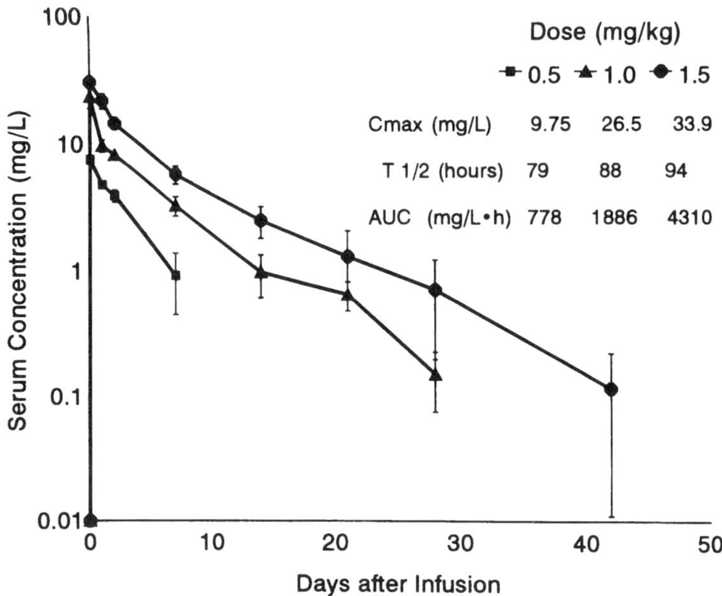

FIGURE 5
Mean (± standard error of the mean) serum concentrations of HAT in patients treated with 0.5 (n = 4), 1.0 (n = 4), or 1.5 mg/kg (n = 12) of this preparation. (From Anasetti, C., et al., *Blood*, 84, 1320, 1994. With permission.)

12.4.2 Pharmacodynamics

Anasetti et al.[62] carried out a limited pharmacodynamic analysis of HAT in patients with GVHD. Tac was saturated by HAT on the cells of all patients who were studied on day 7 following treatment and on the cells of most patients who were studied on day 28. Staining of freshly isolated lymphocytes with an anti-human globulin showed that cells isolated during days 7 through 28 post-treatment were coated with HAT. Expression of IL-2Rα and IL-2Rβ on the surface of circulating lymphocytes did not appear to be influenced by treatment with a single dose of HAT.

12.4.3 Efficacy

12.4.3.1 GVHD

Anasetti et al.[62] evaluated HAT in 20 patients who developed acute GVHD, 5 to 26 days post-BMT, that was resistant to therapy with cyclosporin and methylprednisolone. Patients were treated with single doses of 0.5, 1.0, or 1.5 mg/kg of HAT. Eight patients who experienced a transient improvement following the first HAT infusion received a second dose 11 to 48 days after the first treatment. Overall, improvement of acute GVHD was observed in eight patients. Four patients had complete responses to therapy at day 29 (defined as a resolution of GVHD for all evaluable organs with no additional subsequent treatment for GVHD) and four patients experienced partial responses (defined as improvement in at least one evaluable organ without deterioration in at least one other). Two patients were alive at 529 and 645 days following treatment; 2 patients died after a relapse of leukemia; and 16 patients died of infection or organ failure between 5 and 211 days after treatment.

12.4.3.2 Solid Organ Transplantation

Vincenti et al.[65] have recently reported the results of an open-label phase I trial in which HAT was administered prophylactically to patients receiving either living-related (n = 10) or first cadaveric (n = 2) renal transplants using one of four dosing regimens: 0.5 mg/kg or 1.0 mg/kg either every week or every other week for a total of five doses. All patients also received cyclosporin, azathioprine, and prednisone. Only one patient who received a cadaveric graft (and 0.5 mg/kg of HAT every other week) had a transient rejection episode. At 1-year followup, all patients were alive with functioning grafts. At 12 months post-transplantation, the mean serum creatinine was 1.4 mg/dl. Only one patient developed anti-HAT antibodies, and there were no significant changes in the percentages of T-cell subsets during therapy observed. These encouraging results have prompted the current evaluation of HAT in a phase III clinical trial in renal transplant recipients.

12.4.4 Safety

The results from the study by Anasetti et al.[62] indicate that HAT is well tolerated. Only 2 of 28 antibody infusions in that study were followed by side effects possibly related to HAT. One patient experienced chills and a second patient experienced diaphoresis. No consistent changes in serum chemistry were noted after HAT treatment, nor was there evidence of other toxicities. Vincenti et al.[65] reported no HAT-related adverse events in 12 renal transplant recipients treated with HAT.

12.4.5 Immunogenicity

The immunogenicity of HAT has been evaluated with an enzyme immunologic assay in the patients with GVHD treated by Anasetti et al.[62] At 28 days after treatment, none of these patients had detectable anti-HAT antibody levels. Ten of these patients were also tested 56 days after treatment and, here again, none had detectable anti-HAT antibodies. In addition, none of the six patients who received a second infusion of HAT developed detectable antibodies to this preparation. Vincenti et al.[65] noted that one renal transplant recipient they treated with HAT developed antibodies to this preparation. The lack of immunogenicity of HAT in human patients receiving concomitant immunosuppressive therapy is also consistent with the observation that a second dose of this preparation resulted in a half-life similar to that for the first dose.[63] The lack of immunogenicity of HAT reported by Anasetti et al.[62] and Vincenti et al.[64] contrast sharply with those that have been reported for MAT[41] and other murine anti-IL-2R antibodies.[28,38,44]

12.5 SUMMARY

The results presented in this review indicate that the humanization of a murine MAb directed against the alpha chain of the IL-2R may enhance both the pharmacokinetic profile and therapeutic potential of this preparation. The development of HAT has overcome three important therapeutic limitations of murine MAbs: short serum half-life neutralization by patient immune responses and inability to recruit human immune effector functions.

The HAT antibody is well tolerated and has a much longer half-life than the murine preparation, and it may be efficacious for the treatment of GVHD that is resistant to standard therapy and for prophylaxis against rejection in patients who have received renal allografts. The encouraging results in early trials warrant phase II and phase III studies to define whether HAT is effective in modifying human immune responses in autoimmune diseases and transplantation and in the management of malignancies such as ATL and certain autoimmune diseases.

REFERENCES

1. Waldmann, T. A. and Goldman, C. K., The multichain Interleukin-2 receptor: a target for immunotherapy of patients receiving allografts, *Am. J. Kidney Dis.*, 15(Suppl. 2), 45, 1989.
2. Smith, K. A., Interleukin-2: inception, impact, and implications, *Science*, 240, 1169, 1988.
3. Kaempfer, R., Regulation of the human interleukin-2/interleukin-2 receptor system: a role for immunosuppression, *Proc. Soc. Exp. Biol. Med.*, 206, 176, 1994.
4. Whittington, R. and Faulds, D., Interleukin-2: a review of its pharmacological properties and therapeutic use in patients with cancer, *Drugs*, 46, 446, 1993.

5. Voss, S. D., Leary, T. P., Sondel, P. M., and Robb, R. J., Identification of a direct interaction between interleukin 2 and the p64 interleukin-2 receptor γ chain, *Proc. Natl. Acad. Sci. U.S.A.*, 90, 2428, 1993.
6. Taniguchi, T. and Minami, Y., The IL-2/IL-2 receptor system: A current overview, *Cell*, 73, 5, 1993.
7. Waldmann, T. A., The IL-2/IL-2 receptor system: a target for rational immune intervention, *TIPS*, 14, 159, 1993.
8. Waldmann, T. A., Multichain interleukin-2 receptor: a target for immunotherapy in lymphoma, *J. Natl. Cancer Inst.*, 81, 914, 1989.
9. Giri, J. G., Ahdieh, M., Eisenman, J., Shanebeck, K., Grabstein, K., Kumaki, S., Namen, A., Park, L. S., Cosman, K., and Anderson D., Utilization of the β and γ chains of the IL-2 receptor by the novel cytokine IL-15, *EMBO J.*, 13, 2822, 1994.
10. Kimura, Y., Takeshita, T., Kondo, M., Ishii, N., Nakamura, M., Van Snick, J., and Sugamura, K., Sharing of the IL-2 receptor γ chain with the functional IL-9 receptor complex, *Int. Immunol.*, 7, 115, 1995.
11. Leonard, W. J., Depper, J. M., Uchiyama, T., Smith, K. A., Waldmann, T. A., and Greene, W. C., A monoclonal antibody that appears to recognize the receptor for human T-cell growth factor; partial characterization of the receptor, *Nature*, 300, 267, 1982.
12. Robb, R. J. and Greene, W. C., Direct demonstration of the identity of T cell growth factor binding protein and the Tac antigen, *J. Exp. Med.*, 158, 1332, 1983.
13. Uchiyama, T., Nelson, D. L., Fleisher, T. A., and Waldmann, T. A., A monoclonal antibody (anti-Tac) reactive with activated and functionally mature human T cells, *J. Immunol.*, 126, 1398, 1981.
14. Depper, J. M., Leonard, W. J., Robb, R. J., Waldmann, T. A., and Greene, W. C., Blockade of the interleukin-2 receptor by anti-Tac antibody: Inhibition of human lymphocyte activation, *J. Immunol.*, 131, 690, 1983.
15. Mingari, M. C., Gerosa, F., Carra, G., Accolla, S., Moretta, A., Zubler, R. H., Waldmann, T. A., and Moretta, L., Human interleukin-2 promotes proliferation of activated B cells via surface receptors similar to those of activated T cells, *Nature*, 312, 641, 1984.
16. Siegel, J. P., Sharon, M., Smith, P. L., and Leonard, W. J., The IL-2 receptor β chain (p70) role in mediating signals for LAK, NK, and proliferative activities, *Science*, 238, 74, 1987.
17. Williams, J. M., Kelley, V. E., Kirkman, R. L., Tilney, N. L., Shapiro, M. E., Murphy, J. R., and Strom, T. B., T-cell activation antigens: Therapeutic implications, *Immunol. Invest.*, 16, 687, 1987.
18. Suthanthiran, M. and Strom, T. B., Renal transplantation, *N. Engl. J. Med.*, 331, 365, 1994.
19. Le Mauff, B., Cantarovich, D., Jacques, Y., and Soulillou, J.-P., Monoclonal antibodies against interleukin-2 receptors in the immunosuppressive management of kidney graft recipients, *Transplantat. Rev.*, 4, 79, 1990.
20. Kirkman, R. I., Barrett, L. V., Koltun, W. A., and Diamanstein, T., Prolongation of murine cardiac allograft survival by the anti-interleukin-2 receptor monoclonal antibody AMT-13, *Transplant. Proc.*, 29, 618, 1987.
21. Kirkman, R. I., Barrett, L. V., Gaulton, G. N., Kelley, V. E., Ythier, A., and Strom, T. B., Administration of an anti-interleukin-2 receptor monoclonal antibody prolongs cardiac allograft survival in mice, *J. Exp. Med.*, 162, 358, 1985.
22. Kupiec-Weglinski, J. W., Padberg, W., Uhteg, L. C., Ma, L., Lord, R. H., Araneda, D., Strom, T. B., Diamantstein, T., and Tilney, N. L., Selective immunosuppression with anti-interleukin-2 receptor-targeted therapy: helper and suppressor cell activity in rat recipients of cardiac allografts, *Eur. J. Immunol.*, 17, 313, 1987.

23. Reed, M. H., Shapiro, M. F., Strom, T. B., Milford, E. L., Carpenter, C. B., Weinberg, D. S., Reimann, K. A., Letvin, N. L., Waldmann, T. A., and Kirkman, R. L., Prolongation of primate renal allograft survival by anti-Tac, an anti-human IL-2 receptor monoclonal antibody, *Transplantation*, 47, 55, 1989.
24. Ferrara, J. L. M. and Dreg, H. J., Graft-versus-host disease, *N. Engl. J. Med.*, 324, 667, 1991.
25. Ferrara, J. L. M., Cytokine dysregulation as a mechanism of graft-versus-host-disease, *Curr. Opin. Immunol.*, 5, 794, 1993.
26. Kernan, N. A., Bartsch, G., Ash, R. C., Beatty, P. G., Champlin, R., Filipovich, A., Gajewski, J., Hansen, J. A., Henslee-Downey, J., McCullough, J., McGlave, P., Perkins, H. A., Phillips, G. L., Sanders, J., Stroncek, D., Thomas, E. D., and Blume, K. G., Analysis of 462 transplantations from unrelated donors facilitated by the National Marrow Donor Program, *N. Engl. J. Med.*, 328, 593, 1993.
27. Theobald, M., Nierle, T., Bunjes, D., Arnold, R., and Heimpel, H., Host-specific interleukin-2-secreting donor T-cell precursors as predictors of acute graft-versus-host disease in bone marrow transplantation between HLA-identical siblings, *N. Engl. J. Med.*, 327, 1613, 1992.
28. Anasetti, C., Martin, P. J., Hansen, J. A., Appelbaum, F. R., Beatty, P. G., Doney, K., Harkonen, S., Jackson, A., Reichert, T., Stewart, P., Storb, R., Sullivan, K. M., Thomas, E. D., Warner, N., and Witherspoon, R. P., A phase I-II study evaluating the murine anti-IL-2 receptor antibody 2A3 for treatment of acute graft-versus-host disease, *Transplantation*, 50, 49, 1990.
29. Ferrara, J. L. M., Marion, A., McIntyre, J. F., Murphy, G. F., and Burakoff, S. J., Amelioration of acute graft vs. host disease due to minor histocompatibility antigens by *in vivo* administration of anti-interleukin-2 receptor antibody, *J. Immunol.*, 137, 1874, 1986.
30. Via, C. S. and Finkelman, F. D., Critical role of interleukin-2 in the development of acute graft-versus-host disease, *Int. Immunol.*, 5, 565, 1993.
31. Waldmann, T. A., Goldman, C., Top, L., Grant, A., Burton, J., Bamford, R., Roessler, E., Horak, I., Zaknoen, S., Kasten-Sportes, C., White, J., England, R., Horak, E., Martinucci, J., Tinubu, S. A., Mishra, B., Junghans, R., Dipre, M., Carrasquillo, J., Reynolds, J., Gansow, O., and Nelson, D., The interleukin-2 receptor: a target for immunotherapy, *Ann. N. Y. Acad. Sci.*, 685, 603, 1993.
32. Diamantstein, T. and Osawa, H., The interleukin-2 receptor, its physiology and a new approach to a selective immunosuppressive therapy by anti-interleukin-2 receptor monoclonal antibodies, *Immunol. Rev.*, 92, 5, 1986.
33. Sheibani, K., Winberg, C. D., Van de Velde, S., Blayney, D. W., and Rappaport, H., Distribution of lymphocytes with interleukin-2 receptors (Tac antigens) in reactive lymphoproliferative processes, Hodgkin's disease, and non-Hodgkin's lymphomas, *Am. J. Pathol.*, 127, 27, 1987.
34. Nelson, D. L. and Kurman, C. C., Targeting human IL-2 receptors for diagnosis and therapy, *Proc. Soc. Exp. Biol. Med.*, 206, 309, 1994.
35. Waldmann, T. A., Greene, W. C., Sarin, P. S., Saxinger, C., Blayney, D. W., Blattner, W. A., Goldman, C. K., Bongiovanni, K., Sharrow, S., Depper, J. M., Leonard, W., Uchiyama, T., and Gallo, R. C., Functional and phenotypic comparison of human T-cell leukemia/lymphoma virus positive adult T-cell leukemia with human T-cell leukemia/lymphoma virus negative Sézary leukemia, and their distinction using anti-Tac: monoclonal antibody identifying the human receptor for T-cell growth factor, *J. Clin. Invest.*, 73, 1711, 1984.
36. Uchiyama, T., Hori, T., Tsudo, M., Wano, Y., Umadome, H., Tamori, S., Yodoi, J., Maeda, M., Sawami, H., and Uchino, H., Interleukin-2 receptor (Tac antigen) expressed on adult T cell leukemia cells, *J. Clin. Invest.*, 76, 446, 1985.

37. Maeda, M., Aeima, N., Diatoku, Y., Kashihara, M., Okamoto, H., Uchiyama, T., Shirono, K., Matsuoka, M., Hattori, H., Takasuki, K., Ikuta, K., Shimizu, A., Honjo, T., and Yodoi, J., Evidence for the interleukin-2 dependent expansion of leukemic cells in adult T cell leukemia, *Blood*, 70, 1407, 1987.
38. Soulillou, J.-P., Cantarovich, D., Le Mauff, B., Giral, M., Robillard, N., Hourmant, M., Hirn, M., and Jacques, Y., Randomized controlled trial of a monoclonal antibody against the interleukin-2 receptor (33B3.1) as compared with rabbit antithymocyte globulin for prophylaxis against rejection of renal allografts, *N. Engl. J. Med.*, 322, 1175, 1990.
39. Cantarovich, D., Le Mauff, B., Hourmant, M., Dantal, J., Baatard, R., Denis, M., Jacques, Y., Karam, G., Paineau, J., and Soulillou, J.-P., Prevention of acute rejection episodes with an anti-interleukin 2 receptor monoclonal antibody. I. Results after combined pancreas and kidney transplantation, *Transplantation*, 57, 198, 1994.
40. Hourmant, M., Le Mauff, B., Cantarovich, D., Dantal, J., Baatard, R., Denis, M., Jacques, Y., Karam, G., and Soulillou, J.-P., Prevention of acute rejection episodes with an anti-interleukin 2 receptor monoclonal antibody. II. Results after a second kidney transplantation, *Transplantation*, 57, 204, 1994.
41. Kirkman, R. L., Shapiro, M. E., Carpenter, C. B., McKay, D. B., Milford, E. L., Ramos, E. L., Tilney, N. L., Waldmann, T. A., Zimmerman, C. E., and Strom, T. B., A randomized prospective trial of anti-Tac monoclonal antibody in human renal transplantation, *Transplantation*, 51, 107, 1991.
42. Hervé, P., Wijdenes, J., Bergerat, J. P., Bordigoni, P., Milpied, N., Cahn, J. Y., Clément, C., Béliard, R., Morel-Fourrier, B., Racadot, E., Troussard, X., Benz-Lemoine, E., Gaud, C., Legros, M., Attal, M., Kloft, M., and Peters, A., Treatment of corticosteroid resistant acute graft-versus-host disease by *in vivo* administration of anti-interleukin-2 receptor monoclonal antibody (B-B10), *Blood*, 75, 1017, 1990.
43. Blaise, D., Olive, D., Hirn, M., Viens, P., Lafage, M., Attal, M., Stoppa, A. M., Gabert, J., Gastaut, J. A., Camerlo, J., Mannoni, P., Mawas, C., and Maraninchi, D., Prevention of acute GVHD by *in vivo* use of anti-interleukin-2 receptor monoclonal antibody (33B3.1): a feasibility trial in 15 patients, *Bone Marrow Transplant.*, 8, 105, 1991.
44. Belanger, C., Esperou-Bourdeau, H., Bordigoni, P., Jouet, J. P., Souillet, G., Milpied, N., Troussard, X., Kuentz, M., Hervé, P., Reiffers, J., Demeocq, F., Dauriac, C., Blaise, D., Michallet, M., Fiere, D., Freycon, F., Gratecos, N., Rio, B., Leblond, V., Ifrah, N., Attal, M., Bergerat, J. P., Vilmer, E., Pico, J., Raffoux, C., Caudrelier, P., and Gluckman, E., Use of an anti-interleukin-2 receptor monoclonal antibody for GVHD prophylaxis in unrelated donor BMT, *Bone Marrow Transplant.*, 11, 293, 1993.
45. Blaise, D., Olive, D., Michallet, M., Marit, G., Leblond, V., and Maraninchi, D., Impairment of leukaemia-free survival by addition of interleukin-2-receptor antibody to standard graft-versus-host prophylaxis, *Lancet*, 345, 1144, 1995.
46. Cuthbert, R. J., Phillips, G. L., Barnett, M. J., Nantel, S. H., Reece, D. E., Sheperd, J. D., and Klingemann, H. G., Anti-interleukin-2 receptor monoclonal antibody (BT 563) in the treatment of severe acute GVHD refractory to systemic corticosteroid therapy, *Bone Marrow Transplant.*, 10, 451, 1992.
47. Herbelin, C., Stephan, J. L., Donadieu, J., LeDeist, F., Racadot, E., Wijdenes, J., and Fischer, A., Treatment of steroid-resistant acute graft-versus-host disease with an anti-IL-2 receptor monoclonal antibody (BT 563) in children who received T-cell-depleted, partially matched, bone marrow transplants, *Bone Marrow Transplant.*, 13, 563, 1994.
48. Waldmann, T. A., White, J. D., Goldman, C. K., Top, L., Grant, A., Bamford, R., Roessler, E., Horak, I. D., Zaknoen, S., Kanten-Sportes, C., England, R., Horak, E., Mishra, B., Dipre, M., Hale, P., Fleisher, T. A., Junghans, R. P., Jaffe, E. S., and Nelson, D. L., The interleukin-2 receptor: A target for monoclonal antibody treatment of human T-cell lymphotrophic virus I-induced adult T-cell leukemia, *Blood*, 82, 1701, 1993.

49. Junghans, R. P., Waldmann, T. A., Landolfi, N. F., Avdalovic, N. M., Schneider, W. P., and Queen, C., Anti-Tac-H, a humanized antibody to the interleukin-2 receptor with new features for immunotherapy in malignant and immune disorders, *Cancer Res.*, 50, 1495, 1990.
50. Brown, P. S., Parenteau, G. L., Dirbas, F. M., Garsia, R. J., Goldman, C. K., Bukowski, M. A., Junghans, R. P., Queen, C., Hakimi, J., Benjamin, W. R., Clark, R. E., and Waldmann, T. A., Anti-Tac-H, a humanized antibody to the interleukin-2 receptor, prolongs primate cardiac allograft survival, *Proc. Natl. Acad. Sci. U.S.A.*, 88, 2663, 1991.
51. LuBuglio, A. F., Wheeler, R. H., Trang, J., Haynes, A., Rogers, K., Harvey, E. B., Sun, L., Ghrayeb, J., and Khazaeli, M. B., Mouse/human chimeric monoclonal antibody in man: kinetics and immune response, *Proc. Natl. Acad. Sci. U.S.A.*, 86, 4220, 1989.
52. Henry, R., Begent, J., and Pedley, R. B., Monoclonal antibody administration: current clinical pharmacokinetic status and future trends, *Clin. Pharmacol.*, 23, 85, 1992.
53. Queen, C., Schneider, W. P., Selick, H. E., Payne, P. W., Landolfi, N. F., Duncan, J. F., Avdalovic, N. M., Levitt, M., Junghans, R. P., and Waldmann, T. A., A humanized antibody that binds to the interleukin 2 receptor, *Proc. Natl. Acad. Sci. U.S.A.*, 86, 10029, 1989.
54. Fauci, A. S., Rosenberg, S. A., Sherwin, S. A., Dinarello, C. A., Longo, D. L., and Lane, C., Immunomodulators in clinical medicine, *Ann. Intern. Med.*, 106, 421, 1987.
55. Rubin, L. A., Kurman, C. C., Biddison, W. E., Goldman, N. D., and Nelson, D. L., A monoclonal antibody 7G7/B6, binds to an epitope on the human interleukin-2 (IL-2) receptor that is distinct from that recognized by IL-2 or anti-Tac, *Hybridoma*, 4, 91, 1985.
56. Audrain, M., Boeffard, F., Soulillou, J.-P., and Jacques, Y., Synergistic action of monoclonal antibodies directed at p55 and p75 chains of the human IL-2-receptor, *J. Immunol.*, 146, 884, 1991.
57. Hakimi, J., Ha, V. C., Lin, P., Campbell, E., Gately, M. K., Tsudo, M., Payne, P. W., Waldmann, T. A., Grant, A. J., Tsien, W.-H., and Schneider, W. P., Humanized Mikβ1, a humanized antibody to the IL-2 receptor β-chain that acts synergistically with humanized anti-Tac, *J. Immunol.*, 151, 1075, 1993.
58. Tinubu, S. A., Hakimi, J., Kondas, J. A., Bailon, P., Familletti, P. C., Spence, C., Crittendon, M. D., Parenteau, G. L., Dirbas F. M., Tsudo, M., Bacher, J. D., Kastensportes, C., Martinucci, J. L., Goldman, C. K., Clark, R. E., and Waldmann, T. A., Humanized antibody directed to the IL-2 receptor β-chain prolongs primate cardiac allograft survival, *J. Immunol.*, 153, 4330, 1994.
59. Hakimi, J., Chizzonite, R., Luke, D. R., Familletti, P. C., Bailon, P., Kondas, J. A., Pilson, R. S., Lin, P., Weber, D. V., Spence, C., Mondini, L. J., Tsien, W., Levin, J. L., Gallati, V. H., Korn, L., Waldmann, T. A., Queen, C., and Benjamin, W. R., Reduced immunogenicity and improved pharmacokinetics of humanized anti-Tac in cynomolgus monkeys, *J. Immunol.*, 147, 1352, 1991.
60. Schneider, W. P., Glaser, S. M., Kondas, J. A., and Hakimi, J., The anti-idiotypic response by cynomolgus monkeys to humanized anti-Tac is primarily directed to complementarity-determining regions H1, H2, and L3, *J. Immunol.*, 150, 3086, 1993.
61. Hoffmann-La Roche, Nutley NJ, data on file.
62. Anasetti, C., Hansen, J. A., Waldmann, T. A., Appelbaum, F. R., Davis, J., Deeg, H. J., Doney, K., Martin, P. J., Nash, R., Storb, R., Sullivan, K. M., Witherspoon, R. P., Binger, M.-H., Chizzonite, R., Hakimi, J., Mould, D., Satoh, H., and Light, S. E., Treatment of acute graft-versus-host disease with humanized anti-Tac: an antibody that binds to the interleukin-2 receptor, *Blood*, 84, 1320, 1994.
63. Hoffmann-La Roche, Nutley NJ, data on file.

64. Waldmann, T. A. and Strober, W., Metabolism of immunoglobulins, *Prog. Allergy,* 13, 1, 1969.
65. Vincenti, F., Lantz, M., Birnbaum, J., Garovoy, M., Mould, D., Hakimi, J., and Light, S.E., A phase I trial of humanized anti-interleukin 2 receptor (HAT) in renal transplant recipients, *Transplantation,* in press.

Chapter **13**

PROGRESS WITH A RESHAPED HUMAN MONOCLONAL ANTIBODY, RSHZ19, FOR THE PROPHYLAXIS AND TREATMENT OF RESPIRATORY SYNCYTIAL VIRUS INFECTION

Susan B. Dillon and Terence G. Porter

CONTENTS

0-8493-8547-4/97/$0.00+$.50

13.1 CURRENT AND EMERGING TREATMENTS FOR RSV INFECTION

Respiratory syncytial virus (RSV) is a major cause of bronchiolitis and pneumonia in infants and young children under 2 years of age,[1] and causes annual epidemics which peak during the winter months. Hospitalization due to RSV lower respiratory tract infection occurs in about 1% of normal infants less than 6 months of age, and is more frequent in certain high-risk groups including preterm infants (≤35 weeks gestation), and infants or young children with bronchopulmonary dysplasia or congenital heart disease. Overall, the infant population hospitalized for RSV infection is estimated at approximately 100,000 patients annually in the U.S. alone.[2] Reinfection with RSV is common, and among immunocompetent older children and adults, manifests as mild to severe upper respiratory tract infection that resolves within 1–2 weeks.[3] However, RSV infection can be life threatening in severely immunosuppressed patients of any age.[4] Hospitalization for RSV is expensive due to the requirement for isolation to prevent nosocomial spread of disease to high-risk patients, and the frequent need for respiratory support and intensive care. The only antiviral agent licensed for treatment of RSV disease, ribavirin (Virazole™*), requires aerosolized administration over a period of days and is restricted to use in high risk or severely ill infants.[5] The efficacy of ribavirin still remains controversial, and given additional concerns surrounding safety and cost, this agent has not gained wide acceptance within the medical community.

The ideal approach to RSV disease would be effective vaccination of all infants. A formalin-killed RSV vaccine tested in the late 1960s not only failed to confer protection, but increased the severity of lower respiratory tract illness in vaccinated children who experienced RSV infection (reviewed in References 6 and 7). Despite decades of research and clinical investigation into RSV vaccines, and the advent of purified, subunit vaccines and attenuated live virus vaccine strains, significant development hurdles beyond safety still exist. These include the young age of patients at highest risk (newborn to six months) where pre-existing maternal antibody can interfere with effective immunization, the relatively poor immunogenicity of subunit vaccines tested to date,

* Registered trademark of ICN Pharmaceuticals, Inc., Costa Mesa, CA.

and the need to adequately balance attenuation vs. immunogenicity of candidate live virus vaccine strains.[8]

Currently, administration of passive antibody represents the most promising near-term approach toward preventing or treating serious RSV disease. Several lines of experimental and epidemiologic evidence support the rationale for antibody therapy. Studies comparing RSV neutralization titers in cord blood specimens or in infant serum showed an inverse correlation between antibody titer and both the incidence of RSV infection and severity of disease in infants less than one year of age.[9] Studies in RSV animal models have demonstrated that human serum immunoglobulin preparations selected for high RSV neutralizing titers can reduce or eliminate virus shedding in the lungs when administered either prior to virus challenge, or post-infection (reviewed in References 6 and 10). Recently, the first immunoglobulin product for RSV infection, Respigam™* (RSVIG), was approved by the U.S. Food and Drug Administration (FDA) for seasonal prophylaxis of children under 24 months of age who are at high risk for serious RSV infection due to a history of prematurity or bronchopulmonary dysplasia. Clinical studies demonstrated that prophylactic administration of RSVIG resulted in significantly fewer RSV lower respiratory tract infections and a lower incidence of hospitalization due to RSV infection.[11,12] RSVIG was administered by intravenous infusion once a month throughout the RSV season. The response to treatment was dose dependent, with efficacy demonstrated only in the highest dose group (750 mg/kg) where protective serum RSV neutralizing titers were ≥1:200.

Reshaped human (humanized) IgG monoclonal antibodies (MAbs) specific for RSV are expected to retain the desirable properties of human immunoglobulin products including long serum half-life, distribution to the lungs upon parenteral administration, and the absence of significant immunogenicity, while demonstrating additional clinical advantages. The uniform specificity of MAbs for a protective epitope on the virus is expected to significantly improve potency relative to polyclonal immune globulin preparations allowing significant reduction of intravenous dosing volumes and the potential for development of intramuscular formulations. Higher potency MAbs may also be efficacious for the treatment of established RSV infection, where significantly higher neutralization titers are expected to be required for protection. Further, recombinant MAbs should offer significant safety advantages over the administration of large volumes of human blood-derived products. The most advanced RSV-specific reshaped human antibody currently in clinical development, RSHZ19, is described below.

---

* Registered trademark of MedImmune, Inc., Gaithersburg, MD.

13.2 RSHZ19, A RESHAPED HUMAN ANTIBODY SPECIFIC FOR RSV

Two major surface RSV glycoproteins, F (fusion) and G, are the targets of neutralizing antibodies generated in response to natural RSV infection. The F protein is well conserved antigenically and has ≥90% amino acid sequence homology among RSV strains. In contrast, G protein sequences from various strains differ by as much as 50%, and the consequent antigenic variation defines two major viral subgroups A and B.[13] Antigenic variants with the A and B subgroups have been further defined based on reactivity to a panel of F and G protein-specific MAbs.[14] As both the A and B subgroups can cause RSV infections and epidemics worldwide, it is imperative that a MAb be broadly cross-reactive for all virus strains regardless of antigenic subtype. The majority of F protein-specific MAbs described are cross-reactive for RSV isolates in the A and B subgroups, whereas most G protein-specific MAbs are subgroup specific.[15-17]

The RSV G surface glycoprotein is required for virus attachment to permissive cells while the F and SH surface proteins are required for fusion of virus-infected cells to form multinucleated giant cells, or syncytia. A subset of F or G protein-specific MAbs can neutralize virus infection when the virus and MAb are mixed together prior to co-culture with permissive cells. A further subset of F protein-specific MAbs also inhibit syncytia formation, as measured by inhibition of the formation of multinucleated giant cells when added to cell cultures 24 h post-infection. Examination of a panel of F protein-specific neutralizing MAbs demonstrated that the subset which also inhibited syncytia formation was the most effective *in vivo* when administered to mice either prophylactically, or up to 4 days post-infection with RSV.[16] Thus, the *in vitro* property of fusion-inhibition appears to correlate with the ability of F protein-specific MAbs to inhibit the spread of RSV between infected cells *in vivo*. The mechanistic basis for the protection mediated by G protein-specific MAbs in mouse models is less clear, as the majority of protective MAbs were not neutralizing *in vitro*.[17]

The murine MAb selected for humanization, MAb 19, recognized a defined epitope on the RSV F protein, had potent neutralizing and fusion-inhibiting activity *in vitro*, recognized a panel of RSV subgroup A and B isolates, and both prevented and cleared RSV infection in mice.[16,18] The reshaped human MAb, RSHZ19, was constructed by grafting the antigen-binding hypervariable complementarity determining regions (CDRs) from MAb 19 into human IgG heavy and kappa light chain variable region frameworks.[18] To retain the binding affinity

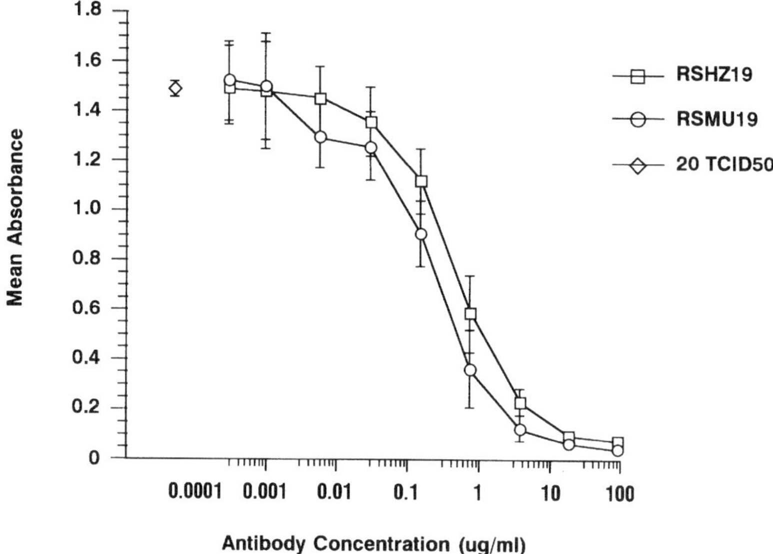

FIGURE 1
Equipotent neutralizing activity of the reshaped human MAb RSHZ19 vs. the parent murine MAb 19. MAbs were titrated against subgroup A RSV Long strain (20 $TCID_{50}$) in a microneutralization assay.[37] Virus growth was determined by ELISA using biotin-labeled anti-F protein antibody and ED_{50}s were calculated as the reciprocal of the dilution which caused a 50% reduction in ELISA signal based on the regression analysis of the sample titration.

for viral antigen observed with the parent murine MAb, minimal alterations were made in the variable region frameworks of RSHZ19 (these are described in detail by Tempest, et al.[18] where RSHZ19 is referred to as HuRSV19HFNSNK). RSHZ19 was recognized by the anti-idiotypic MAbs, B11 and B12, which were raised by immunizing calves with MAb 19,[19] providing evidence that the structural integrity and presentation of the murine CDRs are preserved after transfer to the human frameworks in RSHZ19. The antiviral potency of RSHZ19 was equivalent to the parent murine MAb 19 in viral microneutralization assays (ED_{50}s of approximately 0.5 μg/ml, Figure 1), and retained the property of blocking syncytia formation in RSV-infected cells.[18] RSHZ19 also neutralized a panel of subgroup A and B RSV clinical isolates (ED_{50} 0.1 3 μg/ml)[19] and had equal activity to the original mouse MAb *in vivo*.[18] Thus, in addition to maintaining essential structural elements required for binding to the F protein, RSHZ19 retained the key *in vitro* and *in vivo* antiviral properties of MAb 19. Preclinical and clinical results relating to safety, pharmacokinetics, and potency of RSHZ19 are reviewed below.

13.2.1 Preclinical Characterization of RSHZ19

13.2.1.1 Animal Models of RSV Infection

Prior to being isolated from infants with lower respiratory disease, human RSV was first isolated from chimpanzees with upper respiratory tract infections and was described as "chimp choryza agent."[1] Experimental studies later confirmed that infection of seronegative chimpanzees 9–23 months of age with human RSV caused upper respiratory symptoms including rhinorrhea, mild cough, and sneezing, but no lower respiratory illness or fever.[20,21] The virus replicated to high titer in nasopharyngeal and tracheal lavage samples (peak titers were 10^5–10^6 pfu/ml) and resolved by 8–13 days post-infection. High serum neutralizing antibody titers were present by 4 weeks post-infection. Studies with infant chimpanzees, which might be expected to experience lower respiratory tract disease, have not been published. Cost and the limited availability of seronegative animals have precluded extensive use of chimpanzees.

Cattle are the natural host for bovine RSV, which shares a similar pathogenesis to human RSV, causing severe lower respiratory tract infection in young calves under one year of age. Interestingly, although bovine and human RSV F protein-specific, cross-reactive, neutralizing epitopes have been described,[15,16] infection of chimpanzees with bovine RSV did not elicit protection from subsequent challenge with human RSV.[8]

The most widely used and well-characterized small animal models of RSV infection utilize adult cotton rats (*Sigmodon hispidus*)[22] or Balb/c mice.[23] While cotton rats can be infected with subgroups A and B of RSV, mice are only readily infected with subgroup A of RSV. RSV replicates for about 7–9 days in the upper and lower respiratory tract of these animals (10^4–10^5 pfu/g tissue), causes mild to moderate pulmonary histopathologic changes in the absence of overt upper or lower respiratory tract disease, and induces serum neutralizing antibody titers which correlate with resistance to reinfection. In cotton rats, titers ≥1:350 are required to completely prevent infection. This value roughly correlates to maternally derived antibody titers in young human infants who are relatively resistant to serious RSV infections (reviewed in Reference 6).

Both cotton rats and mice have been used to dissect the immunologic events leading to failure of a formalin-inactivated RSV vaccine preparation tested in the 1960s (reviewed in References 6 and 7). Children who received this RSV vaccine were not protected from RSV infection, and upon natural exposure, experienced more serious RSV disease than did controls. In the cotton rat model, enhanced lung histopathologic changes were seen following experimental RSV infection in animals that had been vaccinated with a similar formalin-inactivated

RSV vaccine preparation.[10] Studies in Balb/c mice demonstrated that CD4+ T cells elicited in response to an RSV formalin-inactivated vaccine were responsible for mediating enhanced lung histopathology.[24]

Studies in cotton rats, mice, and nonhuman primates have demonstrated that passive administration of immune globulin, or of neutralizing antibodies directed to the F or G proteins, results in protection from RSV infection, and does not enhance lung pathology following primary or secondary RSV infection.[19,25-29] In nude mice, which lack a mature thymus and are severely impaired in the ability to generate both T cell and antibody responses, there is prolonged replication of RSV, but no overt disease is observed.[30] Therefore, this model can be used to determine duration of antiviral MAb effects, since virus continues to replicate in untreated animals beyond the time at which antibody has been cleared from the circulation.

13.2.1.2 Activity of RSHZ19 in Rodent Models of RSV Infection

In Balb/c mice, intraperitoneal administration of 5 mg/kg RSHZ19 either prophylactically or therapeutically reduced peak pulmonary virus titers to below detectable levels.[18] To determine if residual, undetectable levels of virus remained in the lungs after MAb treatment, RSHZ19 was administered to immunocompromised nude mice on day 4 post-infection, and groups of mice were sacrificed at various times up to 2 months post-treatment, a time when RSHZ19 had been cleared from the circulation. Despite persistence of virus replication in untreated controls, there was no rebound of virus growth in the lungs of MAb-treated mice two months post-treatment, thus confirming that RSV infection had been eliminated.[17]

In further studies, cotton rats treated with RSHZ19 and challenged with subgroup A or B RSV strains were evaluated for pulmonary virus clearance, the impact on viral-induced pulmonary histopathology, serum concentrations of RSHZ19, and serum antiviral neutralizing titers. Prophylactic administration of 10 mg/kg RSHZ19 1 day prior to challenge with either subgroup A or B RSV strains cleared pulmonary virus from infected cotton rats to below detectable levels (Figure 2a), and reduced lung histopathology scores to control (uninfected) levels.[19] At the time of sacrifice (4 days post-infection), circulating concentrations of RSHZ19 in these animals, were approximately 50 μg/ml. Determination of the MAb concentration in lung lavages demonstrated that the amount in lavage was approximately 1% of the amount in plasma at matched time points.[19] Protective serum neutralization titers were determined to be ≥1:32, a titer significantly lower than that required for protection by polyclonal human serum immune globulin (HSIG) in cotton rats.[10,27] RSHZ19 was also efficacious in reducing lung virus by ≥2.0 $\log_{10}$ when administered on day 4 post-infection. However, in

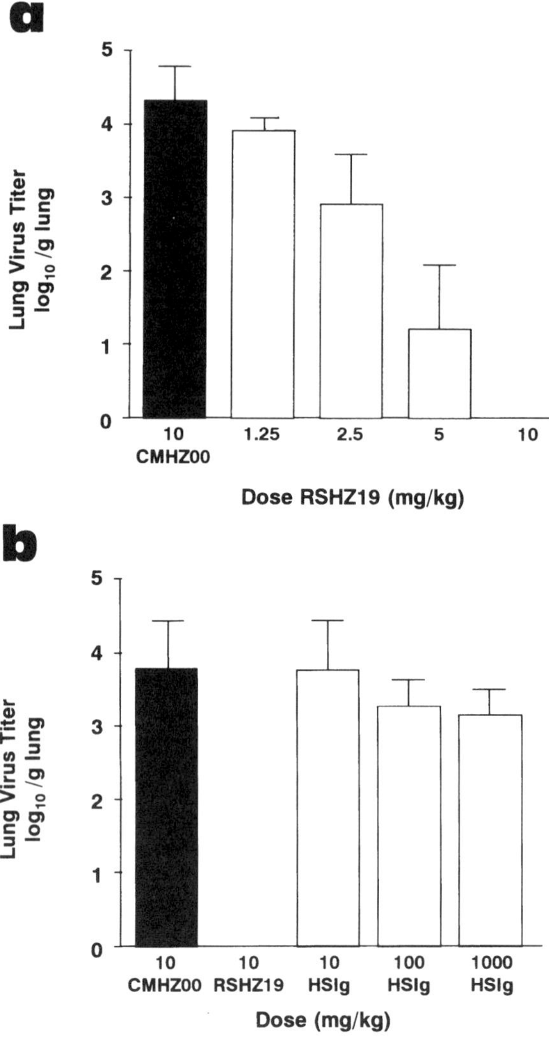

FIGURE 2

Prophylactic activity of RSHZ19 in cotton rats and comparison of activity with human serum immunoglobulin (HSIG). (a) RSHZ19 or CMHZ00 (control) MAbs were administered i.m. 24 h before challenge with RSV subgroup A or B (≥10 animals/dose group). Animals were sacrificed on day 4 post-challenge to determine lung virus titers. (b) RSHZ19, CMHZ00 (control) MAbs or HSIG were administered i.m. 24 h before challenge with RSV subgroup A or B (4 animals/dose group). Animals were sacrificed on day 4 post-challenge to determine lung virus titers. Data adapted from Reference 19.

contrast to studies in which RSHZ19 was administered prophylactically, virus clearance was not complete in all animals in the highest dose group (10 mg/kg). Despite this, pulmonary histopathology scores were reduced to control (uninfected) levels when 10 mg/kg of RSHZ19 was used to prevent or treat RSV infection.[19]

Further studies in cotton rats were done to compare directly the potency of RSHZ19 to polyclonal human immune globulin. A lot of commercially available polyclonal human serum immune globulin (HSIG) which had a relatively high *in vitro* RSV microneutralization titer (1:6400) was selected. The RSV microneutralization assay has been shown by Siber et al.[32] to be the most predictive screen for identification of human plasma samples with maximal potency for clearance of pulmonary virus in mice. The lot of HSIG identified was an intramuscular formulation, therefore, both RSHZ19 and HSIG were administered via this route in a comparative prophylaxis study. Interestingly, the fusion-inhibition titer of the HSIG was reduced fivefold relative to the neutralization titer, whereas the fusion-inhibition and neutralization titers of RSHZ19 were equivalent.[19] A dose of 10 mg/kg of RSHZ19 completely protected the lungs from RSV infection, a comparable dose of HSIG had no significant antiviral effect, while a dose of 1000 mg/kg HSIG only reduced titers by ≤1 log (Figure 2b). Despite 28-fold higher serum concentrations of human IgG in the animals dosed with 1000 mg/kg HSIG vs. 10 mg/kg RSHZ19 (1400 μg/ml vs. 50 μg/ml, respectively), serum neutralization titers in the two groups were comparable (1:64 vs. 1:78, respectively). These results suggested that the neutralizing antibodies in the polyclonal preparation are not uniformly protective *in vivo*, and demonstrated the increased potency of RSHZ19 relative to HSIG.

13.2.1.3 Preclinical and Pharmacokinetic Safety Studies in Nonhuman Primates

Preclinical safety and pharmacokinetic/toxicokinetic studies with RSHZ19 were conducted in nonhuman primates because of the relative sequence similarity between monkey and human IgG.[33] The use of primates therefore allowed for long term monitoring of pharmacokinetics and toxicity, including repeated dosing, in the absence of strong immune responses that would be expected in lower species. Toxicology and pharmacokinetic studies were conducted with RSHZ19 in adult cynomolgus macaques to support phase I clinical studies. An intravenous (i.v.) formulation of RSHZ19 was evaluated to support studies in patients hospitalized for RSV, and an intramuscular (i.m.) formulation was evaluated to support convenient prophylactic administration to high-risk infants and young children in outpatient clinics or physicians offices.

In the pharmacokinetic study, adult male cynomolgus macaques were administered single i.v. doses of RSHZ19. A biphasic decline in plasma concentration of RSHZ19 was observed, with the dominant terminal phase characterized by a half-life of approximately 21 days

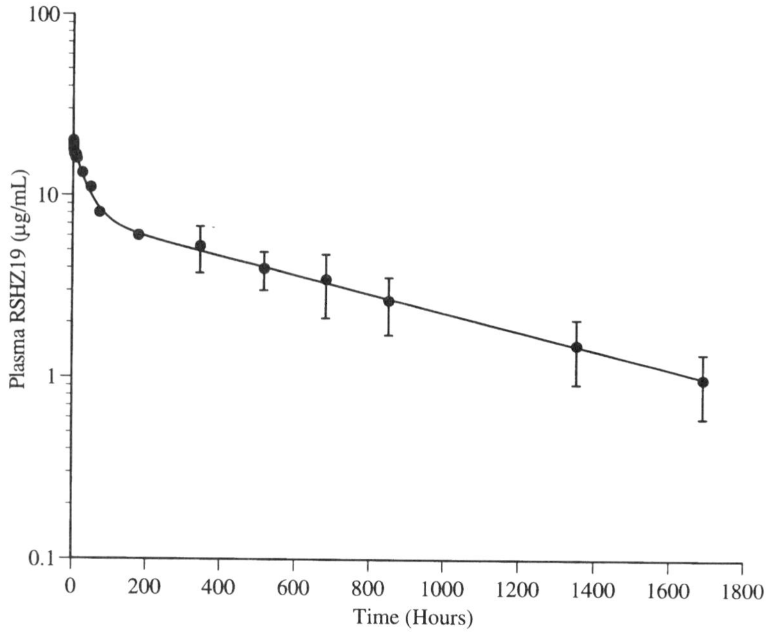

FIGURE 3
Mean (±SD) plasma concentration vs. time profiles following i.v. administration of 1 mg/kg RSHZ19 to male cynomolgus macaques (n = 3). Plasma samples were analyzed by the anti-idiotypic ELISA. The $t_{1/2}$ for the dominant terminal phase was approximately 21 days. Data adapted from Reference 34.

(Figure 3). Western blot analysis of sera from monkeys dosed with RSHZ19 demonstrated that the electrophoretic integrity of RSHZ19 was indistinguishable from that of dosing material up to 8 weeks after i.v. administration.[34] To evaluate the biological potency of RSHZ19 MAb in monkey plasma, fusion-inhibition assays were performed at 1 day, 1 week, and 1 month post-dosing in each of three animals. These studies demonstrated that, in plasma samples taken up to 1 month after i.v. administration, the apparent ED_{50} of plasma RSHZ19 (ED_{50} range of 0.54–1.95 µg/ml; calculated by dividing the MAb concentration by the fusion-inhibition titer) was equipotent to RSHZ19 dosing material.[34] Collectively, these results show that circulating levels of RSHZ19 reflect predominantly intact, biologically active MAb in monkey plasma. In the toxicology studies, the toxicokinetic profiles obtained following single i.v. doses of 50 or 200 mg/kg were consistent with the 1 mg/kg data; with the exception of one monkey from the 200 mg/kg dose group which demonstrated a sudden drop in plasma RSHZ19 concentration at day 56 post-dosing. Anti-RSHZ19 antibodies directed primarily against the human framework of RSHZ19 were detected in this animal coincident with decreases in circulating RSHZ19.[34]

Following a single i.m. administration of 20 or 40 mg/kg, absorption of RSHZ19 into the systemic circulation was essentially complete (bioavailability ≥(82%). Maximal plasma concentrations were obtained 2 to 3 days after dosing and elimination half-lives of 17–27 days were observed. Western blot analysis of plasma from monkeys administered RSHZ19 i.m. demonstrated that intact MAb was absorbed following i.m. dosing. One of three animals that received a single 40 mg/kg dose of RSHZ19 developed an anti-RSHZ19 titer, which resulted in rapid clearance of the MAb from the circulation. As observed following i.v. administration, the antibody responses were directed primarily to the human framework regions of RSHZ19.

To determine if there were any significant differences between the pharmacokinetic behavior of RSHZ19 in adult vs. infant nonhuman primates, or between males and females, studies were conducted in infant baboons.[34] RSHZ19 was administered as a slow i.v. bolus to infant baboons as 5 daily i.v. doses of 10 or 40 mg/kg. A kinetically dominant terminal elimination phase was characterized by a half-life of approximately 23 days for both dose levels. There was no evidence of marked differences in the pharmacokinetic properties of RSHZ19 between the males and females. The total systemic exposure following 5 daily i.v. doses of 10 mg/kg RSHZ19 to infant baboons was approximately the same as that observed following a single i.v. dose of 50 mg/kg to adult cynomolgus macaques suggesting that the overall pharmacokinetics were comparable in infant vs. adult monkeys at equivalent doses. Figure 4 shows computer simulations of the plasma concentration-time profiles expected following 5 daily i.v. administrations of 10 and 40 mg/kg to adult cynomolgus macaques based on the actual measured concentrations determined in animals dosed with 1 mg/kg. Superimposed on this curve, are data points representing the actual mean plasma RSHZ19 concentrations from infant baboons dosed under the same regimen. The accuracy of the simulation suggests that the pharmacokinetics of RSHZ19 in infant and adult monkeys are comparable.[34]

RSHZ19 administered i.v. or i.m. as single or repeated doses was well tolerated in both adult and infant nonhuman primates, and produced no acute or delayed toxicity over periods of approximately 85 days. Doses up to 200 mg/kg, which is 20-fold higher than the maximal clinical dose (10 mg/kg) were found to be uniformly safe and well tolerated.

13.2.2 Results of Phase I Clinical Studies with RSHZ19

An initial phase I clinical study was conducted in healthy adult male volunteers to determine if RSHZ19 dosed i.v. was safe, well tolerated, and had a circulating half-life comparable to that seen in monkeys, and typical for native human IgG. In this study, 0.025 to 10 mg/kg

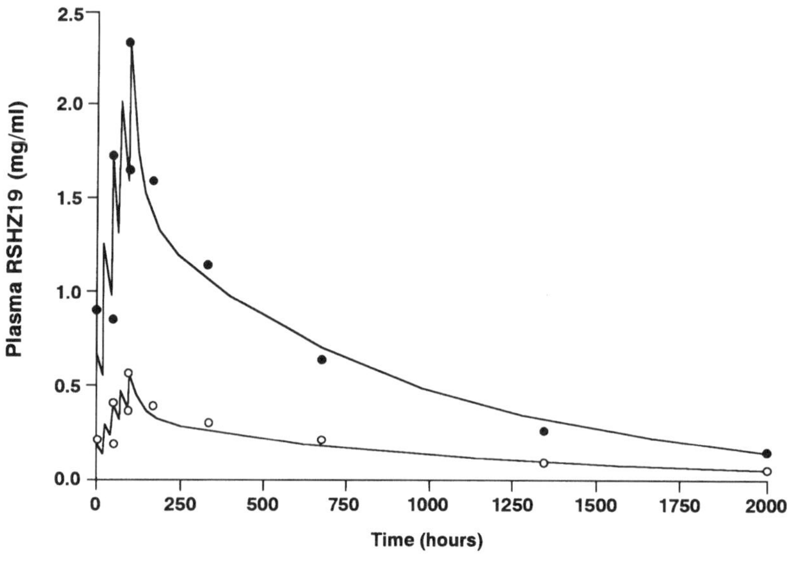

FIGURE 4
Mean (±SD) plasma concentration vs. time profiles following five daily i.v. doses of 10 (○, n = 4) and 40 (●, n = 3) mg/kg to male and female infant baboons. A model derived from single dose i.v. pharmacokinetics at 1 mg/kg in adult male cynomolgus macaques is superimposed on the data points as a solid line. Plasma samples were analyzed by the anti-idiotype ELISA. Data from Davis, C. B., Hepburn, T. W., and Urbanski, J. J., *Drug Metab. Dispos.*, 23, 10, 1028, 1995.)

RSHZ19, or placebo, were infused over 30 min, and volunteers were monitored for 10 weeks after dosing.[35] RSHZ19 was safe and well tolerated in all subjects, and no antibodies reactive with RSHZ19 were detected over the course of the study. Importantly, RSHZ19 demonstrated low plasma clearance with a long half-life of approximately 23 days consistent with endogenous IgG. Modest (threefold) increases in fusion-inhibition titers were detected in 4 of 4 subjects dosed with 10 mg/kg RSHZ19, but the proportion with detectable increases declined at lower doses RSHZ19. Since RSHZ19 serum concentration was measurable at all doses administered, it was assumed that the preexisting anti-RSV fusion-inhibition titers detected in adults precluded detection of fusion-inhibition activity specific for RSHZ19. For example, maximum plasma concentrations of approximately 200 μg/ml would be predicted for a 70-kg adult administered a 10 mg/kg i.v. bolus dose of RSHZ19 (assuming a plasma volume of 3 l). Based on the ED_{50} for RSHZ19 of approximately 1 μg/ml, a plasma RSHZ19 concentration of 200 μg/ml would correspond to a fusion-inhibition titer of 1:200, which would be difficult to detect when superimposed on the background of normal adult titers. Studies with an i.m. formulation of RSHZ19 have also been initiated.[36]

13.3 CONCLUSIONS

Preclinical studies of RSHZ19 in adult cynomolgus macaques were highly predictive of the pharmacokinetic behavior and safety profile observed in normal adults. The lack of immunogenicity of RSHZ19 in adult human subjects to date correlates with the absence of immunogenicity in the nonhuman primates administered comparable doses of RSHZ19 (≤10 mg/kg). Ongoing studies with single and repeat dosing regimens in larger numbers of subjects, and in the appropriate target populations, will further address the question of immunogenicity in humans.

Pharmacokinetic characterization of RSHZ19 was achieved via the use of a highly sensitive ELISA assay based on anti-idiotypic MAbs, which allowed the detection of RSHZ19 in human plasma in the presence of high titers of RSV-specific native IgG. Fusion-inhibition activity due to administered RSHZ19 was more difficult to detect in the context of this background in human plasma, in contrast to a preclinical study in RSV seronegative monkeys. Thus, RSHZ19 serum concentration may provide a more useful and convenient clinical surrogate marker for protective MAb levels than will functional antibody assays.

Comparative studies in cotton rats demonstrated that RSHZ19 is significantly more potent than high titer human immune serum globulin. Lower serum neutralization titers were required for lung virus clearance in animals treated with RSHZ19 vs. those reported for polyclonal globulin preparations (≥1:32 vs. ≥1:250, respectively). This presumably reflects the uniform specificity and potent antiviral activity of the MAb preparation, in contrast to the varied specificity and potencies of antibodies in the polyclonal preparation. The approximately 65-fold lower fusion-inhibition activity of the polyclonal immune globulin vs. RSHZ19 (ED_{50} = 65 μg/ml vs. 1 μg/ml, respectively) may also explain the dramatic difference in potency observed in these studies.

Collectively, the early clinical results described herein are encouraging in terms of safety, tolerability, and pharmacokinetic properties of RSHZ19 administered to normal human adults. Furthermore, as a result of the potency observed in RSV animal models, the doses of RSHZ19 being evaluated in human subjects are ≥75-fold lower than those required for effective prophylaxis with Respigam. Thus, an i.m. formulation will be available which will impact significantly on ease of administration of RSHZ19 for prophylaxis in the outpatient setting. Another consequence of the higher potency MAb will be to substantially reduce the i.v. injection volumes required for treatment of hospitalized patients. Clinical studies are going to evaluate the safety and efficacy of RSHZ19 for prophylaxis and treatment of the RSV infection in infants and young children.

ACKNOWLEDGMENTS

The authors acknowledge Sandra Griego, Charles Davis, Timothy Hart, Danuta Herzyk, Martha Chapeski, Daniel Everitt, Kathleen Thompson (SmithKline Beecham Pharmaceuticals), Geraldine Taylor (Institute for Animal Health, Compton, U.K.), Philip Wyde (Baylor College of Medicine, TX) and Michelle Leland (Southwest Foundation for Biomedical Research, TX) for technical contributions and for reviewing the manuscript. The expert advice and support of Martin Rosenberg (SmithKline Beecham Pharmaceuticals) and William Harris (University of Aberdeen, Scotland) is also gratefully acknowledged.

REFERENCES

1. Collins, P. L., Channock, R. M. and McIntosh, K., Parainfluenza viruses, in *Virology*, Field, B. N., Ed., Raven Press, New York, 1996, 1205.
2. Institute of Medicine, Appendix N: prospects for immunizing against respiratory syncytial virus, in *New Vaccine Development: Establishing Priorities Volume 1: Diseases of Importance in the United States*, National Academy Press, Washington, D.C., 1985, 397.
3. Breese Hall, C., Walsh, E. E., Long, C. E., and Schnabel, K. C., Immunity to and frequency of reinfection with respiratory syncytial virus, *J. Infect Dis.*, 163, 693, 1991.
4. Englund, J. A., Sullivan, C. J., Jordan, M. C., Dehner, L. P., Vercellotti, G. M., and Balfour, Jr., H. H., Respiratory syncytial virus infection in immuno-compromised adults, *Ann. Int. Med.*, 109, 203, 1988.
5. Committee on Infectious Diseases, Use of ribavirin in the treatment of respiratory syncytial virus in infection, *Pediatrics*, 92, 501, 1993.
6. Groothuis, J. R., The role of RSV neutralizing antibodies in the treatment and prevention of respiratory syncytial virus infection in high-risk children, *Antiviral Res.*, 23, 1, 1994.
7. Murphy, B. R., Hall, S. L., Kulkarni, A. B., Crowe, J. E., Jr., Collins, P. L., Connors, M., Karron, R. A., and Chanock, R. M., An update on approaches to the development of respiratory syncytial virus (RSV) and parainfluenza virus type 3 (PIV3) vaccines, *Virus Res.*, 32, 13, 1994.
8. Crowe, J. E., Current approaches to the development of vaccines against disease caused by respiratory syncytial virus (RSV) and parainfluenza virus (PIV). A meeting report of the WHO Programme for Vaccine Development, *Vaccine*, 13, 415, 1995.
9. Glezen, W. P., Paredes, A., Allison, J. E., Taber, L. H., and Frank, A. L., Risk of respiratory syncytial virus infection for infants from low-income families in relationship to age, sex, ethnic group, and maternal antibody level, *J. Pediatr.*, 98, 708, 1981.
10. Hemming, V. G. and Prince, G. A., Respiratory syncytial virus: babies and antibodies, *Infect. Agents Dis.*, 1, 24, 1992.
11. Groothuis, J. R., Simoes, E. A. F., Levin, M. J., Hall, C. B., Long, C. E., Rodriguez, W. J., Arrobio, J., Meissner, H. C., Fulton, D. R., Welliver, R. C., Tristram, D. A., Siber, G. R., Prince, G. A., Van Raden, M., and Hemming, V. G., Prophylactic administration of respiratory syncytial virus immune globulin to high-risk infants and young children, *N. Engl. J. Med.*, 329, 1524, 1993.

12. Groothuis, J. R., Simoes, E. A. F., and Hemming V. G., Respiratory syncytial virus (RSV) infection in preterm infants and the protection effects of RSV immune globulin (RSVIG), *Pediatrics,* 95, 463, 1995.
13. Collins, P. L., The molecular biology of respiratory syncytial virus (RSV) of the genus *pneumovirus,* in *The Paramyxoviruses,* Kingsbury, D. W., Ed., Plenum Press, New York, 1994, 103.
14. Anderson, L. J., Hierholzer, J. C., Tsou, C., Hendry, R. M., Femie, B. F., Stone, Y., and McIntosh, K., Antigenic characterization of respiratory syncytial virus strains and monoclonal antibodies, *J. Infect. Dis.,* 151, 626, 1985.
15. Beeler, J. A. and Van Wyke Coelingh, K., Neutralization epitopes of the F glycoprotein of respiratory syncytial virus: effect of mutation upon fusion function, *J. Virology,* 63, 2941, 1989.
16. Taylor, G., Stott, E. J., Furze, J., Ford, J., and Sopp, P., Protection epitopes on the fusion protein of respiratory syncytial virus recognized by murine and bovine monoclonal antibodies, *J. Gen. Virol.,* 73, 2227, 1992.
17. Taylor, G., The role of antibody in controlling and/or clearing virus infections, in *Strategies in Vaccine Design,* Ada, G. L., Ed., R. G. Landes Co., Austin, 1994, 17.
18. Tempest, P. R., Brenner, P., Lambert, M., Taylor, G., Furze, J. M., Carr, F. J., and Harris, W. J., Reshaping a human monoclonal antibody to inhibit human respiratory syncytial virus infection *in vivo, Bio/Technology,* 9, 266, 1991.
19. Wyde, P. R., Moore, D. K., Hepburn, T., Silverman, C. L., Porter, T. G., Gross, M., Taylor, G., Demuth, S. G., and Dillon, S. B., Evaluation of the protection efficacy of reshaped human monoclonal antibody RSHZ19 against respiratory syncytial virus in cotton rats, *Pediatr. Res.,* 38, 543, 1995.
20. Belshe, R. B., Richardson, L. S., London, W. T., Sly, D. L., Lorfeld, J. H., Camargo, E., Prevar, D. A., and Chanock, R. M., Experimental respiratory syncytial virus infection of four species of primates, *J. Med. Virol.,* 1, 157, 1977.
21. Crowe, J. E., Jr., Bui, P. T., London, W. T., Davis, A. R., Hung, P. P., Chanock, R. B., and Murphy, B. R., Satisfactorily attenuated and protective mutants derived from a partially attenuated cold-passaged respiratory syncytial virus mutant by introduction of additional attenuating mutations during chemical mutagenesis, *Vaccine,* 12, 691, 1994.
22. Prince, G. A., Jenson, A. B., Horswood, R. L., Camargo, E., and Chanock, R. M., The pathogenesis of respiratory syncytial virus infection in cotton rats, *Am. J. Pathol.,* 771, 1978.
23. Taylor, G., Stott, E. J., Hughes, M., and Collins, A. P., Respiratory syncytial virus infection in mice, *Infect. Immun.,* 43, 649, 1984.
24. Connors, M., Kulkarni, A. B., Firestone, C.-Y., Holmes, K. L., Morse, H. C., III, Sotnikov, A. V., and Murphy, B. R., Pulmonary histopathology induced by respiratory syncytial virus (RSV) challenge of formalin-inactivated RSV-immunized BALB/c mice is abrogated by depletion of CD4T cells, *J. Virol.,* 66, 7444, 1992.
25. Walsh, E., Schlesinger, J. J., and Bradriss, M. W., Protection from respiratory syncytial virus infection in cotton rats by passive transfer of monoclonal antibodies, *Infect. Immun.,* 43, 756, 1984.
26. Taylor G., Stott, E. J., Bew, M., Femle, B. F., Cote, P. J., Collins, A. P., Hughes, M., and Jebbett, J., Monoclonal antibodies protect against respiratory syncytial virus infection in mice, *Immunology,* 52, 137, 1984.
27. Prince, G., Hemming, V. G., Horswood, R. L., and Chanock, R. M., Immunoprophylaxis and immunotherapy of respiratory syncytial virus infection in the cotton rat, *Virus Res.,* 1 3, 193, 1985.
28. Hemming, V. G., Prince, G. A., Horswood, R. L., London, W. T., Murphy, B. R., Walsh, E. W., Fischer, G. W., Weisman, L. E., Baron, P. A., and Chanock, R. M., Studies of passive immunotherapy for infection of respiratory syncytial virus in the respiratory tract of a primate model, *J. Infect. Dis.,* 152, 1083, 1985.

29. Graham, B. S., Bunton, L. A., Rowland, J., Wright, P. F., and Karzon, D. T., Respiratory syncytial virus infection in anti-μ-treated mice, *J. Virol.*, 65, 4936, 1991.
30. Cannon, M. J., Stott, E. J., Taylor, G., and Aksonas, B. A., Clearance of persistent respiratory syncytial virus infections in immunodeficient mice following transfer of primed T Cells, *Immunology*, 62, 133, 1987.
31. Taylor, G., Porter, T., Dillon, S., Trulli, J., Ganguly, S., Hart, T., Davis, C., Wyde, P., Tempest, P., and Harris W., Anti-respiratory syncytial monoclonal antibodies show promise in the treatment and prophylaxis of viral disease. *Biochem. Soc. Trans.*, 23, 2063, 1995.
32. Siber, G. R., Leszczynski, J., Pena-Cruz, V., Ferren-Gardner, C., Anderson, R., Hemming, V. G., Walsh, E. E., Bums, J., MacIntosh, K., Gonin, R., and Anderson, L. J., Protective activity of a human respiratory syncytial virus immune globulin prepared from donors screened by microneutralization assay, *J. Infect. Dis.*, 165, 456, 1992.
33. Newman, R., Alberts, J., Anderson, D., Carner, K., Heard, C., Norton, F., Raab, R., Reff, M., Shuey, S., and Hanna, N., "Primatization" of recombinant antibodies for immunotherapy of human diseases: a macaque/human chimeric antibody against human CD4, *Bio/Technology*, 10, 1455, 1992.
34. Davis, C. B., Hepburn, T. W., Urbanski, J. J., Kwok, D. C., Hart, T. K., Herzyk, D. J., Demuth, S. G., Leland, M., and Rhodes, G. R., Pre-clinical pharmacokinetic evaluation of the respiratory syncytial virus-specific virus-specific reshaped human monoclonal antibody RSHZ19, *Drug Metab. Dispos.*, 23, 10, 1028, 1995.
35. Everitt, D., Thompson, K., DiCicco, R., Davis, C., Demuth, S., Herzyk, D. J., Ilson, B., and Jorkasky, D., Safety, pharmacokinetics, antigenicity and fusion inhibition activity of SB 209763, a reshaped human monoclonal antibody to respiratory syncytial virus, *Pediatr. Res.*, 37, 173A, 1995.
36. Thompson, K. A., Everitt, D. E., Chapelsky, M., Miller, A. K., Herzyk, D. J., and Jorkasky, D., Safety, pharmacokinetics and antigenicity of single and repeat in infections of a reshaped human monoclonal antibody (RSHZ19) in healthy volunteers, *Am. Soc. Clin. Pharm. Ther.*, in press.
37. Anderson, L. J., Hieholzer, J. R., Bingham, P. G., and Stone, Y. O., Microneutralization test for respiratory syncytial virus based on an enzyme immunoassay, *J. Clin. Microb.*, 22, 1050, 1985.

Chapter 14

CDP571, An Engineered Antibody to Human Tumor Necrosis Factor

Sue Stephens, Olivia Vetterlein, and Mark Sopwith

CONTENTS

0-8493-8547-4/97/$0.00+$.50

14.1 INTRODUCTION

Tumor necrosis factor α (TNF-α) is a proinflammatory cytokine produced by many cells, including those of the monocyte/macrophage lineage and to a lesser extent T cells, neutrophils, and mast cells. It has a molecular weight of 17,350 and is secreted as a trimer.[1] TNF-α is an important regulatory molecule and interacts with a variety of cells via p55 or p75 TNF-α receptors.[2,3] Excess TNF-α production, however, can have adverse effects, and has been implicated in the pathology of several human diseases, including septic shock,[4,5] rheumatoid arthritis,[6,7] transplant rejection,[8] graft-versus-host disease (GVHD),[9,10] diabetes,[11] multiple sclerosis,[12] and inflammatory bowel disease (IBD).[13] The potential for neutralization of excess TNF-α by the use of monoclonal antibodies (MAbs) has been explored using a variety of animal models.[14-19] Factors contributing to the outcome of these studies are dose and potency of the antibody, the isotype used, the circulating half-life, and immunogenicity. We have taken these points into consideration when developing an engineered antibody to human TNF-α for use in man. This chapter will describe the selection and engineering of a murine antibody, preclinical studies in primates, and early studies in man, including healthy human volunteers and patients with acute and chronic diseases.

14.2 GENERATION OF ENGINEERED HUMAN ANTIBODY (CDP571)

Monoclonal antibodies to recombinant human TNF-α (rhTNF-α) were raised in Balb/c mice and screened in microtiter plates coated with TNF-α. Positive hybridomas were compared for TNF-α neutralizing activity in a cytotoxicity assay using L929 murine fibroblast cells. Genes for the most potent antibody (CB0010), were isolated from a cDNA library and their sequences determined. Complementarity determining regions (CDRs), together with framework residues, defined by a computer graphic model as being capable of affecting antigen-binding activity, were transferred into the framework of the human antibody Eu with human κ light and γ4 heavy chain constant regions.[20] The selection of constant region isotype was based on comparisons of effector functions using murine disease models and chimeric versions of the hamster anti-mouse TNF-α antibody TN3 19.12 expressed with mouse constant regions. In models of lipopolysaccharide (LPS) induced shock or sepsis resulting from *Pseudomonas* infection, the inactive (in terms of complement fixation and Fc receptor binding) mouse isotype (γ1) was more effective in reducing mortality than the active isotype (mouse γ2a).[21] In models of colonic inflammation and collagen-induced arthritis, both isotypes were equally protective.[18,22] In addition, comparisons of human γ4 and γ1 isotypes in an rhTNF-α-induced rabbit pyrexia model showed that immune complexes of TNF-α with γ1 (active) isotype-generated secondary effector functions via Fc receptor binding or complement activation, resulting in increased pyrexia compared with TNF-α/saline controls. The γ4 (inactive) isotype showed a dose-dependent inhibition of pyrexia, confirming the benefit of selection of the inactive isotype.[21]

An expression vector was constructed with a glutamine synthetase selectable marker as described previously[20] and the plasmid was transferred into NS0 myeloma cells and glutamine-independent transfectants isolated. The engineered antibody retained the full binding and biological activity for TNF-α and was demonstrated to cross-react with nonhuman primate TNF-α.

14.3 PRECLINICAL STUDIES WITH CDP571 IN NONHUMAN PRIMATES

CDP571 was investigated for potency in a lethal model of *E. coli*-induced sepsis in baboons.[23] Control animals received saline, followed 2 h later by 2×10^9 log-phase *E. coli*. Animals were maintained under intensive care conditions with instrumentation (for measurement of mean arterial pressure (MAP), pulmonary arterial and wedge pressure, and cardiac output) and fluid replacement when required. Mortality was 87.5% (7/8) within 72 h, circulating TNF-α levels were as high as 15 ng/ml, and IL-6 and IL-8 were also raised. Six animals were pretreated with CDP571 at 1 mg/kg and 6 with 0.1 mg/kg. Mortality was reduced to 0 and 33% respectively, base deficit and plasma lactate levels were reduced, circulating TNF-α was undetectable, and IL-6 and IL-8 levels were substantially decreased. Anti-TNF-α treatment also prevented falls in MAP, cardiac index, and stroke volume ratio and reduced or prevented organ damage in the liver, lungs, adrenals, kidney, and brain, indicating that anti-TNF-α can prevent morbidity and mortality in a baboon model of septic shock.

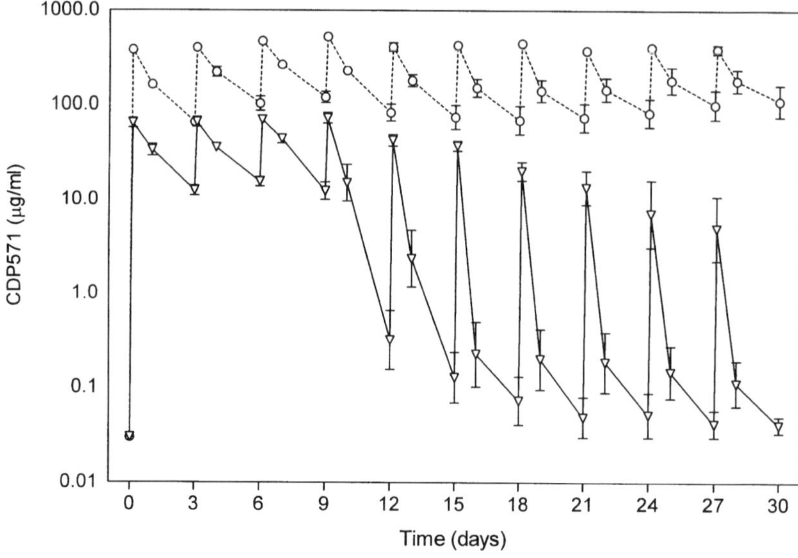

FIGURE 1
CDP571 plasma levels in cynomolgus monkeys following ten infusions at 3-day intervals at the following doses: —∇— 4.0 mg/kg (n = 8) ···○··· 20.0 mg/kg (n = 7).

Preclinical studies of CDP571 were performed in cynomolgus monkeys. In the initial experiments, the engineered antibody was compared with the murine parent (CB0010) for pharmacokinetics and immunogenicity. Following a single dose of 0.1 mg/kg, the half-life of CDP571 was increased from 27 to 66 h and immunogenicity was reduced by more than 90% compared to CB0010. Immune responses to the constant regions were absent and responses to the idiotype were considerably reduced.[20] In a second study, repeated doses of 4 and 20 mg/kg were administered at 72-h intervals for 30 days. The pharmacokinetic profiles (Figure 1) indicate that at 20 mg/kg, peak and trough antibody levels in 7/8 animals remained constant throughout the dosing period and antibodies to CDP571 were low or undetectable. One animal in the 20 mg/kg group mounted a strong anti-CDP571 response. At 4 mg/kg, peak and trough antibody levels declined from the fourth dose onward and this coincided with the development of antibodies to the idiotype and, in some animals, to constant and/or framework regions. This suggests that the non-responsiveness at 20 mg/kg may be due to high dose tolerance.

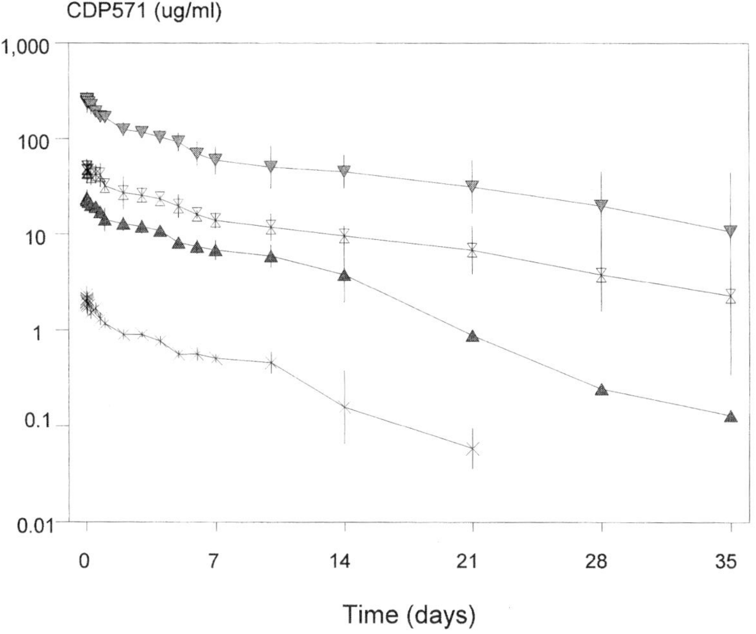

FIGURE 2
CDP571 plasma levels in human volunteers (n = 6) following a single infusion at the following doses: × 0.1 mg/kg ▲ 1.0 mg/kg ⧖ 2.0 mg/kg ▼ 10.0 mg/kg

14.4 SAFETY STUDIES IN HUMAN VOLUNTEERS, PHARMACOKINETICS AND IMMUNOGENICITY OF CDP571

CDP571 was infused into 24 healthy male volunteers in a dose-escalating, placebo-blinded study to examine safety, pharmacokinetics, and immunogenicity of the antibody. All infusions were well tolerated and there was no evidence of any unwanted effects. The antibody was eliminated with a half-life ranging from 5 days at the lowest dose (0.1 mg/kg) to 14 days at higher doses (up to 10 mg/kg; Figure 2). Antibodies to CDP571 were detectable in volunteers receiving lower doses but decreased with increasing dose (Figure 3). These antibodies were predominantly IgM (in contrast to the cynomolgus monkey where there was a switch to IgG) and were directed entirely against the idiotype.[20] Circulating CDP571 remained detectable in the plasma after the fall in titer of these antibodies and was still able to bind TNF-α.

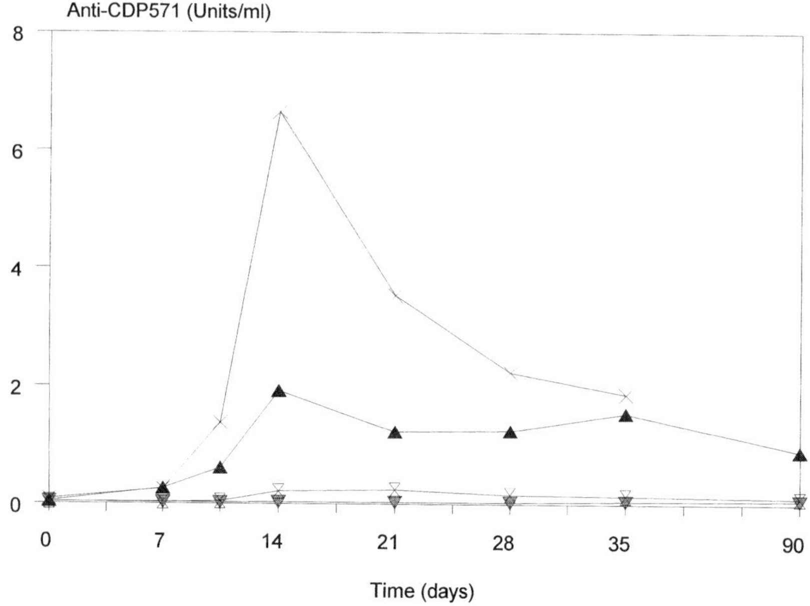

FIGURE 3
Anti-CDP571 antibodies in human volunteers (n = 6) after a single infusion of CDP571 at the following doses: × 0.1 mg/kg ▲ 1.0 mg/kg ⧖ 2.0 mg/kg ▼ 10.0 mg/kg

14.5 SINGLE DOSE PHASE IIa STUDIES IN SEPTIC SHOCK

Sepsis syndrome and septic shock are diseases which present in a wide variety of forms ranging from acute diseases such as meningococcal meningitis to more chronic presentations such as sepsis associated with cancer or surgical trauma. All presentations still have high mortality rates (40 to 60%), in spite of the availability of appropriate antibiotic treatment for gram-positive and -negative infections. Recent trials of therapy with MAbs to endotoxin have been disappointing[24,25] in spite of promising early trials with polyclonal antibodies to endotoxin core glycolipid.[26] The problems with these agents are compounded by the fact that a high percentage of septic shock cases follow infections with Gram-positive organisms,[27] where endotoxin is not implicated and the antibodies will not have therapeutic benefit in these patients (and in fact may have deleterious effects[28]). A more general approach is to neutralize one of the mediators of septic shock. There is now substantial evidence that TNF-α is one of the key cytokines involved in the pathogenesis of the disease. First, TNF-α has been demonstrated in the plasma of patients with septic shock and high levels tend to be prognostic of mortality.[29-32] The symptoms of septic shock, such as fall in systemic blood pressure and multiple organ injury, can be reproduced by injection of TNF-α into animals or humans[5,14] and thirdly, blockade of TNF-α can reduce morbidity and mortality in animal models of septic shock.[33,34] Recent trials in sepsis syndrome with a murine antibody to human TNF-α (BAYX1351) have been encouraging, with a reduction in mortality in patients with shock of 48.7% at 3 days ($p = 0.004$) and 17.1% at 28 days ($p = 0.2$) for the 7.5 mg/kg group.[35] Patients without shock did not show benefit and therefore a further phase III trial is currently in progress including only patients with shock.

CDP571 has been examined in a placebo-controlled safety study of 42 patients with septic shock.[36] The antibody was infused at 0.1, 0.3, 1, or 3 mg/kg, and although there were differences in cytokine levels between groups at entry into the study, CDP571 infusion caused a rapid reduction in circulating TNF-α with concomitant decreases in IL-1β and IL-6 (see Table 1). The numbers in each dose group were too small to show any significant differences in mortality; however, there were no adverse events attributable to administration of the antibody. The elimination half-life was approximately 6 days which is longer than murine antibodies (40–55 h[37]) and also than other cytokine antagonists such as TNF-α receptor-immunoglobulin constructs[38] and IL-1 receptor antagonists[39] currently being evaluated in the clinic. This extended half-life may have the benefit of providing prolonged anti-TNF-α cover during the critical days following the onset of septic shock. Further work is continuing with this indication although it is clear from previous studies that this is a complex, heterogeneous disease and care needs to be taken in prospectively selecting the patients most likely to benefit from intervention.[35,40]

14.6 STUDIES IN INFLAMMATORY BOWEL DISEASE (IBD)

Cytokines, including TNF-α, have been shown to be increased in the plasma,[13] stools,[41] and the lamina propria[42] of patients with IBD compared with normal individuals and are thought to be involved in the pathology of both Crohn's disease and ulcerative colitis. Animal models of these diseases are generally colonic inflammation generated by local application of irritants such as acetic acid[18] or carrageenan, which induce a pathology which is transient and unlike human IBD. However, TNF-α has been detected in these models[43] and anti-TNF-α MAbs can block the induced inflammation.[18] A more relevant model of human IBD can be seen in cotton-top tamarin monkeys, a proportion of which develop a spontaneous colitis which resembles human ulcerative colitis.[44] This disease is characterized by acute inflammation, neutrophil infiltration in the lamina propria, and development of crypt abscesses. This is associated with diarrhea and weight loss and may

TABLE 1

Cytokine Levels in Plasma from Patients with Septic Shock before and after Receiving CDP571

Time relative to CDP571	CDP571 Dose (mg/kg)				
	Placebo	0.1	0.3	1.0	3.0
TNF-α					
Pre	42.2 (17.8–100.4)	142.0 (44.1–456.6)	132.2 (20.2–866.4)	142.4 (76.2–266.1)	27.4 (10.4–71.7)
0.5 h	37.4 (17.4–80.4)	13.3 (4.4–40.3)	7.7 (1.0–57.3)	4.9 (2.2–11.0)	2.2 (1.7–2.9)
% Reduction	11.4	91.6	94.2	96.6	91.8
IL-1β					
Pre	1.29 (0.6–2.7)	1.19 (0.4–3.3)	6.54 (1.0–41.5)	4.24 (1.7–10.9)	0.85 (0.4–1.7)
24 h	1.25 (0.6–2.6)	0.76 (0.4–1.5)	1.83 (0.1–66.0)	1.18 (0.6–2.5)	0.69 (0.4–1.2)
% Reduction	3.1	36.1	72.0	72.2	18.8
IL-6					
Pre	990 (278–3522)	1048 (206–5318)	10352 (469–228418)	7108 (1344–37589)	409 (96–1736)
24 h	562 (185–1709)	471 (188–1180)	1504 (76–29423)	1532 (273–8592)	145 (40–529)
% Reduction	43.2	55.1	85.5	78.4	64.5

Note: Results are expressed as geometric means in pg/ml (± 95% confidence intervals).

result in death if untreated. The current best treatment is olsalazine or prednisolone, although a proportion of animals become resistant to treatment. TNF-α levels in stools of diseased animals are raised compared with healthy controls, and a single dose of CDP571 has been shown to have benefit in reversing the diarrhea.[45] We have now treated 6 animals who developed symptoms of disease with 6 repeated doses of CDP571 at 20 mg/kg given intramuscularly every 6 days. No adverse events were seen following administration of antibody, either locally or systemically. All animals showed a rapid improvement following the first dose, with an increase in body weight, a fall in rectal biopsy score, and improvement in fecal stool quality. Body weight continued to rise throughout the period of therapy and was maintained for the month of followup. Rectal biopsy scores were significantly improved by day 12 ($p < 0.05$) and this was maintained for a further 5 weeks. Of the 6 animals recruited to the study, the majority (4/6) have not required further treatment for the 2 years following the last dose. This response is more rapid than that seen to the established therapy using olsalazine and the prolonged nature of the benefit suggests that the antibody is exerting a disease modifying effect. Clinical studies in Crohn's disease in man with a chimeric anti-TNF-α (cA2) have given encouraging results.[46] CDP571 has now been evaluated as a single dose of 5 mg/kg in 20 patients with active Crohn's disease in a placebo-blinded study.[47] Disease activity was monitored using the Harvey Bradshaw index (HB), Crohn's Disease Activity Index (CDAI), and C-reactive protein (CRP). In the CDP571 treated group, median HB fell from 10 to 5 by week 2 (p <0.001), CDAI fell from 263 to 167 (p <0.001), and CRP fell from 12.5 to 6. Corresponding values for pretreatment and 2-week assessments in the placebo group (n = 10) were HB 6.5 to 6.5, CDAI 253 to 247, and CRP 6 to 7. In the CDP571 group, 6 patients were considered to be in remission (CDAI < 150) and a further 3 patients had CDAI ≤ 156 at 2 weeks, the corresponding numbers for placebo being 0 and 1. Improvements seen were maximal at 2 weeks but some patients continued to show benefit for the 8 weeks of the study.

An additional open study was conducted in 15 patients with mild/moderate ulcerative colitis.[48] Patients were treated with a single i.v. infusion of CDP571 at 5 mg/kg and their disease assessed by Powell-Tuck score, CRP, diary card (number of liquid stools), sigmoidoscopy, and histology. A consistent reduction in disease activity was seen for all parameters. By 1 week, the mean Powell-Tuck score had fallen from 6.4 to 4.7, CRP fell from 20.4 to 9.1, and mean number of stools per day had decreased from 6.1 to 4.8. Sigmoidoscopy was not performed at week 1, but by week 2 the mean score had fallen from 2.3 to 1.2. These benefits persisted for several weeks.

These preliminary studies support the suggestion that anti-TNF-α antibodies have therapeutic potential in IBD and larger studies are now required to confirm this.

14.7 SINGLE AND REPEAT DOSING STUDIES IN PATIENTS WITH RHEUMATOID ARTHRITIS

Within the rheumatoid joint, TNFα is expressed by macrophages, T lymphocytes, cells that have fibroblast characteristics, and by vascular endothelial cells. TNFα expression is increased especially at the pannus-cartilage junction where joint destruction is particularly active.[49,50] Effects which suggest that TNF-α may contribute to the inflammation and joint destruction which characterize the course of the disease are the recruitment of cells into regions of inflammation, upregulation of adhesion molecules (e.g., E-selectin, VCAM, ICAMs, CD18), stimulation of chemokine expression (e.g., RANTES, IL-8, PAF),[51-56] and direct activation of leukocytes.[57] TNF-α also upregulates MHC class I and class II expression and stimulates prostaglandin and nitric oxide synthesis.[58] It is probably through these actions and the upregulation of tissue matrix metalloproteinase expression that TNF-α-mediated osteoclast activation can result in the resorption of cartilage and bone.[59] In promoting cartilage degradation, the activity of TNF-α is increased by IL-1, which in the rheumatoid joint, may itself be under the control of TNF-α.[55] TNF-α activities such as the stimulation of angiogenesis and synoviocyte proliferation[60] suggest a longer term contribution to the disease process. Lastly, TNF-α may contribute to the systemic symptoms and ill-health suffered by patients with rheumatoid arthritis.

Evidence of a more direct kind in favor of TNF-α's participation in joint disease has been obtained in three separate animal models of arthritis, in which antibodies that neutralize the cytokine are able not only to prevent the onset of arthritis but to ameliorate on-going disease.[61-63]

14.7.1 DESCRIPTION OF CLINICAL STUDY

Thirty-six patients with currently active disease were enrolled at two centers in London according to the criteria described previously.[64] Screened patients were infused with CDP571 as a single dose at 0.1, 1, or 10 mg/kg over a period of 1 h. In each group of 12 patients, 8 were randomized in a blinded fashion to receive CDP571 and 4 to receive a matching solution of human serum albumin as placebo. Assessments were conducted 1–3 weeks prior to receiving treatment, and at 1, 2, 4, and 8 weeks after. Disease activity was measured using the European League Against Rheumatism core criteria, which included assessor scores of the number of tender and swollen joints (maximum 28 joints); the duration of early morning stiffness (EMS) and patients' own assessment of pain and disease activity (using visual analog scales); and ESR and CRP. To assess each patient's response to treatment, the Disease Activity Score was calculated from the number of tender and swollen joints, ESR, and patient's own assessment of disease activity. Before the start of the study, the assessors all attended a workshop to standardize their examination technique. Plasma IL-6, circulating CDP571 concentrations, and immune response were also measured. More speculatively, circulating levels of stromelysin (a matrix metalloproteinase whose circulating concentration has been shown to be elevated in patients with rheumatoid arthritis) and the urinary excretion of pyridinoline and deoxypyridinoline (that reflect predominantly the degradation of type I and type II collagen as markers of bone and cartilage degradation, respectively) and of the N telopeptide of type I collagen were measured.

The second part of the study was conducted in open fashion. Patients who had experienced no untoward effect after the first infusion of investigational drug were invited to enter a continuation phase. In this phase 30 patients received either 1 or 10 mg/kg CDP571 and were assessed over 8 weeks as before.

Finally, in response to investigator and patient request, the study was extended beyond the original protocol. Sixteen patients received a third infusion and 14 patients received a fourth infusion, at whichever dosage level of CDP571 had been allocated to each at the second infusion. Concomitant medication was less closely controlled. After third and fourth administrations of CDP571 to this selected patient group, safety monitoring and blood sampling only were undertaken.

A statistical analysis was carried out for the initial randomized, placebo-controlled phase of the study. The analysis was an intent-to-treat analysis. At each time point, the Kruskal-Wallis test was used to compare the median changes from preinfusion between the four groups for the variables measured. If this overall test showed significant or borderline significant differences between the groups, the Mann-Whitney U test was used to compare the median changes from preinfusion in each CDP571 group to the change in the placebo group. The Bonferroni method was used to adjust the p values to take into account the multiple comparisons.

14.7.2 Results of Clinical Study

The results of key variables after the first and second infusions of investigational drug are summarized in Tables 2 and 3.

First infusion — Patients who received placebo did not improve. In contrast, there was a dose-dependent effect of CDP571 treatment with maximum patient responses after 10 mg/kg. After CDP571 10 mg/kg, the median tender joint score was reduced from 16.5 to 10–11 joints at weeks 1–4; and by week 8 the median score of 12 joints was still reduced from baseline. At this dosage, the reduction in median number of tender joints at week 2 was statistically significant vs. the placebo group ($p = 0.048$, adjusted). The median number of swollen joints fell by between 2 and 5 joints for up to 4 weeks, but no difference was statistically significant. All patients who received CDP571 scored a reduction in pain scale by week 1. After 10 mg/kg CDP571, the pain score was reduced by a maximum of 40% by 2 weeks (difference from the placebo group statistically significant, $p = 0.024$, adjusted), with evidence of improvement still at 8 weeks. Patient's global assessment of disease activity showed dose-dependent reductions, the change at week 1 after both 1 and 10 mg/kg being of borderline statistical significance vs. the placebo group ($p = 0.099$ and 0.153, respectively, adjusted). There was a trend to reduction in the duration of early morning stiffness after 10 mg/kg CDP571.

TABLE 2

Results in Rheumatoid Arthritis Patients Following First Infusion of CDP571 at 1 mg/kg or 10 mg/kg or Placebo

	Placebo					1 mg/kg Group					10 mg/kg Group				
Visit	N	Tender Joints	Swollen Joints	Pain (cm)	CRP (mg/l)	N	Tender Joints	Swollen Joints	Pain (cm)	CRP (mg/l)	N	Tender Joints	Swollen Joints	Pain (cm)	CRP (mg/l)
Pre	12	12.5	17.5	6.2	80.0	8	16.0	15.0	5.5	37.0	8	16.5	16.5	8.4	50.5
-infusion		(7–28)	(7–24)	(3.2–8)	(6–142)		(3–28)	(6–22)	(4.1–8.3)	(13–116)		(10–28)	(8–25)	(2.9–9.9)	(3–118)
Week 1	12	13.0	17.0	5.7	68.5	8	17.0	16.5	4.2	10.5	8	11.0	11.5	4.3	11.0
		(7–28)	(5–25)	(1.7–7.8)	(4–135)		(0–24)	(7–20)	(1.6–6.3)	(2–61)		(3–28)	(7–25)	(0.6–9.7)	(2–22)
Week 2	12	14.5	16.0	7.9	59.0	8	14.0	16.0	5.0	12.5	8	11.0	11.5	3.6	12.5
		(9–28)	(7–25)	(0.8–9.5)	(2–104)		(0–27)	(10–23)	(2.0–8.3)	(3–62)		(3–28)	(10–25)	(0.9–9.9)	(1–30)
Week 4	11	16.0	20.0	5.5	55.0	7	15.0	17.0	7.7	41.0	8	10.0	14.0	5.7	19.0
		(4–28)	(0–26)	(1.4–9.1)	(3–118)		(1–21)	(2–24)	(1.4–8.6)	(4–128)		(2–28)	(6–25)	(0.2–9.9)	(1–30)
Week 8	11	20.0	19.0	8.5	31.0	7	13.0	17.0	8.3	37.0	8	12.0	14.5	7.2	27.5
		(2–28)	(2–25)	(0–9.9)	(2–115)		(4–26)	(5–23)	(6.6–9.7)	(11–152)		(2–28)	(8–24)	(0.6–9.5)	(1–47)

TABLE 3

Results in Rheumatoid Arthritis Patients Following Second Infusion of CDP571 at 1 mg/kg or 10 mg/kg

	1 mg/kg Group					10 mg/kg Group				
Visit	N	Tender Joints	Swollen Joints	Pain (cm)	CRP (mg/l)	N	Tender Joints	Swollen Joints	Pain (cm)	CRP (mg/l)
Pre-infusion	17	13.0 (2–28)	18.0 (6–25)	8.3 (0.8–9.8)	48.0 (3–151)	12	20.0 (4–28)	19.5 (3–24)	7.6 (0.5–9.7)	40.0 (2–120)
Week 1	16	9.5 (0–28)	17.5 (2–25)	4.6 (0.3–9.7)	24.0 (2–169)	12	7.0 (1–28)	14.0 (2–22)	3.15 (0–7.5)	5.0 (1–125)
Week 2	15	7.0 (1–28)	16.0 (2–27)	4.1 (0.3–9.8)	20.0 (5–160)	12	6.5 (2–28)	13.5 (5–24)	2.15 (0.2–9.1)	11.5 (1–107)
Week 4	13	11.0 (0–28)	18.0 (4–25)	4.0 (0.3–9.6)	21.0 (1–125)	12	4.0 (0–28)	13.0 (3–23)	1.65 (0.4–9.8)	13.50 (1–192)
Week 8	11	13.0 (1–28)	17.0 (4–26)	5.6 (0–9.9)	34.5 (3–135)	12	11.0 (0–28)	19.5 (0–25)	7.2 (0.2–9.9)	44.5 (2–111)

Of the changes in laboratory variables, the fall in CRP was the most marked. At dosages of 1 and 10 mg/kg of CDP571, median CRP concentrations were reduced at week 1 virtually to within the normal range. These reductions in CRP appeared to be sustained for up to 8 weeks in the 10 mg/kg group. At week 1, the change after CDP571 10 mg/kg was of borderline statistical significance ($p = 0.057$, adjusted).

The changes in ESR were proportionally less great, but after 1 and 10 mg/kg median ESR values were reduced at week 1 and the fall appeared sustained for 4–8 weeks. At week 2, the change in ESR after CDP571 10 mg/kg was statistically significant vs. the placebo group ($p = 0.015$, adjusted). These reductions in acute phase response were paralleled by reductions in circulating IL-6. Finally, after CDP571 there were dose-dependent trends to reduction in circulating stromelysin supported by consistent dose-dependent trends to reduction in urinary excretion of pyridinoline and deoxypyridinoline collagen cross-links and of type I N-telopeptide. After 1 and 10 mg/kg CDP571, the median stromelysin concentration was reduced from baseline by a maximum of 25–45% at weeks 1 and 2; and after 10 mg/kg CDP571 the concentration at week 8 was still less than the value at baseline. In parallel, the urinary excretion of all three collagen degradation fragments was reduced by 20–30% one week after 10 mg/kg CDP571 and their excretion at week 8 was still less than baseline. CDP571 was well tolerated, reports of symptoms during the infusion being of similar frequency in the treated and placebo groups. During followup, fewer adverse events occurred in the CDP571-treated groups than after placebo.

Second infusion — In this open continuation phase, patients received either 1 or 10 mg/kg CDP571. For simplicity, results in Table 3 are presented as the outcome of the two second infusion dosage groups; a more detailed breakdown into small subsets depending on the dosage received as first infusion has not been shown.

Patients' rheumatoid arthritis improved. The reductions noted in assessor endpoints and in patients' own scores were supported by reductions in the laboratory variables ESR and CRP (which in turn were paralleled by a reduction in circulating IL-6). The changes after treatment were somewhat greater after 10 mg/kg than after 1 mg/kg. Inspection of individual patient data over the duration of the first and second infusions suggested that patients who had received 10 mg/kg on both occasions were especially benefited. The maximum reduction in median serum stromelysin was 20–40% at weeks 1 and 2; and after 10 mg/kg CDP571 the stromelysin concentration at week 8 was still less than the value before the second infusion. The urinary excretion of collagen fragments was not measured after the second infusion.

During the course of followup after the second infusion, a total of 8 patients withdrew because disease progression occurred that required modification to their arthritis therapy. Of these 8 patients, 6 had received 1 mg/kg CDP571 and 2 had received 10 mg/kg.

Third and fourth infusions — In this open extension phase a selected group of patients received further infusions of CDP571 in response to their own request and that of the investigator. Clinical assessments were not made, but safety monitoring continued.

After infusions of either 1 and 10 mg/kg, the laboratory variables ESR and CRP were once more reduced. The lowest levels were achieved after repeated administrations of 10 mg/kg CDP571. Again, these diminutions in acute phase response were paralleled by reductions in IL-6. Repeated infusions of CDP571 at these dosage levels were generally very well tolerated.

14.7.3 Pharmacokinetics

Because of the study design (placebo, 0.1, 1 or 10.0 mg/kg in the first phase and then randomization to 1 or 10 mg/kg) and the voluntary nature of the study extension, the numbers of patients receiving the same 4 doses was small. Figure 4 shows the mean elimination profiles for all patients receiving each dose in the relevant cycle, regardless of which dose of CDP571 they received in the first cycle. The overall elimination rate does not change after repeated doses with approximate half-lives calculated as 6 days. Although the low numbers make detailed analysis difficult, some general observations are relevant when examining individual patients (Figure 5). Three patients completed 4 cycles with 10 mg/kg, and a typical pharmacokinetic profile is illustrated in panel a. Consistent or prolonged elimination profiles were observed, with CDP571 still detectable 8 weeks after the fourth infusion. Two of three patients receiving 3 cycles at 10 mg/kg gave similar profiles and the remaining patient had slightly accelerated clearance of CDP571 following the second and third dose (panel b). One patient received 10 mg/kg in the first cycle followed by 3 repeated doses at 1 mg/kg and again showed constant elimination rates (panel c). Patients receiving 1 mg/kg in the first cycle followed by 1 or 10 mg/kg, varied in their responses, with some showing constant elimination rates (panel d) and others showing increased clearance rates (panel e). Those receiving 0.1 mg/kg in the first cycle generally showed accelerated clearance in the second cycle, whether they subsequently received 1 or 10 mg/kg (panel f).

14.7.4 Immunogenicity

Most patients produced detectable antibodies to CDP571 at some time point during their course of therapy, but there was variation in

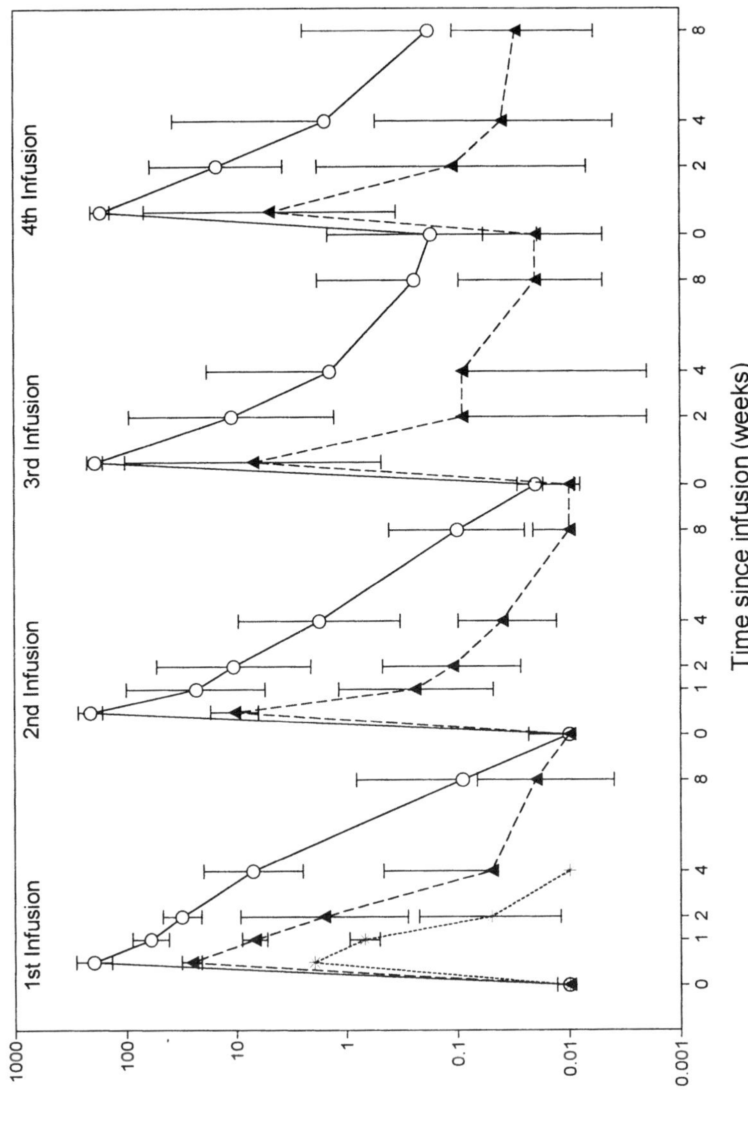

FIGURE 4
CDP571 plasma concentration in patients with rheumatoid arthritis following up to four infusions at the following doses: …*… 0.1 mg/kg - - ▲ - - 1.0 mg/kg —○—10.0 mg/kg.

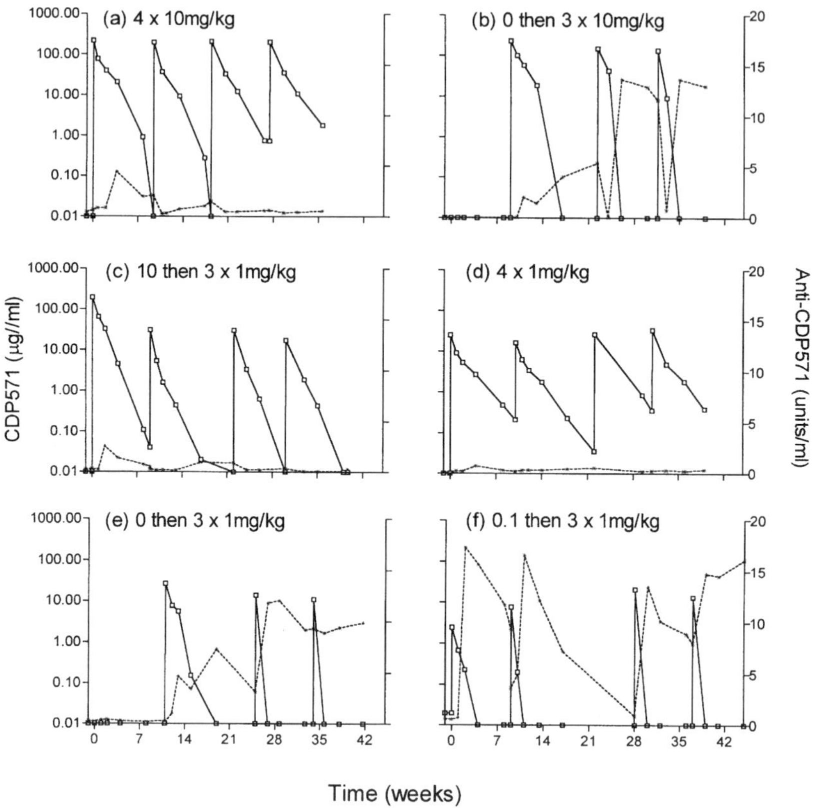

FIGURE 5
Plasma CDP571 (—□—) and anti-CDP571 levels (...*...) in individual rheumatoid arthritis patients given up to four infusions of CDP571.

the levels and the effect that these antibodies had on the clearance of CDP571. The previous single-dose studies described had indicated that the level of antibodies detectable was inversely proportional to the dose of CDP571, although interference of CDP571 in the immune response assay made it uncertain whether this was due to lower antibody production or detection. Following repeated doses, the immune response and pharmacokinetic profiles suggest that at higher doses a state of high dose tolerance is reached, anti-CDP571 antibodies are no longer detectable, and the clearance rate is prolonged (Figure 5, panel a). A single dose at 10 mg/kg may be sufficient to induce tolerance and subsequent lower doses maintain this state (panel c). The class of anti-CDP571 (measured by high performance liquid chromatography; HPLC[20]) produced in these patients is IgM and little or no switch to IgG was detected. In contrast, patients receiving 0.1 mg/kg (and one patient receiving 10 mg/kg) tended to show a class-switch to IgG anti-CDP571 production by 8 weeks following their first dose and subsequent doses of CDP571, whether at 1 or 10 mg/kg, boosted specific IgG production, resulting in increased clearance of CDP571.

One of the diagnostic criteria for rheumatoid arthritis in this study was a positive rheumatoid factor result and it was therefore likely that some anti-IgG antibodies might cross-react with CDP571. In some of these rheumatoid arthritis patients, cross-reacting antibodies were detectable at entry into the study which had not been the case in the volunteer or sepsis studies. Epitope mapping of these cross-reacting antibodies (using excess of related molecules in the immune response assay), indicated that they were directed both against $\gamma4$ constant regions and against the CDP571 idiotype (Figure 6a). However, their presence was not predictive of subsequent development of a specific immune response. In addition, in those patients who did make a specific response to CDP571, the antibodies were directed against the idiotype and there was no evidence of any increase in antibodies to the $\gamma4$ constant regions (Figure 6b). Another concern regarding the therapeutic use of recombinant antibodies produced in a xenogeneic host cell line, is that the pattern of glycosylation might be abnormal and hence give rise to immunogenic epitopes. The lack of cross-reactivity of the antibodies directed against CDP571 with an unrelated murine antibody to TNF-α, also produced in NS0 cells (CB0006, Figure 6b), confirms that there are no antibodies which are directed against the carbohydrate moiety.

14.7.4.1 Clinical Summary

CDP571 caused improvement in patients' joints, whether assessed by an investigator or by the patients themselves. The clinical improvements were supported by changes in objective laboratory measurements. These showed reductions in the acute phase response accompanied by reductions in circulating concentrations of IL-6, a cytokine important in the mediation of the biological actions of TNF-α. The effects of CDP571 occurred rapidly, especially after 10 mg/kg, with patients reporting benefit within 24–48 h. Maximum benefit occurred after 2–4 weeks, with trends to improvement from baseline still evident at 8 weeks. Based on the Disease Activity Score, 4 of the 8 patients who received a single 10 mg/kg infusion of CDP571 fulfilled the criterion for a significant clinical improvement.

Not captured by the standard assessments used in this study, but nevertheless striking, were the unsolicited reports by patients that they felt a much improved sense of well-being beginning soon after the infusion.

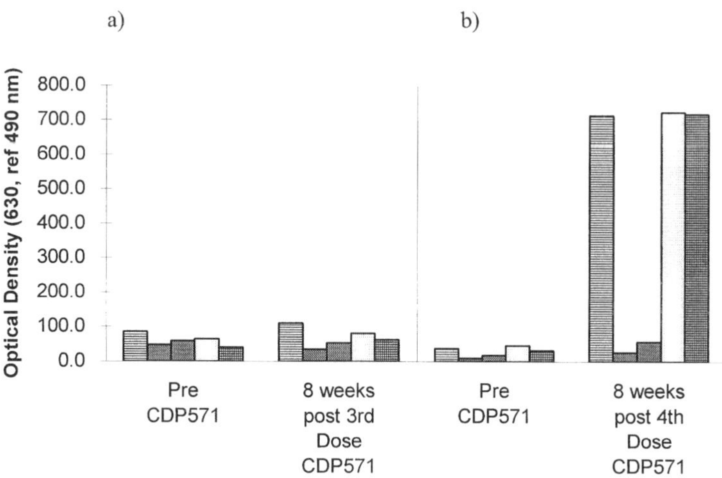

FIGURE 6

Epitope mapping of anti-CDP571 response. (a) Non-responding patient showing baseline cross-reacting antibodies. (b) Responding patient showing specificity of antibodies for CDP571 idiotype. Results are expressed as optical density in the presence of the following molecules: ▤ Buffer ▩ CDP571 ▩ CB0010 □ CB0006 ▦ gB72.3 where CB0010 is the murine parent antibody to CDP571; CB0006 is a murine anti-TNF-α with unrelated idiotype and gB72.3 has human γ4 and κ constant and Eu framework regions in common with CDP571, but unrelated idiotype.

CDP571 was well tolerated in single or repeated infusions. In the subset of patients who received repeated doses of 10 mg/kg, especially, there appeared to be cumulative benefit of the antibody; although from the second infusion onward the study was open and no longer placebo-controlled.

During the study as a whole, there were nine infectious events after CDP571 administration. Two of these sporadic events involved bacterial infection: the first was mild, short-lived parotitis and the second was salmonella trochanteric bursitis that required antibiotic therapy. Both events occurred after 10 mg/kg CDP571. Whether neutralizing TNF-α in patients with rheumatoid arthritis is associated with any increased incidence of infection can only be determined by larger experience; however, in this small study, infectious events did not increase in incidence with repeated dosing of the antibody. The emergence of autoantibodies to double-stranded DNA (dsDNA) has been reported in clinical studies of another anti-TNF-α antibody.[65] In the study of CDP571 described here a total of two patients developed antinuclear antibodies during the course of repeated treatments. In one case the target remained unidentified; in the other, anti-dsDNA antibodies were detected but were not accompanied during the study or afterward to date by attributable clinical sequelae.

Reductions in ESR and CRP in response to a therapy have previously been held to suggest modification of rheumatoid arthritis disease progression, although the ability of any currently available intervention genuinely to slow joint destruction is controversial. With the use of anti-cytokines such as CDP571 it remains possible that the reduction observed in acute phase response reflects systemic neutralization of TNF-α rather than amelioration of disease activity within the joint. The trends to reduction in circulating stromelysin and in the urinary excretion of specific collagen degradation fragments are therefore provocative. Stromelysin is a tissue matrix metalloproteinase whose expression is upregulated by TNF-α.[66] It is highly active *in vitro* against cartilage aggrecan. Enzyme activity is greatly increased in the rheumatoid joint, and its elevated concentration can be detected in the circulation of patients with the disease.[67] The consistent trends to reduction in the enzyme and in bone and cartilage degradation markers found following CDP571 treatment suggest that TNF-α neutralization may not only improve the pain and inflammation suffered by patients with rheumatiod arthritis but may actually slow disease progression.

The study suggests that it is safe and practicable to administer CDP571 repeatedly, and that repeated dosing obtains repeated or sustained benefits. It is remarkable that neutralization of a single cytokine should have so clear-cut a clinical effect. However, the outcome of this study is supported by the positive results of studies in which another anti-TNF-α antibody, the chimeric cA2, has been used.[65,68]

14.8 CONCLUSIONS

The involvement of TNF-α in pathogenesis of acute and chronic diseases is now beyond question. In addition to the indications discussed in this chapter, TNF-α has been implicated in diseases such as cerebral malaria,[69] pneumonia,[70] transplant rejection,[8] ischemia/reperfusion damage,[71] GVHD,[9] and multiple sclerosis.[12] The evidence that neutralizing TNF-α in animal models of these diseases is beneficial is also accumulating rapidly. Indeed several of these clinical conditions have been targets for therapy with murine antibodies to TNF-α.[72,73]

We have demonstrated that administration of an engineered human neutralizing TNF-α antibody to volunteers and patients is safe and that the long half-life obtained with engineered antibodies provides not only prolonged circulating neutralizing capacity but also allows repeated dosing without any of the adverse events associated with HAMA responses. We have also demonstrated clear clinical benefit in rheumatoid arthritis and IBDs. The potential for therapy in the other indications remains and these early successes should encourage further studies.

ACKNOWLEDGMENTS

The authors wish to thank all the investigators involved in the clinical studies. In particular, for the sepsis study, Professor J.-F. Dhainaut (Cochin Port-Royal Hospital, Paris) and Professor J.-L. Vincent (L'Hopital Erasme, Brussels); for the rheumatoid arthritis studies at the Middlesex Hospital. Dr. Elizabeth Rankin, Professor David Isenberg, and at Guy's Hospital Dr. Ernest Choy, Dr. Dimitris Kassimos, Dr. Gabrielle Kingsley, Professor Gabriel Panayi; and for the IBD studies Professor C. Hawkey (Nottingham), Dr. M. Kamm (St. Mark's Hospital, London), and Professor J. M. Rhodes (University of Liverpool).

REFERENCES

1. Eck, M. J. and Sprang, S. R., The structure of tumor necrosis factor-a at 2.6Å resolution. Implications for receptor binding, *J. Biol. Chem.*, 264, 17595, 1989.
2. Seckinger, P., Isaaz, S., and Dayer, J.-M., A human inhibitor of tumor necrosis factor-α, *J. Exp. Med.*, 167, 1511, 1988.
3. Dembic, Z., Loetscher, H., Gubler, U., Pan, Y. C., Lahm, H.-W., Gentz, R., Brockhaus, M., and Lesslauer, W., Two human TNF receptors have similar extracellular, but distinct intracellular, domain sequences, *Cytokines*, 2, 231, 1990.
4. Tracey, K. J., Beutler, B., Lowry, S. F., Merryweather, J., Wolpe, S., Milsark, I. W., Hariri, R. J., Fahey III, T. J., Zentella, A., Albert, J. D., Shires, G. T., and Cerami, A., Shock and tissue injury induced by recombinant human cachectin, *Science*, 234, 470, 1986.
5. Michie, H. R., Manogue, K. R., Spriggs, D. R., Revhaug, A., O'Dwyer, S., Dinarello, C. A., Cerami, A., Wolff, S. M., and Wilmore, D. W., Detection of circulating tumor necrosis factor after endotoxin administration, *N. Engl. J. Med.*, 318, 1481, 1988.
6. Hopkins, S. J. and Meager, A., Cytokines in synovial fluid: II. The presence of tumour necrosis factor and interferon, *Clin. Exp. Immunol.*, 73, 88, 1988.
7. Brennan, F. M., Chantry, D., Jackson, A., Maini, R., and Feldmann, M., Inhibitory effect of TNFα antibodies on synovial cell interleukin-1 production in rheumatoid arthritis, *Lancet*, ii, 244, 1989.
8. Maury, C. P. and Teppo, A. M., Raised serum levels of cachectin/tumor necrosis factor alpha in renal allograft rejection, *J. Exp. Med.*, 166, 1132, 1987.
9. Piguet, P.-F., Grau, G. E., Allet, B., and Vassalli, P., Tumour necrosis factor/cachectin is an effector of skin and gut lesions of the acute phase of graft-vs-host disease, *J. Exp. Med.*, 166, 1280, 1987.
10. Garside, P., Bunce, C., Tomlinson, C., Nichols, B. L., and Mowat, A. McI., Analysis of enteropathy induced by tumour necrosis factor α, *Cytokine*, 5, 24, 1993.
11. Hotamisligil, G. S., Shargill, N. S., and Spiegelman, B. M., Adipose expression of tumor necrosis factor-α: direct role in obesity-linked insulin resistance, *Science*, 259, 87, 1993.
12. Beck, J., Rondot, P., Catinot, L., Falcoff, E., Kirchner, H., and Wietzerbin, J., Increased production of interferon gamma and tumor necrosis factor precedes clinical manifestation in multiple sclerosis: do cytokines trigger off exacerbations?, *Acta Neurol. Scand.*, 78, 318, 1988.

13. Murch, S. H., Lamkin, V. A., Savage, M. O., Walker-Smith, J. A., and MacDonald, T. T., Serum concentrations of tumour necrosis factor-α in childhood chronic inflammatory bowel disease, *Gut*, 32, 913, 1991.
14. Tracey, K. J., Fong, Y., Hesse, D. G., Manogue, K. R., Lee, A. T., Kuo, G. C., Lowry, S. F., and Cerami, A., Anti-cachectin/TNF monoclonal antibodies prevent septic shock during lethal bacteraemia, *Nature*, 330, 662, 1987.
15. Imagawa, D. K., Millis, J. M., Seu, P., Olthoff, K. M., Hart, J., Wasef, E., Dempsey, R. A., Stephens, S., and Busuttil, R. W., The role of tumor necrosis factor in allograft rejection. III. Anti-TNF antibody therapy prolongs allograft survival in rats with acute rejection, *Transplantation*, 51, 57, 1991.
16. Grau, G. E., Vesin, C., De Groote, D., Delacroix, D., Gysler, C., Piguet, P.-F., and Lambert, P. H., Prevention of human TNF-induced cutaneous Schwartzmann reaction and acute mortality in mice treated with anti-human TNF monoclonal antibodies, *Clin. Exp. Immunol.*, 84, 411, 1991.
17. Stevens, H. P. J. D., van der Kwast, T. H., van der Miede, P. H., Vuzevski, V. D., Buurman, W. A., and Jonker, M., Synergistic immunosuppressive effects of monoclonal antibodies specific for interferon-gamma and tumor necrosis factor alpha. A skin transplantation study in the rhesus monkey, *Transplantation*, 50, 856, 1990.
18. Ward, P. S., Woodger, S. R., Bodmer, M., and Foulkes, R., Anti-tumour necrosis factor α monoclonal antibodies (anti-TNF MAb) are therapeutically effective in a model of colonic inflammation, *Br. J. Pharmacol.*, 110, 77P, 1993.
19. Keffer, J., Probert, L., Cazarlis, H., Georgopoulos, S., Kaslaris, E., Kioussis, D., and Kollias, G., Transgenic mice expressing human tumor necrosis factor: a predictive genetic model of arthritis, *EMBO J.*, 10, 4025, 1991.
20. Stephens, S., Emtage, S., Vetterlein, O., Chaplin, L., Bebbington, C., Nesbitt, A., Sopwith, M., Athwal, D., Novak, C., and Bodmer, M., Comprehensive pharmacokinetics of a humanized antibody and analysis of residual anti-idiotypic responses, *Immunology*, 85, 668, 1995.
21. Suitters, A. J., Foulkes, R., Opal, S. M., Palardy, J. E., Emtage, J. S., Rolfe, M., Stephens, S., Morgan, A., Holt, A. R., Chaplin, L. C., Shaw, N. E., Nesbitt, A. M., and Bodmer, M. W., Differential effect of isotype on efficacy of anti-tumor necrosis factor α chimeric antibodies in experimental septic shock, *J. Exp. Med.*, 179, 849, 1994.
22. Ward, P. S., Boden, T., Woodger, R., and Foulkes, R., Isotype variation of TNF monoclonal antibodies. Is there a therapeutic difference in rheumatoid arthritis? *Br. J. Rheumatol.*, 34 (Suppl.), 294, 1995.
23. Foulkes, R., Schlag, G., Redl, H., van Vuuren, C., Davies, J., Stephens, S., and Bodmer, M., A humanized monoclonal antibody to human TNFα improves survival and organ failure in a lethal septic model in baboons, *Eur. Cyt. Netw.*, 3, 218, 1992.
24. Ziegler, E. J., Fisher, C. J., Sprung, C. L., Straube, R. C., Sadoff, J. C., Foulke, G. E., Wortel, C. H., Fink, M. P., Dellinger, R. P., Teng, N. N. H., Allen, I. E., Berger, H. J., Knatterud, G. L., LoBuglio, A. F., Smith, C. R., and the HA-1A Sepsis Study Group, Treatment of gram-negative bacteremia and septic shock with HA-1A human monoclonal antibody against endotoxin. A randomised, double-blind, placebo-controlled trial, *N. Engl. J. Med.*, 324, 429, 1991.
25. Bone, R. C., Balk, R. A., Fein, A. M., Perl, T. M., Wenzel, R. P., Reines, H. D., Quenzer, R. W., Iberti, T. J., Macintyre, N., Schein, R. M. H., and the E5 Sepsis Study Group, A second large controlled clinical study of E5, a monoclonal antibody to endotoxin: results of a prospective multicenter, randomized, controlled trial, *Crit. Care Med.*, 23, 994, 1995.
26. Ziegler, E. J., McCutchan, J. A., Fierer, J., Glauser, M. P., Sadoff, J. C., Douglas, H., and Braude, A. I., Treatment of gram-negative bacteremia and shock with human antiserum to a mutant *Escherichia coli*, *N. Engl. J. Med.*, 307, 1225, 1982.

27. Schlievert, P. M., Shands, K. N., Dan, B. B., Schmid, G. P., and Nishimura, R. D. Identification and characterisation of an exotoxin from *Staphylococcus aureus* associated with toxic shock syndrome, *J. Infect. Dis.*, 143, 509, 1981.
28. Anonymous, The French National Registry of HA-1A (Centoxin) in septic shock. A cohort study of 600 patients. The National Committee for the Evaluation of Centoxin, *Arch. Int. Med.*, 154, 2484, 1994.
29. Waage, A., Halstensen, A., and Espevik, T., Association between tumour necrosis factor in serum and fatal outcome in patients with meningococcal disease, *Lancet*, i, 355, 1987.
30. Girardin, E., Grau, G. E., Dayer, J.-M., and Roux-Lombard, P., The J5 Study Group, and Lambert, P.-H., Tumor necrosis factor and interleukin-1 in the serum of children with severe infectious purpura, *N. Engl. J. Med.*, 319, 397, 1988.
31. Debets, J. M. H., Kampmeijer, R., van der Linden, M. P. M. H., Buurman, W. A., and van der Linden, C. J., Plasma tumor necrosis factor and mortality in critically ill septic patients, *Crit. Care Med.*, 17, 489, 1989.
32. Calandra, T., Baumgartner, J.-D., Grau, G. E., Wu, M.-M. Lambert, P.-H., Schellekens, J., Verhoef, J., Glauser, M. P., and The Swiss-Dutch J5 Immunoglobulin Study Group, Prognostic values of tumor necrosis factor/cachectin, interleukin-1, interferon-α, and interferon-γ in the serum of patients with septic shock, *J. Infect. Dis.*, 161, 982, 1990.
33. Opal, S. M., Cross, A. S., Kelly, N. M., Sadoff, J. C., Bodmer, M. W., Palardy, J. E., and Victor, G. H., Efficacy of a monoclonal antibody directed against tumor necrosis factor in protecting neutropenic rats from lethal infection with *Pseudomonas aeruginosa*, *J. Infect. Dis.*, 161, 1148, 1990.
34. Hinshaw, L. B., Tekamp-Olson, P., Chang, A. C. K., Lee, P. A., Taylor, F. B. J. R., Murray, C. K., Peer, G. T., Emerson, Jr., T. E., Passey, R. B., and Kuo, G. C., Survival of primates in LD_{100} septic shock following therapy with antibody to tumor necrosis factor (TNF-α), *Circ. Shock*, 30, 279, 1990.
35. Abraham, E., Wunderink, R., Silverman, H., Perl, T. M., Nasraway, S., Levy, H., Bone, R., Wenzel, R. P., Balk, R., Allred, R., Pennington, J. E., and Wherry, J. C., for the TNF-α MAb Sepsis Study Group, Efficacy and safety of monoclonal antibody to human tumor necrosis factor α in patients with sepsis syndrome. A randomised, controlled, double-blind, multicentre clinical trial, *J. Am. Med. Assoc.*, 273, 934, 1995.
36. Dhainaut, J.-F. A., Vincent, J.-L., Richard, C., Lejeune, P., Martin, C., Fierobe, L., Stephens, S., Ney, U. M., Sopwith, M., and the CDP571 Sepsis Study Group, CDP571, a humanized antibody to human TNF-α: safety, pharmacokinetics, immune response and influence on cytokine levels in patients with septic shock, *Crit. Care Med.*, 23, 1461, 1995.
37. Exley, A. R., Cohen, J., Buurman, W., Owen, R., Hanson, G., Lumley, J., Aulakh, J. M., Bodmer, M., Riddell, A., Stephens, S., and Perry, M., Monoclonal antibody to TNF in severe septic shock, *Lancet*, 335, 1275, 1990.
38. Peppel, K., Crawford, D., and Beutler, B., A tumor necrosis factor (TNF) receptor-IgG heavy chain chimeric protein as a bivalent antagonist of TNF activity, *J. Exp. Med.*, 174, 1483, 1991.
39. Fisher, Jr., C. J., Dhainaut, J. F., Opal, S. M., Pribble, J. P., Balk, R. A., Slotman, G. J., Iberti, T. J., Rackow, E. C., Shapiro, M. J., Greenman, R. L., Reines, H. D., Shelly, M. P., Thompson, B. W., LaBrecque, J. F., Catalano, M. A., Knaus, W. A., and Sadoff, J. C., Recombinant human interleukin-1 receptor antagonist in the treatment of patients with sepsis syndrome. Results from a randomised, double-blind, placebo-controlled trial, *J. Am. Med. Assoc.*, 271, 1836, 1994.
40. Fisher, Jr., C. J., Opal, S. M., Lowry, S. F., Sadoff, J. C., LaBrecque, J. F., Donovan, H. C., Lookabaugh, J. L., Lemke, J., Pribble, J. P., Strommatt, S. C., Vigers, G. P., Russel, D. A., and Thompson, R. C., Role of interleukin-1 and the therapeutic potential of interleukin receptor antagonist in sepsis, *Circ. Shock*, 44, 1, 1994.

41. Braegger, C. P., Nicholls, S. W., Murch, S. H., Stephens, S., and MacDonald, T. T., Tumour necrosis factor alpha in stool as a marker of intestinal inflammation, *Lancet*, 339, 89, 1992.
42. Murch, S. H., Braegger, C. P., Walker-Smith, J. A., and MacDonald, T. T., Location of tumour necrosis factor α by immunohistochemistry in chronic inflammatory bowel disease, *Gut*, 34, 1705, 1993.
43. Neilly, P. J. D., Campbell, G. R., Anderson, N. H., Gardiner, K. R., Kirk, S. J., and Rowlands, B. J., Faecal and systemic tumour necrosis factor in experimental inflammatory bowel disease, *Intensive Care Med.*, 20, A277, 1994.
44. Madara, J. L., Podolsky, D. K., King, N. W., Sengal, P. K., Moore, R., and Winter, H. S., Characterization of spontaneous colitis in cotton-top tamarins (*Sanguinus oedipus*) and its response to sulphasalazine, *Gastroenterology*, 88, 13, 1985.
45. Warren, B. F., Watkins, P. E., Foulkes, R., Ward, P., Stephens, S., and Bodmer, M., Anti-TNF alpha treatment of a model of human ulcerative colitis, *Gut*, 35, (Suppl. 2), 850, 1994.
46. Van Dullemen, H. M., van Deventer, S. J. H., Hommes, D. W., Bijl, H. A., Jansen, J., Tytgat, G. N. J., and Woody, J., Treatment of Crohn's disease with anti-tumor necrosis factor chimeric monoclonal antibody (cA2), *Gastroenterology*, 109, 129, 1995.
47. Stack, W., Mann, S., Roy, A., Heath, P., Sopwith, M., Freeman, J., Holmes, G., Long, R., Forbes, A., Kamm, M., and Hawkey, C., The effects of CDP571, an engineered Human IgG_4 anti-TNF antibody in Crohn's Disease, Abstract, submitted.
48. Evans, R. C., Clark, L., Heath, P., and Rhodes, J. M., Treatment of ulcerative colitis with an engineered human anti-TNF-α antibody CDP571, Abstract, submitted.
49. Maini, R. N., Brennan, F. M., Williams, R., Chu, C. Q., Cope, A. P., Gibbons, D., Elliott, M., and Feldmann, M., TNF-α in rheumatoid arthritis and prospects of anti-TNF therapy, *Clin. Exp. Rheum.*, 11 (Suppl. 8), S173, 1993.
50. Chu, C. Q., Field, M., Feldmann, M., and Maini, R. N., Localization of tumor necrosis factor α in synovial tissues and the cartilage-pannus junction in patients with rheumatoid arthritis, *Arthritis Rheum.*, 34, 1125, 1991.
51. Adams, D. H. and Shaw, S., Leucocyte-endothelial interactions and regulation of leukocyte migration, *Lancet*, 343, 831, 1994.
52. Windsor, A. C. J., Walsh, C. J., Mullen, P. G., Cook, D. J., Fisher, B. J., Blocher, C. R., Leeper-Woodford, S. K., Sugarman, H. J., and Fowler, III, A. A., Tumor necrosis factor-α blockade prevents neutrophil CD18 receptor upregulation and attenuates acute lung injury in porcine sepsis without inhibition of neutrophil oxygen radical generation, *J. Clin. Invest.*, 91, 1459, 1993.
53. Rathanaswami, P., Hachicha, M., Sadick, M., Schall, T. J., and McColl, S. R., Expression of the cytokine RANTES in human rheumatoid synovial fibroblasts. Differential regulation of RANTES and interleukin-8 genes by inflammatory cytokines, *J. Biol. Chem.*, 268, 5834, 1993.
54. van Deventer, S. J. H., Hart, M., van der Poll, T., Hack, C. E., and Aarden, L. A., Endotoxin and tumor necrosis factor-α-induced interleukin-8 release in humans, *J. Infect. Dis.*, 167, 461, 1993.
55. Bussolino, F., Camussi, G., and Baglioni, C., Synthesis and release of platelet activating factor by human vascular endothelial cells treated with tumor necrosis factor or interleukin 1α, *J. Biol. Chem.*, 263, 11856, 1988.
56. Yuo, A., Kitagawa, S., Kasahara, T., Matsushima, K., Saito, M., and Takaku, F., Stimulation and priming of human neutrophils by interleukin-8: cooperation with tumor necrosis factor and colony-stimulating factors, *Blood*, 78, 2708, 1991.
57. Chavin, K. D., Bromberg, J. S., Kunkel, S. L., Naji, A., and Barker, C. F., Effects of a polyclonal anti-TNF antibody on cell-mediated immunity *in vivo*, *Transplant. Proc.*, 1, 847, 1991.

58. Mantovani, A., Bussolino, F., and Dejana, E., Cytokine regulation of endothelial cell function, *FASEB J.*, 6: 2591, 1992.
59. Henderson, B. and Pettipher, E. R., Arthritogenic actions of recombinant IL-1 and tumour necrosis factor α in the rabbit: evidence for synergistic interactions between cytokines *in vivo*, *Clin. Exp. Immunol.*, 75, 306, 1989.
60. Alvaro-Gracia, J. M., Zvaifler, N. J., and Firestein, G. S., Cytokines in chronic inflammatory arthritis. V, *J. Clin. Invest.*, 86, 1790, 1990.
61. Piguet, P. F., Grau, G. E., Vesin, C., Loetscher, H., Gentz, R., and Lesslauer, W., Evolution of collagen arthritis in mice is arrested by treatment with anti-tumour necrosis factor (TNF) antibody or a recombinant soluble TNF receptor, *Immunology*, 77, 510, 1992.
62. Williams, R. O., Feldmann, M., and Maini, R. N., Anti-tumor necrosis factor ameliorates joint disease in murine collagen-induced arthritis, *Proc. Natl. Acad. Sci. U.S.A.*, 89, 9784, 1992.
63. Henderson, B., Foulkes, R., Blake, S., Lewthwaite, J., Brown, D., Andrew, D., and Stephens S., TNF and related cytokines in lapine antigen-induced arthritis, *Eur. Cyto. Netw.*, 3, 261, 1992.
64. Rankin, E. C. C., Choy, E. H. S., Kassimos, D., Kingsley, G. H., Sopwith, A. M., Isenberg, D. A., and Panayi, G. S., The therapeutic effects of an engineered human anti-tumour necrosis factor alpha antibody (CDP571) in rheumatoid arthritis, *Br. J. Rheumatol.*, 34, 334, 1995.
65. Elliott, M. J., Maini, R. N., Feldmann, M., Long-Fox, A., Charles, P., Bijl, H., and Woody, J. N., Repeated therapy with monoclonal antibody to tumour necrosis factor α (cA2) in patients with rheumatoid arthritis, *Lancet*, 344, 1125, 1994.
66. MacNaul, K. L., Chartrain, N., Lark, M., Tocci, M. J., and Hutchison, N. I., Discoordinate expression of stromelysin, collagenase, and tissue inhibitor of metalloproteinases-1 in rheumatoid human synovial fibroblasts. Synergistic effects of interleukin-1 and tumor necrosis factor-alpha on stromelysin expression, *J. Biol. Chem.*, 265, 17238, 1990.
67. Baker, T., Tickle, S., Wasan, H., Docherty, A., Isenberg, D., and Waxman, J., Serum metalloproteinases and their inhibitors: markers for malignant potential, *Br. J. Cancer*, 70, 506, 1994.
68. Elliott, M. J., Maini, R. N., Feldmann, M., Kalden, J. R., Antoni, C., Smolen, J. S., Leeb, B., Breedveld, F. C., Macfarlane, J. D., Bijl, H., and Woody, J. N., Randomised double-blind comparison of chimeric monoclonal antibody to tumour necrosis factor α (cA2) versus placebo in rheumatoid arthritis, *Lancet*, 344, 1105, 1994.
69. Kwiatkowski, D., Hill, A. V. S., Sambou, I., Twumasi, P., Castracane, J., Manogue, K. R., Cerami, A., Brewster, D. R., and Greenwood, B. M., TNF concentration in fatal cerebral, non-fatal cerebral and uncomplicated *Plasmodium falciparum* malaria, *Lancet*, 336, 1201, 1990.
70. Moussa, K., Michie, H. J., Cree, I. A., McCafferty, A. C., Winter, J. H., Dhillon, D. P., Stephens, S., and Brown, R. A., Phagocyte function and cytokine production in community acquired pneumonia, *Thorax*, 49, 107, 1994.
71. Colletti, L. M., Burtch, G. D., Remick, D. G., Kunkel, S. L., Strieter, R. M., Guice, K. S., Oldham, K. T., and Campbell, D. A., The production of tumor necrosis factor alpha and the development of a pulmonary capillary injury following hepatic ischemia/reperfusion, *Transplantation*, 49, 268, 1990.
72. Kwiatkowski, D., Molyneux, M. E., Stephens, S., Curtis, N., Klein, N., Pointaire, P., Smit, M., Allan, R., Brewster, D. R., Grau, G. E., and Greenwood, B. M., Anti-TNF therapy inhibits fever in cerebral malaria, *Q. J. Med.*, 86, 91, 1993.
73. Herve, P., Flesch, M., Tiberghien, P., Wijdenes, J., Racadot, E., Bordigoni, P., Plouvier, E., Stephan, J. L., Bourdeau, H., and Holler, E., Phase I-II trial of a monoclonal anti-tumor necrosis factor alpha antibody for the treatment of refractory severe acute graft-versus-host disease, *Blood*, 79, 3362, 1992.

Chapter **15**

The Therapeutic Potential of a PRIMATIZED®, Nondepleting Anti-CD4 (IDEC-CE9.1) Monoclonal Antibody in Rheumatoid Arthritis

Alan M. Solinger, Alemseged Truneh, John A. Lipani, and Roland A. Newman

CONTENTS

0-8493-8547-4/97/$0.00+$.50

15.1 INTRODUCTION

Current evidence suggests that a number of autoimmune diseases, including rheumatoid arthritis (RA), are driven by CD4+ T cells. In RA there is clear evidence that activated T cells predominate in the synovial lesion. One strategy of intervention in RA is to develop reagents that short circuit the inflammatory condition by denying the T cells the capacity to be continuously activated. Several groups have used monoclonal antibodies (MAbs) against the CD4 molecule to inhibit such T-cell activity and experiments using animal models of autoimmunity have shown that anti-CD4 MAbs can arrest or reverse disease progression. The use of CD4 MAbs for selective intervention in RA is a modality gaining in potential. Described in this review is the approach we have taken using a PRIMATIZED®* CD4 MAb for the treatment of this disease.

15.2 CONCEPT AND BACKGROUND

The use of MAbs for immunomodulatory intervention in human diseases is not new. However, many of the earlier studies employed murine antibodies and suffered from the development of anti-xenogeneic responses in recipients.[1,2] The development of human anti-murine antibody responses (HAMA) has severely limited the use of murine antibodies in human trials, particularly those directed against chronic conditions, because neutralizing HAMA can rapidly bind newly injected MAbs, and thus impair therapeutic efficacy. Several strategies to circumvent these problems have been investigated, including the development of human/mouse chimeric antibodies, humanized antibodies or various techniques to produce nonimmunogenic murine antibodies, such

* Registered trademark of IDEC Pharmaceuticals Corporation, San Diego, CA.

as antibody veneering. Humanization of murine antibodies replaces murine framework regions with an appropriate human framework but retains the original complementarity determining region (CDR) of the mouse. However, several framework residues from the mouse must be retained in order to conserve CDR orientation and antigen-binding activity. The re-introduction of "murine" residues into the human framework, therefore, may still contribute to the immunogenicity of the molecule in a human host. Although humanized antibodies have clearly been an improvement over murine antibodies, their efficacy and immunogenicity in clinical trials remains to be determined.

There is a clear need for a high-affinity antibody directed against human antigens that is structurally similar to, or indistinguishable from, human immunoglobulins, and therefore immuno-silent. The approach we have used to address this need is the development of PRIMATIZED® antibodies.[3] These antibodies consist of variable regions from cynomolgus macaques and constant regions from humans (Figure 1). The cynomolgus macaque was chosen in this study because its immunoglobulin genes are highly homologous to those of humans, and it is phylogenetically distant enough that it should mount a strong immune response against human antigens. Chimpanzees, by contrast, are more closely related to humans, and may at first seem a better choice, but they do not respond well to human antigens.

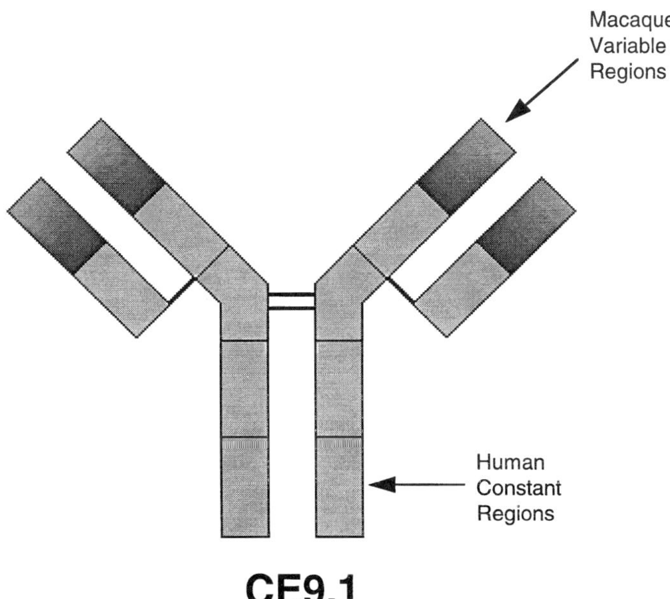

FIGURE 1
Structure of PRIMATIZED® IDEC-CE9.1.

A number of cynomolgus monkey heavy- and light-chain variable region immunoglobulin genes spanning five heavy-chain and three-light chain families were cloned and sequenced.[3] Comparison of their framework regions to human consensus sequences showed that they ranged in homology from 85–98%. This is the same range of homologies seen within an immunoglobulin gene family from different human individuals. No monkey-specific motifs or residues were seen that could not be found in human immunoglobulins. Thus, sequences of human and cynomolgus macaque immunoglobulins were essentially indistinguishable. After establishing that cynomolgus macaque immunoglobulin genes showed a high degree of homology to those of humans, we examined whether they were able to respond to human antigens that are functionally conserved between species. As the immunoglobulin genes of cynomolgus macaques and humans were similar, it is likely that other cell-surface antigens, with conserved functions (e.g., CD4, CD8, CD3, etc.), may also have highly conserved sequence homology and thus elicit a poor immune response. To test this possibility, cynomolgus monkeys were immunized with soluble CD4. Using heterohybridoma technology to immortalize the monkey B cells, we were able to produce several anti-CD4 antibodies. The most highly characterized of these, IDEC-CE9.1, was shown to have a relative affinity binding (Scatchard analysis) to the CD4+ human T cell line Sup-T1 of 3×10^{-11} *M*. When tested on a variety of CD4+ cells from a number of different species, IDEC-CE9.1 was shown to be specific only for human and chimpanzee CD4.[3] Thus, cynomolgus monkeys are capable of recognizing the human-specific epitopes on CD4 that differ from those present on cynomolgus CD4. In addition, these epitopes must be very similar between human and chimpanzee, supporting the notion that chimpanzees are phylogenetically too closely related to humans to be able to mount strong immune responses against conserved antigens such as CD4.

The macaque/human chimeric or PRIMATIZED® antibodies combine a high degree of homology to human immunoglobulin sequences with the ability of cynomolgus monkeys to produce high-affinity antibodies to human antigens. These antibodies, therefore, are ideal reagents for the immunotherapeutic treatment of a number of autoimmune and other diseases, particularly those of a chronic nature that require repeated antibody administration in which immunogenicity would be a significant handicap.

15.3 ANTIBODY CONSTRUCTION

Antibody variable regions were isolated from heterohybridomas using a reverse transcriptase/polymerase chain reaction (RT-PCR).

mRNA isolated from clones producing the desired antibody was converted to cDNA using an oligo-dT primer and reverse transcriptase. Aliquots of the cDNA were then amplified by PCR using a series of primer pairs. Primer sets were designed to amplify members of heavy-chain families (V_H1-V_H6) and kappa or lambda light-chain families. 5′ and 3′ PCR primers were designed to bind to the leader sequence and J regions, respectively, and incorporate restriction enzyme sites to facilitate cloning. Care was taken to select restriction sites that would introduce cloning sites into the DNA sequence without changing the amino acid sequence of the expressed antibody.[3]

Variable region fragments were cloned into a mammalian expression vector; heavy- and light-chain macaque variable regions were cloned upstream of a human heavy-chain γ1 constant region and κ or λ constant regions, respectively. The expression vector has been previously described[3,4] and consisted of the following major elements: a cassette for antibody expression including CMV promoter/enhancers and polyadenylation elements; a neomycin transferase gene; a dihydrofolate reductase (DHFR) gene; and elements required for replication and selection in bacteria. The recombinant antibody construct was electroporated into DHFR-negative Chinese hamster ovary (CHO) cells grown in serum-free medium and selected by growth in geneticin (G418). CHO cells were cloned directly after electroporation and G418 resistant clones producing the most antibody were taken for amplification. Amplification was performed by rounds of selection in increasing concentrations of methotrexate, and antibodies produced were screened for their ability to bind CD4. CHO cell production lines were then established for large-scale manufacture of antibody.

15.4 PRECLINICAL DATA

15.4.1 Fc Receptor Binding Activity

Interferon-γ (IFN-γ) will induce upregulation of Fc receptors (FcRs) on monocytes or certain monocytic cell lines *in vitro*. An assay was established using either free monocytes from peripheral blood, or a monocytic cell line (THP-1) stimulated with IFN-γ and loaded with a fluorescent dye. A second cell line, an adherent mouse fibroblast transfected with human CD4, was also used in this assay. Thus, an antibody which possesses both FcR binding and anti-CD4 activity will bridge these two cell lines and the quantitation of fluorescence will be a measure of the number of FcR-expressing cells bound via the antibody. IDEC-CE9.1 showed binding of fluorescent-loaded THP-1 cells in a dose-dependent manner, demonstrating the FcR binding properties of the antibody.[5] This binding was completely abolished in the presence of soluble CD4 and, as expected, $F(ab')_2$ fragments of IDEC-CE9.1 were negative in this assay. A direct binding assay was also used in which IDEC-CE9.1 showed binding to a fibroblast cell line transfected with FcγRII.

15.4.2 Antibody-Dependent Cell-Mediated Cytotoxicity (ADCC)

Using IL-2 stimulated polymorphonuclear cells (PMNs) from peripheral blood as the effector cell, and the radiolabeled CD4+ cell line Sup-T1 as a target, the ability of IDEC-CE9.1 to effect ADCC was measured. Maximal lysis was seen at a concentration of approximately 6 μg/ml. IDEC-CE9.1, therefore, was considered a very effective antibody in binding to FcRs and killing CD4+ cell lines.

15.4.3 Complement Fixation by IDEC-CE9.1

Despite the fact that IDEC-CE9.1 contains a human heavy-chain constant region of the γ1 subtype, it showed only minimal binding of C1q. A flow cytometry analysis that measured the amount of C1q binding to IDEC-CE9.1 after the antibody interacted with a CD4+ cell line was negative. Control murine anti-CD4 antibodies, for example, the antibody 4D9 of IgG2a isotype, strongly bound C1q as expected over the same concentration range. Similarly, IDEC-CE9.1 failed to lyse CD4+ target cells in the presence of complement. Again, the murine antibody 4D9 lysed target cells as expected.[5] It is unclear why IDEC-CE9.1 failed to bind C1q, and hence was ineffective in a CDC assay. Insufficient antigen density on the target cell is an unlikely explanation, as other anti-CD4 antibodies were capable of lysing the same target cells. The γ1 constant region in this construct contains all the sequence motifs reported necessary for C1q binding. In fact, when the same constant region is grafted onto a murine anti-CD20 antibody, it binds C1q normally.[4] The reason why IDEC-CE9.1 is a non-C1q binder is not apparent and may involve steric interactions of which we are currently not aware.

15.4.4 Inhibition of Immune Function by IDEC-CE9.1

The CD4 molecule plays an important role in the generation of a strong immune response to T-dependent antigens. The T-cell receptor interacts with the class II molecule on the antigen-presenting cell. The CD4 molecule plays a role in both stabilizing and strengthening this interaction and also in generating intracellular T-cell signaling.[6-9] Any agent disrupting this interaction, therefore, would subsequently abolish the T-cell response to the presented antigen. An anti-CD4, providing it was directed against the appropriate epitope, and had the appropriate affinity, would prevent the activation of antigen-specific T cells.[10,11] IDEC-CE9.1 was assayed for its inhibitory properties *in vitro* using a mixed lymphocyte reaction (MLR). As described previously, IDEC-CE9.1 bound only to human and chimpanzee CD4 molecules and, therefore, cells from these two sources were utilized in a MLR to examine the inhibitory properties of the antibody. The dose of IDEC-CE9.1 causing 50% maximal inhibition of thymidine incorporation (IC_{50}) was between 1 and 10 ng/ml in both human and chimpanzees. This value demonstrated the potent inhibitory properties of IDEC-CE9.1, and furthermore, confirmed that the chimpanzee was the appropriate animal model for subsequent *in vivo* experiments.

15.4.5 *In Vivo* Animal Models

In a single-dose, dose-ranging study in chimpanzees, IDEC-CE9.1 had no effect on CD4+ T-cell counts until a level of 0.3 mg/kg was given and a transient reduction of CD4+ cell levels was seen. At a level of 1 mg/kg, a reduction in CD4+ cell count to approximately 5% of baseline levels was observed immediately after dosing, but the count returned to normal level within 10 days.[5]

A second study involving six animals (two animals in each of three groups) was designed to measure the effects of multiple higher level (10 mg/kg) doses of IDEC-CE9.1. One group received a 10 mg/kg dose of IDEC-CE9.1 on day 0 and further doses only after their CD4+ cell levels had returned to within 30% of baseline. A second group received the same initial dose and further doses only after their CD4+ cell counts had returned to within 70% of baseline. A control group received saline infusions. A maximum of three treatment cycles were given to animals on this study. Immediately following antibody administration, the CD4+ cell counts dropped and returned to within the normal range in approximately ten days. The CD8+ cell count remained unchanged throughout the experiment although daily variability was observed. No adverse events or infusion-related problems (cytokine release syndrome) were observed with any animals after any of the doses given, nor were any unusual blood chemistries seen.

By examining the (CD3+-CD8+) lymphocyte numbers, a theoretical measure of the number of CD4+ cells was calculated. When these data were plotted and compared with total CD4+ cell counts, it became clear that the drop in (CD3+-CD8+) cells was not as dramatic as those observed using CD4+ cell numbers alone. These data were interpreted as reflecting cell-surface modulation of CD4 molecules. Thus, the actual numbers of CD4+ cells removed from circulation were minimal and the apparent reduction in CD4+ cell count could be accounted for almost entirely by surface modulation. Long-term followup of the animals over 150 days showed that CD4+ cell numbers had returned close to baseline and that no-long term effects on the animals were evident.

In conclusion, IDEC-CE9.1 was shown to possess a remarkable safety profile. Unlike studies utilizing other anti-CD4 antibodies, this antibody did not deplete CD4+ cells but did modulate CD4 molecules from the cell surface. Although an ADCC assay could be performed with IDEC-CE9.1 *in vitro,* depletion by FcR binding may not be a significant mechanism *in vivo.* The lack of depletion of CD4+ cells may be explained by the inability of IDEC-CE9.1 to fix complement.

15.5 CLINICAL DATA

The goal of our first single-dose, dose-rising study was to evaluate the safety and clinical activity of the PRIMATIZED® IDEC-CE9.1 in patients with seropositive RA and to study immunologic changes in peripheral blood (PB).

15.5.1 Patients

Patients were recruited from three rheumatology practices. All of the patients fulfilled the 1987 American College of Rheumatology's criteria for diagnosis of RA.[12] They had failed at least one, but no more than four disease-modifying anti-rheumatic drugs (DMARDs) and had active disease. DMARDs were stopped 4 weeks prior to treatment in all patients. During this period, the dosage of nonsteroidal anti-inflammatory drugs was not changed. Concurrent oral steroid usage was allowed if the dose was stable and less than 10 mg of prednisone per day. Patients were treated in seven cohorts of three and one cohort of four (highest dose) (0.03-4.0 mg/kg) over a 4-h infusion. Two weeks post-infusion, patients were allowed to begin treatment with DMARDs. Written consent was obtained from all patients after they had been informed, both orally and in writing, of the possible risks of treatment.

15.5.2 Clinical Efficacy

RA disease activity was measured by the modified Ritchie tests, the duration of early morning stiffness, swollen joint count, tender joint count, and patient's and physician's global assessment of disease activity (each graded from 1–5).[13] All disease activity measurements were carried out at the start of therapy (week 0) and at weeks 2, 4, 8, and 12.

Evidence of clinical response was seen at two weeks, with maximal clinical response typically seen 4 weeks after infusion. At 2 weeks, 5 of 25 patients had achieved a significant clinical response as demonstrated by a >20% improvement in swollen and tender joint count as well as improvement in at least one other clinical efficacy criterion. At 4 weeks, 7 of 25 patients had achieved a similar >20% response, which appeared to be dose related.

In addition, at 4 weeks, only 1 patient had dropped out due to lack of efficacy in the group that received ≥0.5 mg/kg vs. 8 of 12 patients in the group that received less antibody. Eight patients did not elect to start treatment with a slow-acting anti-rheumatic drug during the full 3-month duration of observation.

In most patients receiving ≥0.12 mg/kg, a clinical response occurred within 24 h after the infusion. The response was characterized by a decrease in pain and swelling. This immediate response frequently diminished by 72 h post-infusion and generally corresponded with decreasing IDEC-CE9.1 blood levels.

15.5.3 Clinical Laboratory Tests

Full blood count, differential white blood cell count, blood chemistry profile, erythrocyte sedimentation rate (ESR), C-reactive protein (CRP), and rheumatoid factor (RF) were measured before the start of treatment and at each clinical assessment thereafter. In addition, full blood count, differential white blood cell count, and blood chemistry profile were measured at 24 and 72 h post-infusion.

15.5.4 Immunologic Assessment

Circulating PB lymphocyte and monocyte subsets were measured by immunofluorescence and analyzed by flow cytometry using MAbs detailed in Table 1. Immunofluorescence was performed on whole blood samples by standard methodology. IDEC-CE9.1 and Leu3a compete for binding to the CD4 molecule and react with closely related epitopes on the D1 domain, in contrast to OKT4 which recognizes an epitope on the D4 domain. Therefore, the binding activity of IDEC-CE9.1 was measured by comparing binding of OKT4 and Leu3a MAbs. Results were analyzed at weeks 0, 1, 2, 4, 8, and 12, and mouse immunoglobulin conjugated to fluorescein and phycoerythrin was used as negative controls. In addition, peripheral blood mononuclear cells were isolated using Ficoll-Hypaque cushioning, proliferation assays to the mitogens PHA, PWM, and Con A, as well as the soluble recall antigens *Candida*, trichophyton, streptodornase, and tetanus toxoid.

TABLE 1

Flow Cytometry Reagents

Determinant	Specificity
CD4	T cells (helper/inducers)
CD3	Pan-T-cells (associated with T-cell receptor)
CD8	T cells (cytotoxic/suppressor)
CD20	B cells (after pro-B-cell stage)
CD25	IL-2 receptor
HLA-DR	Class II MHC
CD45Ro	T cells (naive)
CD45Ra	T cells (memory)

Overall, the maximum reduction from baseline in CD4+ T cells was 62.8% (median). All counts recovered within 7 days. Prolonged CD4+ cell reduction did not occur in any patients during the 3-month period. However, using the mean fluorescence intensity (MFI) of CD8 staining as a stable internal control, a reduction in CD4 antigen on the surface of CD4+ cells was observed for approximately 1 week after infusion. This decrease in CD4 intensity was dose related and was not associated with CD4+ cell depletion.

Flow cytometric analysis revealed no significant changes in the number of CD8+, CD3+, or CD20+ cells. Measurement of CD25, HLA-DR, CD45Ro, and CD45Ra expression revealed that neither CD45Ro+CD4+ or CD45Ra+CD4+ cell populations changed significantly during the course of treatment or during the followup. However, the number of CD25+CD4+ cells decreased significantly in some patients. This decrease in the number of CD25+CD4+ cells was positively associated with clinical response and a similar clinical association was noted with the number of HLA-DR+CD3+ cells.

Both mitogen and antigen proliferation decreased approximately 4 weeks after treatment and the degree of suppression was dose related. This suppression was not correlated with clinical response and was maintained for 4 to 8 weeks. Three patients who demonstrated hypoproliferation to both mitogens and antigens prior to treatment actually increased their proliferation responses for up to 4 weeks before reverting to their pretreatment hypoproliferative levels. This proliferative change was not associated with a positive clinical response.

15.5.5 IDEC-CE9.1 Serum Levels

Using an antigen capture technique for assay of serum IDEC-CE9.1 levels, no detectable levels were noted at single doses <0.25 mg/kg. At doses of 2 to 4 mg/kg, multiple data points per patient allowed for preliminary estimates of serum half-life — approximately 18 h post-infusion equilibration. In 3 of the 4 patients in the 4 mg/kg dosing group, IDEC-CE9.1 was no longer detectable 5 days post-infusion. These estimates are based on only limited time points in a small number of patients. None of the samples obtained showed quantifiable levels of anti-IDEC-CE9.1 human anti-chimeric antibody (HACA) levels during the 3-month duration of the study.

15.5.6 Adverse Experiences

No infusion-related adverse experiences occurred in this trial. Unlike trials with previous MAbs, no patients experienced systemic reactions such as fevers, chills, hypotension, tachycardia, gastrointestinal upset, and headaches, or local effects such as rashes or local reactions at the venous site from a single infusion. Post-infusion minor reactions thought to possibly be related to study drug during the 3-month observation period included grade I diarrhea in one patient, a *Candida*-like rash under the breast of one patient, and a viral upper respiratory tract-like infection in two patients. Elevated liver enzymes in one patient occurring after restarting Imuran®* therapy. This latter adverse experience was attributed to the Imuran®.

15.6 DISCUSSION

Single infusions of IDEC-CE9.1 into seropositive rheumatoid arthritis patients with active clinical disease was associated with only transient reductions in CD4+ cell count and dose-related CD4 antigenic modulation without cellular depletion. The CD4+ cell counts returned to baseline within 7 days in all patients. Twenty-eight percent of treated patients achieved a positive, dose-related clinical response that was maximal at 4 weeks post-treatment and was associated with a decrease in CD25+CD4+ cells in PB.

Therapy with previous anti-CD4 MAbs has been associated with significant and prolonged CD4+ cellular depletion that did not correlate with positive clinical responses.[14,15] In addition, previous anti-CD4 MAb therapy in RA produced significant infusion-related reactions. In contrast, treatment with IDEC-CE9.1 was not accompanied by infusion-related side effects or any adverse experiences.

In the present trial, CD4 antigen down modulation was dose related and was not associated with a clinical response but did parallel a decreased proliferative response to both mitogens and recall antigens. This effect was not coupled with significant infections or evidence of

* Registered trademark of Burroughs Wellcome, Research Triangle Park, NC.

immune suppression and was reversible by 12 weeks after infusion. The changes in proliferation did not appear to be immune suppression. Some patients who were previously poor proliferators, in fact, increased their proliferative responses. This suggests that the effect on CD4 molecular expression and mitogen/antigen proliferation was modulatory rather than suppressive.

Results of this trial indicate that IDEC-CE9.1 is nondepleting with immunomodulatory effects on several immune parameters but without major negative immunologic effects. Pharmacokinetics data demonstrated rapid clearance of the IDEC-CE9.1 antibody, which suggests that the antibody is rapidly metabolized either by the CD4 lymphocytes or by the reticuloendothelial system interacting with antibody-coated cells. Apparently, this interaction produced CD4 molecular modulation rather than CD4+ cell death. In initial *in vitro* studies with IDEC-CE9.1, antibody binding alone led to suppression of CD4 functions, such as a one-way mixed lymphocyte response or recall antigen proliferation.[3]

A single infusion of IDEC-CE9.1 antibody resulted in positive dose-related clinical effects. Data suggest that IDEC-CE9.1 is a high-affinity antibody that does not lead to significant cell death but produces significant immunomodulation and positive clinical effects. These results are not associated with significant clinical adverse experiences. Further studies, especially using multiple administrations of this antibody, are needed to fully understand its clinical and immunological effects. An ongoing multi-dose study with IDEC-CE9.1 in patients with RA shows continued clinical activity with an excellent safety profile. Therefore, CD4 cell depletion does not appear to be an important factor in obtaining a positive clinical response to such therapy. Further, more extensive, controlled trials are needed to develop optimal regimens for use of this antibody in the therapy of RA.

REFERENCES

1. Herzog, C., Walker, C., Muller, W., Rieber, P., Reiter, C., Riethmuller, G., Wassmer, P., Stockinger, H., Madic, O., and Pichler, W. J., Anti-CD4 antibody treatment of patients with rheumatoid arthritis: I. Effect on clinical course and circulating T cells, *J. Autoimmun.*, 2, 627, 1989.
2. Walker, C., Herzog, C., Rieber, P., Riethmuller, G., Muller, W., and Pichler, W. J., Anti-CD4 antibody treatment of patients with rheumatoid arthritis: II. Effect of *in vivo* treatment on *in vitro* proliferative response of CD4 cells, *J. Autoimmun.*, 2, 643, 1989.
3. Newman, R., Alberts, J., Anderson, D., Carner, K., Heard, C., Norton, F., Raab, R., Reff, M., Shuey, S., and Hanna, N., "Primatization" of recombinant antibodies for immunotherapy of human disease: a macaque/human chimeric antibody against human CD4, *Bio/Technology*, 10, 1455, 1992.

4. Reff, M. E., Carner, K., Chambers, K. S., Chinn, P. C., Leonard, J. E., Raab, R., Newman, R. A., Hanna, N., and Anderson, D. R., Depletion of B cells *in vivo* by a chimeric mouse human monoclonal antibody to CD20, *Blood*, 83, 435, 1994.
5. Anderson, D. et al., *In vitro* and *in vivo* characterization of a PRIMATIZED MAb to human CD4: MAb causes CD4 receptor modulation but not CD4 T cell depletion in chimpanzees, in preparation.
6. Straus, D. B. and Weiss, A., Genetic evidence for the involvement of the lck tyrosine kinase in signal transduction through the T cell antigen receptor, *Cell*, 70, 585, 1992.
7. Greenstein, J. L. and Burakoff, S. J., The role of L3T4 (CD4) in T cell activation, *Ann. Inst. Pasteur Immunol.*, 138, 134, 1987.
8. Eichmann, K., Boyce, N. W., Schmidt-Ullrich, R., and Jonsson, J. I., Distinct functions of CD8(CD4) are utilized at different stages of T-lymphocyte differentiation, *Immunol. Rev.*, 109, 39, 1989.
9. Janeway, C. A., Jr., Rojo, J., Saizawa, K., Dianzani, U., Portoles, P., Tite, J., Haque, S., and Jones, B., The co-receptor function of murine CD4, *Immunol. Rev.*, 109, 77, 1989.
10. Engleman, E. G., Benike, C. J., Glickman, E., and Evans, R. L., Antibodies to membrane structures that distinguish suppressor/cytotoxic and helper T lymphocyte subpopulations block the mixed leukocyte reaction in man, *J. Exp. Med.*, 154, 193, 1981.
11. Shizuru, J. A., Gregory, A. K., Chao, C. T., and Fathman, C. G., Islet allograft survival after a single course of treatment of recipient with antibody to L3T4, *Science*. 237, 278, 1987.
12. Arnett, F. C., Edworthy, S. M., Bloch, D. A., McShane, D. J., Fries, J. F., Cooper, N. S., Healey, L. A., Kaplan, S. R., Liang, M. H., Luthra, H. S., Medsgere, T. A., Jr., Mitchell, D. M., Neustadt, D. H., Pinals, R. S., Schaller, J. G., Sharp, J. T., Wilder, R. L., and Hunder, G. G., The American Rheumatism Association 1987 revised criteria for the classification of rheumatoid arthritis, *Arthritis Rheum.*, 31, 315, 1988.
13. Ritchie, D. M., Boyle, J. A., McInnes, J. M., Jasani, M. K., Dalakos, T. G., Grieveson, P., and Buchanan, W. W., Clinical studies with an articular index for the assessment of joint tenderness in patients with rheumatoid arthritis, *Q. J. Med.*, (New Series) 37, 393, 1968.
14. Moreland, L. W., Pratt, P. W., Bucy, R. P., Jackson, B. S., Feldman, J. W., and Koopman, W. J., Treatment of refractory rheumatoid arthritis with a chimeric anti-CD4 monoclonal antibody. Long-term followup of CD4+ T cell counts, *Arthritis Rheum.*, 37, 834, 1994.
15. Jonker, M., Slingerland, W., Treacy, G., van Eerd, P., Pak, K. Y., Wilson, E., Tam, S., Bakker, K., Lobuglio, A. F., Rieber, P., Riethmuller, G., Daddona, P. E., and Iuliucci, J., *In vivo* treatment with a monoclonal chimeric anti-CD4 antibody results in prolonged depletion of circulating CD4+ cells in chimpanzees, *Clin. Exp. Immunol.*, 93, 301, 1993.

INDEX

INDEX

A

D

E

F

K

L

N

O

P